The Person as Patien

Other titles in the Series

Bovell *et al., Principles of Physiology: A Scientific Foundation of Physiotherapy*
Burns and MacDonald, *Physiotherapy and the Growing Child*
Holey and Cook, *Therapeutic Massage*
Kitchen Bazin, *Clayton's Electrotherapy* 10th edition
McColl and Bickenbach, *Introduction to Disability*
Pickles *et al., Physiotherapy with Older People*
Pitt-Brooke, *Rehabilitation of Movement*
Sapsford *et al., Women's Health: A Textbook for Physiotherapists*
Wilton, *Hand Splinting*

To order any of these titles contact your local bookseller
or call Customer Services on +44 (0) 181 308 5710.
Find us on the web at http://www.hbuk.co.uk

The Person as Patient
Psychosocial Perspectives for the Health Care Professional

Edited by

Elsa Ramsden BS EdM EdD PT

Professor and Scholar in Residence,
School of Human Service Professions, Institute of Physical Therapy Education,
Widener University, Chester, Pennsylvania, USA

WB Saunders Company Ltd
London • Philadelphia • Toronto • Sydney • Tokyo

WB Saunders
An imprint of Harcourt Brace and Company Limited
24-28 Oval Road,
London NWI 7DX, UK

Harcourt Brace and Company,
Robert Stevenson House,
I-3 Baxter's Place, Leith Walk,
Edinburgh EHI 3AF, UK

The Curtis Center,
Independence Square West,
Philadelphia, PA 19106-3399, USA

Harcourt Brace and Company,
55 Horner Avenue,
Toronto, Ontario, M8Z 4X6, Canada

Harcourt Brace and Company, Australia,
30-52 Smidmore Street,
Marrickville,
NSW 2204, Australia

Harcourt Brace and Company - Japan,
Ichibancho Central Buliding,
22 - I Ichibancho,
Chiyoda-ku, Tokyo 102, Japan

First published 1999

A catalogue record for this book is available form the British Library.

ISBN 0 7020 2230 6

Printed in China
NPCC / 01

Contents

Contributors   vii

Preface   ix

SECTION 1: Growth and Development through the Lifespan

1. Of Systems and Theories   1

   ELSA RAMSDEN

2. A System of Ecology   10

   ELSA RAMSDEN

3. Development Through Life: Fundamental Patterns   24

   ELSA RAMSDEN

4. Normal Growth and Development in the Infant and Young Child   43

   ELSA RAMSDEN

5. The Adolescent Years   67

   PAMELA HANSFORD

6. The Adult Years   99

   LENA NORDHOLM

7. Normal Aging   123

   SHULAMIT WERNER

8. Aging with Illness   148

   CECELIA EALES

9. Long-Term Care: Living with Chronic Illness   169

   CHERYL COTT

SECTION 2: The Patient and the Health Professional

10. Self-Efficacy   186

    MONICA LEHMAN and BETH A ROLLER

11. The Relationship Between Health Practitioner and Patient   197

     JUDITH FADLON and SHULAMIT WERNER

12. Bioethics   212

     JAN BRUCKNER

13. The Process of Making Judgments   230

     ELSA RAMSDEN

14. Communication in the Therapeutic Context   244

     ELSA RAMSDEN

     Glossary of Terms   263

     Index   269

Contributors

Jan Bruckner PhD PT
Associate Professor, Bouvé College of Pharmacy
and Health Sciences,
Department of Physical Therapy,
Northeastern University,
Boston, USA

Cheryl A Cott BPT MSc PhD
Assistant Professor,
Department of Physical Therapy and
Graduate Department of Rehabilitation Science,
Faculty of Medicine, University of Torornto,
Toronto, Canada

Cecelia Eales MSc
Acting head, Physiotherpapy Department,
Deputy Dean of the Allied Medical Disciplines,
University of the Witswatersrand,
Johannesburg, South Africa

Judith Fadlon MA
Lecturer, Sackler School of Medicine and
Ben Gurion School of Medicine,
Tel Aviv, Israel

Pamela K Hansford DipPhysio (UCT) BA (Unisa)
Private Practitioner,
Claremont, Cape Town, South Africa

Monica Lehman BS MS PT
Physical Therapist,
Manor Care Nursing and Rehabilitation Center,
York, Pennsylvania, USA

Lena A Nordholm Fil. Kand. MA PhD
Associate Professor and Head of Department,
Department of Rehabilitation,
Goteborg University, Sweden

Elsa Ramsden BS EdM EdD PT
Professor and Scholar in Residence
School of Human Service Professions,
Institute of Physical Therapy Education,
Widener University, Chester, Pennsylvania, USA

Beth A Roller BS MS PT
Physical Therapist,
Muhlenberg Rehabilitation Center,
Bethlehem, Pennsylvania, USA

Shulamit Werner MA RPT
Senior Lecturer, Department of Physical Therapy,
School of Health Professions, Tel Aviv University,
Tel Aviv, Israel

Preface

My first foray into the clinical environment as a student in physical therapy brought me face to face with a conundrum. What I was learning in the curriculum had not prepared me to deal with the patients' questions and concerns about their future and their potential ability to resume a normal or near-normal life. I did not know how to respond to their overt and covert expressions of fear and anxiety, depression and anger, hopelessness and helplessness. That realization led me to graduate school (where I expected to find the answers to those questions, but of course did not) and a career I had never imagined.

A book such as this one has been on my mind for many years. Colleagues have encouraged me to

'... do a book. We need the behavioral science perspectives in our curriculum and we don't have a good text.'

It seemed a daunting task. The themes incorporated in the book have been part of courses I've taught since I first began working with health professional students after finishing graduate school. The intervening years have added three children to our family; now as adults, they have children of their own. They and their children have taught me lessons that would have been impossible to learn any other way; they have contributed directly and indirectly to my courses over the years, and to this book.

Perspective

The authors of this book work from the premise that each of us is the product of many factors that influence our lives. They begin with the fundamental grounding that physical, intellectual, social, and emotional growth are interdependent at every stage of life. The development of the individual is viewed as a function of genetic resources, maturation in a societal context, and self-initiated factors. The quantity of information is formidable. This book touches only the surface of the immense amount of material related to these topics. We hope the reader will be stimulated and challenged to read further.

The psychosocial framework is a useful perspective when we try to analyze human behavior and come to some understanding of the individual. The relationship of early stages to later growth and development is a helpful framework, as is the impact of current life events upon the groundwork of earlier stages. The cyclical nature of these factors contributes to the complexity that is the human being, adds drama to the human experience, and excitement to the analysis process that leads to understanding.

Organization

The book is organized in two parts: Part 1 deals with growth and development through the life span; Part 2 deals with special topics associated with the role of the health professional working with patients in the clinical setting. The introductory chapter identifies some of the assumptions; the foundation for common understanding is laid through definitions of key terms, and the basic concepts are introduced that will be discussed later. The philosophy behind the discussions throughout the book hinges on an appreciation of ecology with interrelatedness among factors that have an impact on the human being.

Overview

Following Chapter 1, which is an introduction, Chapter 2 describes in greater detail the theory of ecology and the several systems that operate within it. Chapter 3 begins the series of discussions on development through life, with general principles that operate in all of us: adaptation, psychosexual development, cognitive development, learning, and social roles. Chapter 4 looks at normal growth and development in the infant and young child. It begins with genetic contributions; developmental tasks are considered and associated with the sensory, perceptual, and motor functions. The evolution of emotion, beginning with responses to basic needs in the new born and the development of attachment with the caregiver enhances our understanding of Erikson's model of psychosocial development in Chapter 2.

In Chapter 5, Pamela Hansford of South Africa draws upon her extensive clinical experience with adolescents in her discussion of the second decade of life. She uses the stories of several of her patients to describe the percep-tions and thoughts of these young people who have a physical disability. Through their stories we learn about the psychosocial dilemmas and crises they experience. In Chapter 6 Lena Nordholm of Sweden moves the discussion into the adult years. She applies Erikson's theory and introduces other theories to enhance our understanding of this stage of life. The developmental tasks of adults included in this chapter are parenthood, work and leadership, and coping. She distinguishes between the life patterns of men and women, and looks at health problems in adulthood.

Shulamit Werner of Israel has provided Chapter 7 on normal aging beginning with an overview of several theoretic approaches. The terms normal aging, successful aging, and pathologic aging are contrasted. She concludes with a brief discussion of impairment and disability that provides the link to the following chapter by Cecelia Eales of South Africa. Chapter 8 looks at illness and aging, beginning with demographic information that puts aging around the world into perspective for us. She also contrasts aging in the developing nations with that in western countries. Common illness and common problems of people in this older age group are discussed.

Cheryl Cott of Canada provides a discussion of role theory in Chapter 9, framed within the perspective of chronic disease and illness. She contrasts two theoretic views, functionalism and interactionism, and then integrates them in a complementary fashion to enhance our appreciation and understanding of the chronic illness experience.

The second part of the book focuses on several topics related to the health professional in relationship with the patient, beginning with a discussion of the key concept of patient self-efficacy. It then continues with attention to role theory, models of relationship, and beliefs, values, and the moral sphere. The book concludes with two chapters related to interpersonal relationships: the process of making judgments, and communication in the therapeutic context.

Chapter 10 begins with a discussion of an important theoretic construct called self-efficacy, developed by Albert Bandura. Monica Lehman and Beth Roller of the United States frame the discussion within the context of a case study of an older patient with a fear of falling. Self-efficacy is defined and discussed along with related concepts to provide the background for the case study. This concept has recently received a great deal of attention with respect to health care outcomes and progress of a patient in rehabilitation.

In Chapter 11 Judith Fadlon and Shulamit Werner of Israel look at the interpersonal relationship between the health practitioner and the patient. They outline the sociologic theory of social role and status and apply it to the interaction in health care. The content of Chapter 12 by Jan Bruckner of the United States takes relationship issues to a deeper level through discussion of beliefs, values, and moral reasoning. Basic terms and concepts are defined and discussed, followed by an exploration of basic ethical principles. These are applied to clinical examples, which in turn help to focus a discussion contrasting different methods of ethical decision making.

The process of making judgments is the linchpin in clinical decision making and in establishing relationships. This process is described in Chapter 13 by Elsa Ramsden of the United States, using the Inference model she developed to organize the large amount of information that bears on the topic. In the final chapter, communication in the therapeutic context is contrasted with that in the social context. Communication processes that arise in treatments that involve patients and health professionals are identified. Deliberate communication strategies are described that may be responsive to different kinds of content.

The editor and contributors to this volume thank all those who have helped to make the publication of this book possible. There are too many colleagues to name who have read earlier drafts and made suggestions, but their help was invaluable, and family and friends have offered support and encouragement all along the way. In particular I would like to thank the contributors who were patient and tolerant with my queries, suggestions, and time schedules. Without their support the effort would not have been possible. Finally, kudos goes to the editorial staff at W.B. Saunders and the talented direction of Miranda Bromage. She demonstrated amazing tolerance in this process of my first venture into the world of publication.

Elsa Ramsden

Dedication

To all those students who have challenged us over the years. And to the colleagues who encouraged us to continue our efforts to teach about human behavior, in cultural and psychological perspectives, in those who happen to be patients.

In memory of
Elsa Harbeck Boedecker, a Swedish-American physiotherapist who first taught me about what it means to care about people, and to be in a caring relationship with people, some of whom are ill and disabled.

1

Of Systems and Theories

Elsa Ramsden

What We're About
•
A Scientific Process
•
Components of Theory
•
Philosophy
•
Psychosocial Perspective
•
Disability
•
Paradigm

What We're About

A common human tendency is to try to analyze how or why it is that some other person has done a particular thing. We frequently base our analysis on our own experience of human behavior and popular or 'lay' theory found in the general press and television programming. In our own mind, we probably have a way of organizing people into groups and categories. This 'system' helps us deal with people who are not well known to us, and helps us relate to those we know perhaps too well. Comments that betray such systems sound similar to these statements: 'Oh well, what can you expect? He's just an excitable type of person!' or 'With more self confidence, she could do a whole lot better'. Some of our ideas about people and how they come to behave as they do emanate from reading the theories of scientists, and from all kinds of informal and formal observations. These classifications we create help us to make sense of our world and the people in it, including even ourselves.

These systems we develop are not the real maps of personhood; they merely try to deal with a small piece of the map, and they certainly do not describe the real territory. Our system may not translate very well to the understanding of another person, and would run into serious problems with those of different ages and from other cultures. We can really only know a limited amount about others or even ourself. Our thoughts are available to us incompletely; what is 'on our mind' at any given moment may be available, but of what is literally *in* our mind, only a small portion is known to us.

In this book we offer an approach based on principles of ecology to understand some of the behavior of people, and particularly those who are patients. We provide basic information from several behavioral science disciplines including psychology, social psychology, anthropology, and sociology based on a set of assumptions. These assumptions are, that we all observe and make judgments constantly; our judgments are informed by our experience of life and our education; we work with human beings who bring their own personal history with them to treatment; and as health professionals we treat the whole person, not just arms and legs and back, stomach or head.

Each of us can influence what actions we take; we are not robots, acting at the whim of another who is in control. Based on this fact, we assume that our intent as health professionals is to do good, to bring about some improvement in the condition of the patient, and to do no harm in the process of reaching that goal. Having said that, we need to include the patient's psyche as well as their body when we think about doing no harm. The intentionality of our therapeutic interventions are the focus of the professional training programs and are well documented in the treatment plans of each health professional discipline. We consider the intentionality of our interpersonal communication with patients in the treatment setting much less. Many of our communicative behaviors are initiated in the belief that they will accomplish a particular outcome, but they may instead result in outcomes that are neither desired nor positive, and may in fact be harmful to the patient's psyche. The primary aim of this book is to provide information from the behavioral sciences in an integrated manner, to inform our judgements about behavior, in order that we may be consciously intentional in our interactions with patients, and more likely to accomplish the desired outcomes.

A Scientific Process

The information contained in the following chapters was thoroughly researched by each of the contributors. Some innovations are introduced, firmly grounded in existing theory. Citations to the scientific literature are extensive. What is this scientific process that we rely upon and how does it pertain to the behavioral sciences? Primarily the scientific process is a methodology that results in new information, using procedures that can be replicated, to demonstrate that they are accurate. Several logical steps characterize the scientific processes. These are outlined below.

The process begins with an observation that causes one to pause to consider how that could have come about. One looks for causes and explanations to deal with the puzzling event. A variety of related thoughts may come to mind explaining it. Words used by scientists to describe these ideas include *assumptions*, *predictions*, and *hypotheses*; these lead to the development of a theory. The theory is not the end of the process, but is rather the beginning. It is a place to start. For example, eucalyptus trees imported from Australia to the west coast of California at the beginning of the twentieth century grew in a twisted manner, in a counter clockwise direction. These same trees grew perfectly straight in their native habitat, which is why they were imported for use in building the railroad in California. What caused them to grow in this strange manner? Is there any relationship between this phenomenon and the fact that water runs down the bathtub drain in a counter clockwise direction in the southern hemisphere? These are the observations and the beginning of related ideas, the beginning of a theory that may be tested logically.

Testing a theory requires that one observe the phenomenon and create experimental conditions to examine and measure it closely without extraneous factors entering the process that might influence the result. This is called operationalizing the concepts of the theory. With the observation above, one might decide to plant new seedlings of eucalyptus trees from Australia, observe them carefully, and measure their growth and rotation, if any. In the meantime we may want to consult with colleagues in geophysics and horticulture to understand underlying principles that may pertain. The steps in the scientific process described above are outlined in Figure 1.1.

Many theories are identified and applied to the clinical environment throughout this book. Most of these began with an *inductive process* as in Figure 1, starting with an observation and moving to the creation of a principle, rule, or fact. The *deductive process* works in the reverse order, beginning with the rule and applying it appropriately to a set of empirical observations. Health professionals routinely work with both of these logical processes in the course of working with patients, building

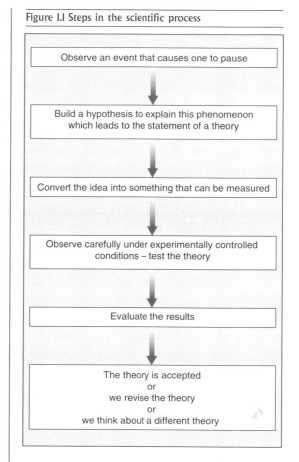

Figure 1.1 Steps in the scientific process

Observe an event that causes one to pause

Build a hypothesis to explain this phenomenon which leads to the statement of a theory

Convert the idea into something that can be measured

Observe carefully under experimentally controlled conditions – test the theory

Evaluate the results

The theory is accepted
or
we revise the theory
or
we think about a different theory

a hypothesis informally from a set of observations, and applying a rule or law of effect by identifying empirical observations.

For example, using the inductive process one may observe the non-verbal behavior of a patient, consisting in part of a slumped posture, bland affect, eyes cast downward, lack of variation in voice quality. We might hypothesize that he or she is depressed. We might then ask a few key questions to validate or invalidate that hypothesis. We have made observations, considered related ideas, gathered information, and come to a conclusion. We would use the deductive process, for example, when one knows that a particular disease process characteristically presents with certain neurologic signs. While examining a patient, who has a tentative diagnosis of this disease, we will gather information through careful observation to deduce whether these signs are present, and whether the tentative diagnosis is valid.

We have become accustomed to the formal logical processes of induction and deduction in the physical sciences throughout our entire education, and particularly in professional curricula. On the other hand, most of us are students of human nature through lifelong habits of observing the behavior of others and making 'guesses' about what that behavior means. Our limited study of psychology and sociology frequently fails to condition us to apply a process of logical analysis to a habit we have practiced for many years. We often fail to learn and apply important theoretic material to inform our judgments and alter our behavior accordingly. In this volume the authors have taken theory from the behavioral sciences and applied it to clinically relevant situations in an effort to make the theory more meaningful. The logical next step would be to add the theory to the information stored in our brain related to human behavior, and to draw on it appropriately with our patients.

Components of Theory

Several words related to theory development have been used in this discussion and will continue to be used regularly. We would do well to define and describe some of these words in order to have a common understanding among us as we move forward. A *theory* is an interrelated system of concepts with a logical organization that provides a framework for organizing, interpreting, and understanding observations, with the goal of explaining and predicting behavior (Newman and Newman, 1995). The infrastructure of theory is *concepts*. A concept is a label. We apply it to objects, behavior, or processes that permit identification and discussion. 'Mother' is a concept, or 'father', or 'food', or 'play', and thousands of other words that imply a complex set of features. We learn these concepts as part of our sensory and musculoskeletal experience throughout life. They help us define and understand our perception of reality. For example the words 'parallel bars' refer to a concept that separates these two words from our conception of other bars with different functions, such as window bars, bars on doors in prison, bars where we have a drink, and so on.

Not all concepts refer to an item we can see or feel, that which is tangible. A concept that refers to something intangible, not able to be seen or felt, is called a *construct*. This refers to words that some have agreed upon to represent that which cannot be seen, such as depression. We can't see it directly, but we infer it from a set of observable behaviors that are related to one another. The description above of the nonverbal behaviors of the patient might lead one to infer that he is depressed. The list of these constructs is very long; it includes words such as intelligent, harassment, and glorious. We cannot see or touch these, but the word conveys a meaning that is known to others. 'It is a glorious day' communicates meaningfully to those who know the language.

In our professional lives we work with very complex concepts which defy our comprehension. For example, the concept of deoxyribonucleic acid (DNA) may intimidate one. The model of the double helix communicates a meaning that represents the extremely complex nature of DNA. The double helix is a *model*, an analogy for the real thing; the muscle spindle is a model frequently used to talk about how the neuromuscular system works. The word 'model' is used many times in these chapters to explain a complex set of phenomena in human behavior individually or in groups. Erikson's psychosocial model of development through the span of life is another example. In this case the model represents a process rather than an object.

We encounter and consider a wide variety of theories, and implicitly or explicitly evaluate whether they can be applied usefully for our purposes. We probably have standards or criteria against which we evaluate each new perspective. Scientists have evolved a set of criteria that characterize a well-developed theory: a good theory should provide a logical and rational explanation of observed phenomena; it should explain the relationship of relevant related variables; and it should allow one to develop deductions that serve as the basis for testing hypotheses. A good theory is also economical, in that it is free of unnecessary complexity. A theory should have some importance, evaluated as significant by others who may use it. Finally, a good theory needs to be consistent with the facts as they have been observed, and by the body of knowledge available in the field.

We will apply some of the criteria in the following discussion of a good theory related to the construct of personality and the development of that theory over time. Psychoanalytic theory is responsible for the view that the personality of an individual is affected and shaped by the experiences in one's life, and that particular stress or trauma could have a negative effect on development. This followed the concept that there is a 'normal' developmental sequence of psychosocial maturation. [The beginning of a description of concepts related to the theory] Though many aspects of psychoanalytic theory as developed by Freud and his students are difficult or impossible to prove, it has served as an important influence on the evolution of theory in psychology and our understanding of personality and behavior. [Testing of hypotheses of a theory, and importance of the theory]

Many theories have experienced popularity over the years with their accompanying jargon persisting in lay language, though the theory may have disappeared from major discussion and research in the disciplines of psychology and sociology. For example, we frequently hear traits of a person discussed, such as 'he is honest ... or trustworthy,' or 'she is joyful ... or a high achiever'. Originally traits were identified as relatively enduring aspects of one's personality that exist in combination, and vary from one person to another. But trait theory proved to be inadequate as a theory of personality or human behavior. [Usefulness of a theory] While we believe traits may derive from some genetic disposition as well as experiences in the family and society, the research available causes them to be of less interest to health professionals than other behavioral variables that may be more easily altered.

The term 'personality' took on special meaning following the early scholarly work of Gordon Allport (1961) which served to move the casual use of the word into a term with some shared meanings among psychologists. [Importance] Some of these meanings, or constructs, which continue in use include distinctive personal qualities, and selfhood. Allport's (1961) definition was the standard for many years:

'Personality is the dynamic organization within the individual of those psychophysical systems that determine his unique adjustments to his environment.'

Over time the definition has seen many modifications and new constructions by various theorists, so that today we must clarify what was intended in the use of the word with the speaker. [Theory defined] Personality is a cognitive construction of human beings. You and I have a personality only because we say that we do, just as we have other constructions created by human kind, such as a love, an anger, creativity, or extroversion. In conclusion, we can see that the theory of personality has altered over the years, that many have contributed to our present understanding of what it is, and we don't all agree on a single definition yet.

In research we often hear people speak of testing a theory, though this is not really possible. What is meant is that the hypotheses derived from the theory will be tested. These hypotheses are deduced from the theory, based upon observations of particular phenomena that the theory describes. For example, Piaget watched his own children grow from infancy. Based upon his carefully recorded observations he formulated his theory of cognition, discussed later in Chapter 3. From both the theory and the observations, he developed hypotheses which he could test, as could others who followed him.

Philosophy

The philosophy inherent in this volume is based on a system of ecology, which suggests that all factors that have an impact on an individual are interrelated. The individual we see before us is a product of his biologic heritage, the family system, and the social and cultural systems. This construct of an ecosystem is meant to imply that all these components act upon the developing human being, and interact with each other to have a formative impact upon the individual. In *The Origin of the Species*, Charles Darwin studied the relationship between red clover and the bumblebees which pollinate this plant (Darwin, 1872, 1979). The following humorous effort was directed to explain the intricate and elaborate nature of ecological systems. Peter Farb identifies this story as an 'ecological classic' (Farb, 1963).

Darwin discovered that bumble bees, because of their long tongues, are the only insects which can effectively pollinate the deep red clover flowers. From this he argued that the success of red clover in England can be attributed to the fact that bumble bees are so prevalent there. He then went on to quote an authority who had found that there were more bumblebees' nests in the vicinity of villages and towns than elsewhere because field mice, which eat bumblebee combs and larvae, are scarce around towns. And why are field mice scarce? Because towns usually harbor large numbers of cats which prey upon the field mice and keep the population down. Here a German scientist took up the argument: cats, he said, were thus proved responsible for the prevalence of red clover in England; red clover, a staple food of British cattle, could be ecologically linked to the British navy, whose staple diet was bully beef; hence cats could be given ultimáte credit for Britain's dominance as a world power. Thomas Huxley then went even one step further: he suggested, half humorously, that since old maids were well known to be the principal protectors of cats throughout England, the fact that Britannia ruled the waves might logically – and ecologically – be traced right back to the cat-loving tendencies of her many spinsters.

This story is obviously overdrawn, and suggests a one-way cause and effect relationship of the components. However, it does serve to illustrate, in a humorous manner, the interconnections and the far-reaching interrelationships the various components have with each other. All the components, and their connections, are bound together in an ecological system. So too in the human individual, all components are interrelated, and are bound together in an ecological system.

Psychosocial Perspective

Psychosocial theory is not the only theoretical framework by which one may examine human development. There are several other approaches that may illuminate our understanding of this very complex process, such as biological evolution, cultural theory, psychosexual theory, cognitive theory, social role theory, and learning theory to name but a few. Many of these are considered at various points throughout the book. Each serves as *a way*, a perspective, through which to view human development. The psychosocial perspective serves as an organizing framework for the early chapters in the book devoted to development through the span of life.

This framework assumes that the human individual is not totally at the mercy of his biological heritage, or of the environmental influences upon his life. It builds a structure to suggest that at each stage of development the individual has the capacity to influence the direction of physical and psychological growth, and to utilize one's experience to direct that course. This theory also assumes that one's culture has a strong impact upon the rate and direction of growth and development because the goals, expectations, and wishes held by a society for its members has an impact on the individual. We see this expressed in cultural patterns of parenting, value systems, styles of education, and role functions expressed in children and adults. The construct of 'maturity' has different meanings in different cultures.

Psychosocial theory is based upon six organizing constructs which are considered together and separately in succeeding chapters. These six begin with the notion of stages of development, followed by specific tasks related to different stages, a psychosocial crisis that stimulates development from one stage to the next, a process for resolving these crises at each stage, the importance of significant relationships in one's life, and the developing ability to cope with adversity.

Disability

Two major conceptual frameworks dominate the field of disability research, treatment, and prevention: the International Classification of Impairments, Disabilities, and Handicaps (ICIDH) (Pope & Tarlov, 1991) and the functional limitation framework of Saad Nagi. The former is a supplement to the International Classification of Diseases developed by the World Health Organization. Several European countries have adopted the ICIDH for use in administration and clinical settings in their national health programs. Celia Eales refers to this in her chapter on illness in the elderly.

The ICIDH and Nagi models each have four basic concepts that describe its dimensions. The four in the ICIDH model are: disease, impairment, disability, and handicap. The four in the Nagi model are: pathology, impairment, functional limitation, and disability. Each of the models specifies that more than the characteristics of the individual are involved in performance of a socially expected activity; the larger social system and physical environments are also key components in determining the nature of the function impairment, and the extent of disability.

These models are the result of efforts to conceptualize disability in order to deal with questions such as: What is it? How does it happen? How do people respond to it? What does a society do about it? Each of our nations deals with disability in its population somewhat differently in terms of health care at the local level and national policy (Howards et al, 1980). Each also defines it and describes it somewhat differently. When discussing disability, one health professional can only know what another is talking about when they understand the model that serves as the basis for the discussion. Beyond that, we also need to have clear definitions of the concepts involved in the models, such as disease or pathology, impairment, disability or functional limitation, and handicap or disability. In the minds of their creators, there is a difference between disease and pathology, and between disability and functional limitation.

Paradigm

The work of the authors in this volume is directed toward an underlying assumption that the information and perspectives will lead to the development of a different view of persons, and particularly persons who are patients. Information ultimately can lead to a different perspective on the people with whom we work and has the potential to create new courses of action. *Paradigm* is the word that describes this phenomenon. The word 'paradigm' was originally used by Thomas Kuhn (Kuhn, 1970) in his monograph called *The Structure of Scientific Revolutions*. He intended it to mean a change in the way we see things, a change in our view on how to deal with a situation or problem. Through the years of use, the word has taken on an additional, somewhat altered meaning similar to that of 'model'.

With the original meaning in mind, it is our fervent hope that the information contained in this volume will inform our judgements, and lead us toward a new way to view people who are patients, so we may be more effective in clinical decision making.

References

Allport, G (1961) *Pattern and Growth in Personality*. New York: Holt, Rinehart & Winston.

Darwin, C (1872,1979) The illustrated *Origin of the Species*. Abridged and introduced by Richard E. Leakey. New York: Hill & Wang.

Farb, P (1963) *Ecology*. New York: Time, Inc.

Howards, I, Brelm, HP, Nagi, S (1980) *Disability, from Social Problem to Federal Program*. New York: Praeger.

Kuhn, T (1970) *The Structure of Scientific Revolutions*. Chicago: University of Chicago Press.

Newman, BM, Newman, PR (1995) *Development through Life*, p. 737. Pacific Grove: Brooks/Cole Publishing Company.

Pope, A, Tarlov, AR (eds) (1991) *Disability in America*: Toward a national agenda for prevention. Washington, DC: National Academy Press.

2

A System of Ecology

Elsa Ramsden

Introduction
•
Biological System
•
Psychosocial Theory
•
Societal System
•
Summary

Introduction

The human individual enters the world full of a potential for growth and development to maturity that depends upon the family into which it is born, the culture of the community and the conditions of the nation where it resides, and the genetic heritage it received from its parents. Each one of these dimensions is very complex in itself, but in combination with each of the other dimensions the complexity becomes almost overwhelming. Behavioral scientists have been working for years separating out some of the factors within each dimension to gain understanding about potential impact on development and

health. Now they are tackling some of the difficult combinations between factors within one dimension, and among factors in different dimensions.

In this chapter we will look at three systems that have an impact on the developing individual: biological, psychological, societal, and some of the relationships among them that combine to constitute the dimensions of family, culture, and genetic heritage. Our objective is to establish the groundwork to gain greater understanding about human behavior. Ultimately we need to know enough about human behavior in order to tailor our treatment intervention to the needs and abilities of each individual patient.

When a health professional faces a new person who has come for treatment in any clinical context, such as the emergency room, intensive care unit, clinic, outpatient facility, or home, a rapid series of judgments is made about that individual. The judgments relate to *who* is this person, *what* are they like as a human being, *where* is the problem, and *how* can the development of this relationship be guided most effectively to meet the patient's needs. The nature of the clinical context will determine the priority of those questions. In the emergency room, 'where is the problem' is paramount. In the rehabilitation facility or home care context, 'how to guide the relationship' may be most important. The judgments we make hinge on our knowledge of the factors that contribute to human behavior, experience in our personal life, professional experience with other patients like this one, and on our ability to put that knowledge into an applied form along with our professional skills.

Biological System

Genes and inheritance

The monk Gregor Mendel was the father of modern genetics. He studied inherited characteristics of plants and is probably best known for his work with garden peas (Mendel, 1866). The 'laws' he formulated occurred long before we knew anything about the biochemical materials that make up genes and chromosomes. The Human Genome Project in the 20th century is a little like the discovery of the periodic table of elements in the preceding century. That process resulted in a systematic identification of all atoms and their relationship to one another in terms of similarities and differences. The objective of the Human Genome Project is to identify the biological corollary of the chemical periodic table, with its 100,000 genes in a tree structure organizing ancestral and functional relationships among them. The interaction of genes and families of genes has become the premier research of today, rather than a focus on the character of single genes, as was the case just a few years ago.

Each individual is the result of genetic combinations from two sexually mature adults of each gender. The contributions of each may produce a variety of genetically distinct children. Some of the individual variations that are genetically determined are individual personality traits and intelligence, the rate of development, psychosocial development, and abnormalities of many kinds. How the individual with a given complement of inherited genes matures has long been the focus of study and debate. The 'nature or nurture' or inheritance versus environment controversy set the biologists and psychologists on opposite sides for decades. We now know that it isn't a simple either/or dilemma, but an intricate interweaving of the two. The experience of an individual affects the expression of inherited characteristics, and will influence adaptation to the events of life and development of the person over time. For example, all individuals are born with a potential for thought, but not all infants receive sufficient nourishment to sustain the growth and development of brain cells. Prolonged starvation will result in limited intellectual capacity, as well as physical illness and if irreversible, death.

The evolution of human beings was a theoretical formulation developed by Charles Darwin as he tried to explain how adaptation occurs. His term 'natural selection' appeared in 1859 in his publication *Origin of the Species* (Darwin, 1968). This theory along with the development of modern day genetics has led to our theory of evolution. The ability of a species to adapt to the conditions in the environment determines the survival and the quality of that survival. The concept of adaptation is basic to our understanding of evolution. Our use of the term 'adaptation' with respect to patients in rehabilitation is quite different, taking on meanings similar to coping and adjusting of a single individual as opposed to a species. We call this behavioral adaption and it is learned behavior. This concept will be discussed further in the next chapter.

Fundamental to adaptation is the human brain, which evolved more extensively than other human organs over hundreds of millions of years. The key to human adaptation is the ability of abstract thought, making it possible to adjust to varying topography, geography, and climate. This capacity makes it possible for the individual to transcend our inherited biological limitations. Our genetic inheritance has a strong influence on who we are and what we become. The research of the subdiscipline of quantitative genetics, which focuses on the contributions to individual differences that genetic and environmental factors affect, suggests that the genetic factors account for between twenty and sixty percent of variance. The effect of genetics is strong but not overpowering

(Plomin *et al.*, 1997). The gene is the basic unit that determines some fixed traits at the time of conception, and affects dispositions of the individual depending on factors in the environment and experience. Our biological capacities together with the environment within which we live interact in a way that results in individual behavior. Some of the factors involved include the nature of the parenting for the infant and young child, the kinds and quality of the resources available to the child and family, the competing interests of other members of the family for attention and resources, and the positive or negative qualities of the cultural climate within which the infant is nurtured. The complexity of these ingredients and the interactions among them helps to explain how two children, close in age in the same family, may grow up one to be a criminal and the other a priest. Figure 2.1 represents these influences in summary form.

Figure 2.1 Major components of the biological system. (Based on Newman and Newman (1995).

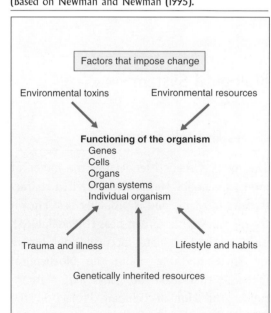

Psychosocial Theory

The body of psychosocial theory tries to explain the development of the human individual in terms of an interaction among the needs and abilities of the person, set within a societal context that has expectations and rules. Students and researchers of human behavior in psychology and sociology have demonstrated that the growth and changes people experience are systematic and predictable, not haphazard. As they grow they acquire and internalize knowledge and values transmitted by older generations. Psychosocial theories frequently are posed in the form of stages or organizing concepts. The underlying psychosocial framework in this volume is based on the work of Eric Erikson (1950, 1963, 1982).

The theorists look at human behavior across the span of life, identify the key components and describe it in terms of stages in the growth from infancy through old age. The theory is based on the premise that we are not merely victims of our biological heritage nor the influences of our environment. At least in a general way these theorists suggest that at every stage in life a potential exists to organize and integrate our experiences that contribute to individual psychological development. Culture plays an important role in individual growth; it sets the rules that guide our lives, the expectations for behavior, and provides opportunities for expression of individuality within the community.

The stages of development are described in basically similar fashion by different theorists, though the number of stages varies among them. Each theory incorporates a set of key concepts that guide its organization. Stage theories present a specific order and direction for development, with each successive stage dependent upon the work accomplished at the preceding level, incorporating the gains made into the work to be done at the new level (Davison et al., 1980; Miller, 1993). Each stage explains a wide range of newly acquired abilities, and the potential for problems in one's life that may lead to conflict. When we observe young children of different ages with a stage theory in mind, the differences we see are quickly apparent: the two year old plays beside but not with another, while three and four year old children play in pairs and threes. The three year old is possessive and holds on to the toy, while the child of five may try to negotiate or trade articles of importance. A little later, young people in their early teen years tend to congregate in groups for social activities, while older teens move off in pairs. And so the stages evolve throughout life.

Stages of development

Erikson (1950, 1963) identified eight stages in his theory of psychosocial development. He arrived at his configuration in part influenced by the earlier work of Freud and in part through his observations and analyses. A summary of these eight stages appears in Table. 2.1. Newman and Newman (1995) propose an eleven stage theory that adds prenatal, middle adulthood, and very old age. These theories share the assumption that psychosocial development at each stage has important effects on all the stages that follow. The sequence is predictable but the work, or tasks accomplished at each stage are not.

Table 2.1
Erikson Theory of Psychosocial Development

Stage	Age range	Developmental Task
Trust versus Mistrust	0 to 12 months	From birth to about one year of age, this stage serves as the basis for all future development in the psychosocial domain. Trust develops from feelings of physical comfort in combination with minimal fear and uncertainty. The quality of the relationship with the mother or surrogate is of prime importance, surpassing even that of food or demonstrations of love. The sensory experience of the infant with its own body is associated with social interaction for the baby, and provides the basis for psychological trust. These issues of trust or mistrust are not resolved for all time, but arise again during succeeding stages of development. These later encounters with trust issues may threaten the basic trust, or provide more opportunities for development.
Autonomy versus Shame and Doubt	2 to 4 years	As the child engages with the world around, it discovers that behavior brings response; the child learns how to use this with increasing effectiveness. Out of these experiences evolves a growing sense of autonomy and control. This is inevitably accompanied by some conflicts related to asserting oneself or remaining dependent. Exploring the environment is a major goal of this being who is developing increasing coordination and physical strength. Staying in one place is more and more difficult. Activities involving holding on to, letting go, and manipulating objects are prominent. The child is occupied in making friends and expressing oneself verbally and physically. Bodily functions become interesting to the child as well as to the parent. Control and regulation of behavior is tested in a variety of ways. Mastery leads to a greater sense of responsibility and self-understanding. In the presence of over-control by the care givers, shame and doubt may result.
Initiative versus Guilt	4 to 5 years	Language and motor development are now at a level to give expression to imagination. Play activities are more creative and interesting; peers are joined for companionship. At this age curiosity is expressed verbally and physically, including sexual curiosity, and comparison with others' skills and size provides new understanding

Table 2.1 (contd.)
Erikson Theory of Psychosocial Development

Stage	Age range	Developmental Task
		of self. It is important to be the biggest and the best compared to some other person. The child seeks attention in a wide variety of ways. The manner in which this curiosity is handled by the caregivers will reinforce the initiative or thwart it, perhaps resulting in shame and guilt. The child has an insatiable curiosity and active imagination. Negative reinforcement of their expression may result in guilt for the thoughts alone, and for activities which no one observed. A healthy identification with authority figures as well as peers leads to resolving some of the guilt
Industry versus Inferiority	6 to 11 years	At this age in western societies the child engages in increased competition with others and begins to separate work and play activities. With school attendance and wider contacts with peers the child feels the impact of many others who influence the developing sense of self. New lessons in work activities are frequently interrupted by retreats into play for comfort and reassurance. Reinforcement by significant others of effort and achievement leads to the developing industry and sense of worth. If the child learns that other things have an impact on identity, such as color of skin and background of parents, or the designer label in the clothes worn, the child may identify worth with those things rather than the self. These first four stages serve as the groundwork upon which the work of the adolescent is based in developing identity.
Identity versus Identity Diffusion	12 to 18 years	Throughout this period the young person strives to be themselves and tries to share with others singly and in groups. Separating from the influence of parents becomes an important agenda with increasing need to be in charge of their own affairs and to be free of the earlier dependency. Emerging new abilities are tested to determine their nature and level, and they seek recognition and acknowledgement from important adults related to these abilities. This is accompanied by the fear that somehow they will not meet the expectations of adulthood.

Table 2.1 (contd.)
Erikson Theory of Psychosocial Development

Stage	Age range	Developmental Task
		Time perspective and time diffusion poses a dilemma at this age. Appropriate timing of responsibilities with abilities to execute, as well as the desire to accomplish the tasks is key to resolving some of the issues of time perspective, rather than resulting in frustration, a sense of urgency, and hopelessness. The accomplishments of earlier stages reappear again in the now more able individual to expand the sense of self (autonomy versus shame and doubt). Timely adult reinforcement builds self esteem; its absence may lead to feelings of inferiority and fears of not achieving much in life. New roles are tried and initiative is expressed in new ways. If limited in this regard, they may seek to resolve conflict through behavior disapproved of by family and community. This results in a less desirable identity, but that is preferred to one that is diffused – no identity. It appears there is an increase in psychic energy at this stage, which may be used to try new experiences and new skills. Some energy may be used to resolve feelings from uncompleted tasks in earlier stages and appears as introspection. These tasks of adolescence may require many years beyond age 18 to accomplish.
Intimacy versus Isolation	18 to 35 years	The young adult works on sexual and psychological intimacy between two people while at the same time maintaining a sense of their own identity. The explorations of adolescence take on new meaning and new dimensions during this time through the formation of friendships at various levels, explorations with leadership, new achievements in athletics, new experiences with travel to more distant places. If one is unwilling or unable to form intimate relationships, not necessarily physical intimacy, a resulting distancing from others relieves the potential threat to identity. Willingness and ability to share in mutual trust with another characterizes achievement at this time, along with regulation of work, time to play, and participation in community activities in ways that satisfy themselves.

Table 2.1 (contd.)
Erikson Theory of Psychosocial Development

Stage	Age range	Developmental Task
Generativity versus Stagnation	35 to 65 years	The main agenda of these years is finding and settling into the right role in life, and guiding the next generation through parenting, employment, and recreation. Through an examination of the journey of one's life, each assesses whether it was satisfying and whether it was good. A self-absorbed turning in on one's self may lead to stagnation.
Integrity versus Despair	65 to advanced old age	The psychosocial task of these years is to arrive at the conclusion that one has done the best one could under the circumstances and to feel OK about that – accepting oneself and one's life. Numerous opportunities exist to feel overwhelmed, disappointed, and frustrated. One confronts a wide variety of feelings and experiences and works to maintain equilibrium throughout it all, which leads to ego integrity. When one has had what feels like a full life, it is possible to give it up with integrity. When one feels little good has come of it and few prospects remain, a sense of despair may result, along with a fear of death.

Progression through the stages is a function of chronologic age, physical and emotional maturation, and the social environment. Different cultural contexts place different demands and expectations on individuals. Those presented here reflect a post-industrial society, and would not necessarily apply to a tribal society or that of a developing country.

Change occurs in the individual in several different areas simultaneously at each psychosocial stage throughout life. Our developmental tasks take place in the physical, emotional, social, and intellectual areas, at the same time that we evolve a sense of who we are, our self-concept. This self-concept undergoes alteration on a constant basis, influenced by newly acquired abilities and knowledge in the early years, and declining abilities and a wealth of experience and knowledge later in life. Mastery of developmental tasks is achieved by coping effectively with the stresses and strains imposed by our own biological clocks and the forces imposed by the social context. These forces are referred to as psychosocial crises in these theories.

For example, the young child of two to three years engages in explorations that frequently encounter restrictions to the activity. The struggle for 'me do it' confronts the needs of the parent or care taker to prevent harm. The child's striving for independence exists in the absence of experience and knowledge of the potential risks involved. The manner in which these stresses are managed will have a direct effect on the evolving sense of self. This 'crisis' may be resolved to produce a sense of responsibility, or shame and doubt.

The psychosocial agenda in late adolescence continues the process of striving for independence, with very different physical and emotional resources. This crisis is posed by the need to be one's own self, and the need to be with one or more others in a give and take relationship. Separation from parents is coincidental with this process. Successful resolution of these stresses results in taking on new responsibilities and having new privileges with a stronger sense of identity.

We can see from Table 2.1 and from the illustrations above that the crises in each of the stages are described with reference to the polarities, for example, Initiative versus Guilt in the four to five year old, and Integrity versus Despair in the elderly. This psychosocial theory suggests that as one moves into a new stage one experiences the pushes and pulls of both ends of the spectrum within that stage. The discrepancy between the individual's ability that is available at the beginning of the stage is in contrast to the expectations set by society for a new level of function at the end. This creates at least a mild experience of tension suggested by the negative label at the end of the spectrum within each stage. So the adolescent may experience some anxiety while developing new mastery and control of affairs, and simultaneously becoming less dependent upon the parents who have provided nurturance and support up to that point.

The resolution of the crises in each stage results as one finds a balance between the internal and external forces at the two extremes, the forces that push and the forces that pull toward new growth. The movie industry created a llama-like animal with two heads at either end of one body that intrigued Dr Dolittle as it represented the 'push me–pull you' dilemmas. The developmental tasks become more and more complex at each successive stage, making it more likely that one will encounter more difficulty in accomplishing the goals, and will be more likely to experience more resistance from society in the efforts to grow. The efforts result in new personal growth, a stronger sense of self, and new personal resources to approach the next stage. Figure 2.2 represents in summary form the major components of the psychosocial system and the key processes involved.

Figure 2.2 Major components of the psychological system. (Based on Newman and Newman (1965).

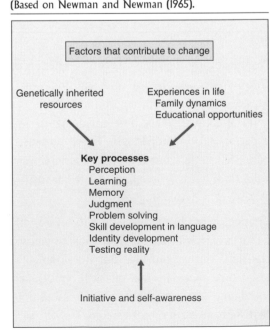

Societal System

Culture

Each of us is a product of one or more cultures, languages, and ethnic groups. Edward Tylor (1874) proposed a definition of culture which continues to be popular,

'...that complex whole which includes knowledge, belief, art, morals, law, custom, and any other capabilities and habits acquired by man as a member of society.'

Culture is the framework that provides the guidelines and boundaries of our actions. This cultural framework evolves over time, is shaped and reshaped as we grow in knowledge and understanding (Anderson and Fenichel, 1989).

People who share a cultural heritage may share many traditions and beliefs, but not all, and their behavior may be similar, or it may be quite different. The social forces we experience within our culture as well as environmental forces contribute in important ways to who we are and how we function in our world. Some of these factors are the nature of that culture, the area we live in such as a neighborhood, the composition of the community or demographics of the population, and the options available to us for play and work in this setting. Whether we grow up rich or poor, native to the country or immigrant or refugee, resident of urban or rural communities, all of these ingredients contribute in powerful ways to who we are.

Cultural determinism

We may say as a more general approach that culture provides a world-view in that it supplies the context within which to make meaning of the events that occur around us, such as the relationships we form and the objects that make up our homes and cities. An early cultural anthropologist (Benedict, 1934, 1950) maintains that the direction and course of human development is primarily the product of cultural expectations. We humans do not carry coding for language or religion or social order in our genes, as is true for the ant of the insect species.

Some experiences are universal among human beings, such as the passage from dependent child to independent adult. The route one takes on that journey, however, varies markedly from one culture to another. Benedict's theory was formative to the theory of psychosocial stages of development. Cultures that have age-related expectations for behavior at different times throughout life also have public ceremonies to mark specific transitions, and other rites of passage from one stage to the next.

Ethnic subcultures

Modern societies have shared cultural characteristics as well as many which are not shared because of the ethnic subcultures that coexist within the nation. Ethnicity is a general concept that encompasses the entirety of shared experience that includes racial similarities as well as religion, social structure, and definitions of gender roles (See and Wilson 1988).

An ethnic group is defined as

'a collectivity within a larger society having real or common ancestry, memories of a shared historical past, and a cultural focus on one or more symbolic elements defined as the epitome of their peoplehood' (Schermerhorn, 1978).

Members within an ethnic group may differ in the degree to which they identify with the group, but usually share some of the values, beliefs, and norms for behavior, and some degree of loyalty. This loyalty may be dormant for prolonged periods, but when the group is threatened in some way, the loyalty may become heightened and find expression in a variety of ways.

These features of the dominant culture of a society and the subculture of the ethnic group may exist in harmony or there may be some tension between them for any given individual. Disharmony may pose particularly difficult situations for the individual in the social institutions of school, employment facility, and in the political arena (Horowitz, 1985). Negative ethnic stereotypes may have an effect on the evolving self-concept of the members of the oppressed group. In some communities the ethnic prejudice produces a separation of ethnic groups that reduces the type and amount of contact members of the groups have to have with one another. It is common in these circumstances to find an increased ethnocentrism, a belief among members of the dominant group that they are somehow superior to those in the other groups. A general lack of tolerance exists, based upon poor or inaccurate knowledge and understanding of the values and beliefs of those in other subcultures.

Culture and human development

Our cultural experience has a major impact on shaping a sense of self and individual identity. For example, many cultures, such as Asian, African, and Latin American, place emphasis on the connections and interdependence between and among members. The self is defined in terms of relatedness to others, particularly one's family. In North American middle-class cultures and some western-European middle-class cultures, the self is defined in terms of internal attributes, suggesting the world-view of self as independent (Berry et al., 1992).

The transition events that mark our lives are viewed differently in different cultures. For example, in some societies people fear menstruation and believe it is dangerous to be in the young woman's company. In other societies, the female is believed to have great power or magic at this time of the month, and believe her behavior will have an influence on her future and the future of the tribe. In some societies sex is perceived as shameful and anything connected with sexuality is hidden from view, kept secret, and not discussed. It would be very different to grow up a female in these three different kinds of belief systems.

Belief systems of cultures and subcultures incorporate a wide variety of behaviors that are distinctive and may be or may not be observed. For example, when we leave our home and expect to be absent for some time, what are our habits associated with departure? In one Native American community, an elderly gentleman was seen to place a large stick against his lockless door as he departed. When asked, he said that was to let others know that he was not at home, and that they should not enter. All members of that community behaved in this manner (Rotter, 1954). At this level of participation in a practice, we would identify the behavior not just as a habit, but more a cultural trait or perhaps a cultural universal.

When we consider psychosocial development, the cultural context is crucial to our understanding of stages, normal behavior, and the personal qualities considered appropriate or inappropriate under given conditions. Standards of talent, beauty, and leadership are culture specific. The timing of particular events in life such as dating, courtship, sexual relationships, marriage, and education are set in the expectations of the society. When one chooses to stray from the established guidelines of the culture, one runs a grave risk of alienating members of the group and one's family. The Amish of Pennsylvania and the eastern United States continue a tradition of

Figure 2.3 Major components of the societal system. (Based on Newman and Newman (1995).

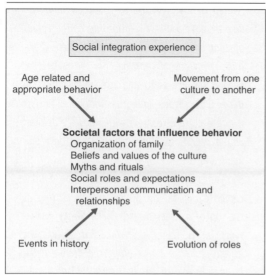

'shunning' the individual who strays from the groups' norms. That person is ignored, not spoken to by anyone including members of one's family, and may not participate in religious activities or any other activities in the community. Any who violate the rule of shunning are themselves punished. This seems extreme behavior in the context of the dominant culture of North America which espouses tolerance for individual differences and diversity in the population. This example has many corollaries in other cultures around the globe. Figure 2.3 presents in summary form some of the components in the societal system that influence behavior.

Ecology

Values inherent in all cultures have the potential for profound impact on individual health and the health of the society as a whole. Ecology is a sub-field within the discipline of biology that deals with relationships between living organisms and their environment. Many believe the survival of the planet and its inhabitants depends on responsible use of resources and appropriate use of the by-products from the use of those resources.

The advent of the industrial revolution and mass production changed the way people produced goods for living and foods for human and animal consumption. The introduction of the automobile, chemicals into production processes, and pest control for large- and small-scale farming has resulted in airborne particulates and smog in urban areas, and polluted waterways everywhere. The increases in population with an expected doubling of the world population over the next 40 years threaten to overwhelm small efforts at pollution control and destruction of natural resources in both the developed and developing nations. We know now that pollutants have a significant negative impact on our genes, organs, and organ systems.

The chemical industries along the Love Canal in Niagara Falls, New York and the heavy industries along the Rhine River in Austria, as elsewhere, found it economically prudent to dump waste material into the local waterways. Years after this process began in Niagara Falls, mothers noticed that children in their community who lived along the Love Canal (the irony in the name is sad) had a much higher incidence of certain kinds of cancer than the rest of the nation. They traced the problem to the chemical waste that had been dumped into the canal. These chemicals had leached into the adjacent soil along which homes and schools had been built. The mothers went to the industries, the state, and finally to the federal government. Twenty years of debate, negotiation, and litigation brought resolution to the problem, but did not bring back the lives of the children. This case was one of the earliest in the new ethics category of 'compensatory justice'. We have learned from this situation, and many others like it, that the by-products and waste products of production and the chemical residue of pesticides lead to genetic changes, illness, and death.

Over the past twenty-five years, the industrial town of Kalundborg in Denmark has created a complex system of symbiosis to use the by-products of production economically (Gertler and Ehrenfeld, 1996). The project was stimulated by increasing governmental regulations to protect the environment. This community found ways to use the heat and steam from the production of electricity used in other industrial processes, to heat the homes and businesses of the entire town, and to run the fish farm. This resulted in markedly reduced oil consumption and clean air. They found that solid waste from the fish ponds could be sold as fertilizer. Many other symbiotic and synergistic relationships evolved in this community. The story is much too involved and complex than this telling can convey, but it serves to illustrate how a society examined its values, reordered some of its priorities, and found economy of scale and financial rewards that resulted in improved health and welfare for its population. It also illustrates well the interconnections of biology, psychology, and culture.

Summary

We have identified three systems that have an impact on the psychosocial development of the individual: biological, psychological, and societal, and have considered some of the relationships among them. Health and illness are related to the structure of a society and frequently have a direct relationship to the values of that society. The individual's genetic heritage provides a portion of the resources needed for access to and use of resources in the environment. And the individual exists within a cultural context with rules, guidelines, and expectations that influence the development and identity of the self.

We can visualize the child's toy, the Slinky, composed of tightly wound spirals, sitting at the top of a series of steps. The Slinky represents in its tight, interconnected spirals the genetic material found along the double helix, intimately related to the psychological devel–

opment process of the self, within the cultural context. The steps upon which the Slinky is poised represent the stages of psychosocial development through the life cycle. Sitting at the top step, the Slinky is full of potential. A bit of energy from outside itself, in the form of a push, will send it down the steps and stages. Succeeding chapters will deal with the journey of the individual through the stages.

References

Anderson, PP, Fenichel, ES (1989) *Serving Culturally Diverse Families of Infants and Toddlers with Disabilities*. Washington, DC: National Center for Clinical Infant Programs.

Benedict, R (1950) *Patterns of Culture*. New York: New American Library.

Berry, JW, Poortinga, YH, Segall, MH, & Dasen, PR (1992) *Cross–cultural Psychology: Research and Applications*. Cambridge, England: Cambridge University Press.

Darwin, C (1968) *On the Origin of Species*. New York: Penguin Books (original work published 1859).

Davison, ML, King, PM, Kitchener, KS, Parker, CA (1980) The stage sequence concept in cognitive and social development. *Developmental Psychology* 16: 121–131.

Erikson, EH (1963) *Childhood and Society*. New York: Norton.

Erikson, EH (1982) *The Life Cycle Completed: A review*. New York: Norton.

Gertler, N, Ehrenfeld, J (1996) A down-to-earth approach to clean production. *Technology Review*, February / March.

Horowitz, D (1985) *Ethnic Groups in Conflict*. Berkeley: University of California Press.

Mendel, G (1866) Experiments with plant hybrids. *Proceedings of the Brunn Natural History Society*, Germany.

Miller, PH (1993) *Theories of Developmental Psychology*, 3rd edn. New York: W.H. Freeman.

Newman, BM, Newman, PR, (1995) *Development through Life: A Psychosocial Approach*. London: International Thomson-Publishing Europe.

Plomin, R, DeFries, J, McClearn, G, Rutter, M (1997) *Behavioral Genetics*, 3rd edn. New York: W.H. Freeman.

Rotter, JB (1954) *Social Learning and Clinical Psychology*. Englewood Cliffs, NJ: Prentice-Hall.

Schermerhorn, RA (1978) *Comparative Ethnic Relations: A Framework for Theory and Research*. Chicago: University of Chicago Press.

See, KO, Wilson, WJ (1988) Race and ethnicity. In Smelser, NJ (ed) *Handbook of Sociology*, pp. 223–242. Newbury Park, CA: Sage.

Tylor, EB (1874) *Primitive Culture: Researches into the Development of Mythology, Philosophy, Religion, Language, Art and Custom*. New York.

3

Development Through Life: Fundamental Patterns

Elsa Ramsden

Introduction
•
Adaptation
•
Cultural Context
•
Cognitive Development
•
Learning and Learning Theory
•
Memory

Introduction

This chapter builds on the information in the preceding chapter by exploring in greater depth some of the fundamental issues involved in the growth and development of an individual throughout the span of life. It provides the groundwork for more specific attention to the young child in the next chapter, the adolescent in Chapter 5, and so on.

In Chapter 1 we described the process by which a theory comes into being. Then in the second chapter we introduced the theory of individual psychosocial development through a discussion of the several systems that bear on that process. In this chapter we will explore psychosocial development further by using several theoretic constructs to describe different aspects of human behavior. The focus of our effort is to understand what that behavior is about. Behavior does not happen in a vacuum. Where does the behavior come from? To what purpose is it directed? These theories deal with the concepts of adaptation, psychosexual development, cognitive development, learning, and social roles.

Adaptation

Adaptation refers to the ability of an organism to change or adjust in order to survive in its environment. It is a process that takes place over generations in the species to develop characteristics that enable it to thrive. This attribute may exist at the biological level, the physical level, the behavioral level, and at the social level. Behavioral adaptation is a characteristic of an individual which is learned, not transmitted through genetic material from generation to generation. We may communicate information about behavioral adaptation from adult or parent to child in the course of child rearing practices, education experiences, and social groups. Human beings have the ability to adapt to a wide range of environmental conditions and still survive. We can modify our behavior to suit the need. For example, when it is very cold, we design suitably warm clothing to protect against the elements, as do any of the native inhabitants of regions near the North Pole. When confronted with overwhelming adversity, the human psyche adapts to the stress through remarkable life-saving strategies to conserve emotional energy and preserve sanity. We could cite a long list of adverse life experiences such as famine, natural disasters, war, concentration camps, and terrorist activities that test our being.

The word adaptation was used by Piaget (1936, 1952) to represent the process by which knowledge develops. It involves taking in new information and comparing it to schemes that already exist, making some kind of sense of the new. The result is a more fully developed scheme, or a new scheme that will take on its own configuration. Human beings constantly strive for equilibrium in their lives. The unknown imposes a condition of disequilibrium.

'It is by adapting to things that thought organizes itself, and it is by organizing itself that it structures things' (Piaget, 1952, pp. 7–8).

The process of adaptation has two parts: assimilation and accomodation. Assimilation may be understood in both biological and intellectual dimensions as the integration of information into an evolving set of structures. For example, imagine visiting a rehabilitation facility in a different country for the first time, without information about the health care system, patient care, education, or the political process. What one sees and hears is familiar in some respects but very different in other respects. As we see things that we do not understand we ask questions to elicit information about how patient care is conducted, how the health care system works in this country, what the political process is and its impact on health care, and what the education of the country is that produces the health care professionals and the consumers of health care. Each answer we receive to a question posed is compared with what we know about the comparative information in our own system in order to understand the new information. We gradually build a new data set or scheme related to each area of questions that we ask. Within a few days or weeks we find that new information is taken directly in to the new scheme, no longer using the step of comparison to our earlier scheme.

Accommodation involves a process of modifying a scheme to account for the new information that alters the dimensions of the scheme. For example, imagine that you are visiting a patient who has experienced a cerebral vascular accident (CVA) and has moderate spasticity in both right upper and lower extremities. We have read about spasticity, learned about the neurologic mechanisms that produce it, learned about the impact on muscular coordination, but have never seen it in a person, nor felt it with our hands. This first contact with the patient provides extensive new information to add to our scheme or data set about spasticity. We now have visual and tactile information to incorporate with the knowledge and limited understanding that existed before. The new material enhances the earlier information, enriching it as well as expanding it. Further experience in treatment with people having spasticity will expand the scheme even further along the dimensions of evaluation and treatment.

The combined processes of assimilation and accommodation lead to knowledge acquisition throughout life. With each new experience we take in information and relate it to previously acquired data residing in a scheme, according to Piaget, or a cognitive map according to Tolman (1932, 1948) and Festinger (1954). We distinguish between what is familiar and what is unknown in the mass of data absorbed by our sensory systems. If the existing schemes do not account for some of the data our cognitive processes find ways of dealing with it. The data may be ignored if it is not crucial to interpreting the situation; we may adjust the schemes to accommodate the new information; or we may adjust the reality so it will fit the scheme we have stored. We will consider this process again in the discussion of cognitive development later in this chapter, and in Chapter 13 as part of a discussion of the process of making judgments.

Cultural Context

As we mentioned earlier in Chapter 2, the cultural context is the framework within which behavior develops. That behavior can be understood only in terms of the cultural context that shapes it. In some cultures activities of children and adults are not graded by age-appropriate standards. The child may do those things it has the ability to perform and is not restricted or pushed by standards set by the society. These societies do not produce stage development categories by age. When the culture is more permissive and flexible, development is more gradual and flowing, with responsibilities of maturity appearing earlier than the western concept of adulthood. For example, a girl of eight initially surprised her neighbors in a suburban community of northeast America when she said she took care of her infant brother after school, did laundry, and helped to prepare the evening meal. Upon questioning the mother the neighbors found this to be true. These responsibilities did not fit their expectations for eight-year-old children in their community. The mother commented that the child was fully capable to do those things, and enjoyed the responsibility. These kinds of activities would not be remarkable in most developing nations or tribal societies.

Our knowledge about human development gained from scientific research is handicapped by a lack of cultural perspective. Much of the research and theory was developed in Western nations, North America, Canada, and Europe in particular. It has been difficult to identify universal principles that span the cultures of the world. Conclusions drawn from scientific observations must be tempered by the knowledge that the cultural context may be limited and quite specific (Nsamenang, 1992).

When one identifies with the norms and values of the subculture to which one belongs a potential exists for them to have a strong impact on behavior, in addition to the norms and values of the dominant culture. How much impact the subculture has on the developing individual's behavior is a function of several factors: how intensely do the individual and family identify with the subculture; how much time do family members spend with others in the same ethnic group, and with members of other groups; how is this subcultural group viewed by members of the dominant culture?

The family structure and ethos is instrumental in shaping the quality of our lives. Relationships between members and among several participants in family dynamics have long-lasting effects on emotional and intellectual development. They affect the way we view ourselves in the world, our coping behavior in daily problem solving and times of crisis, and the motivation energies applied to achieve our goals. The family has the potential to be a strong positive influence in one's life, but it also may have a profound negative impact on the growth and development of the child.

'Families provide the context for some of the most severe violence in our society and for long-term patterns of physical and emotional abuse that can have dire effects on the mental health of adults and children.' (Basic Behavioral Science Task Force, 1996).

A study conducted in Finland demonstrated that children, whose parent had schizophrenia, are at far greater risk to develop the disorder if raised in a dysfunctional adoptive family, than if raised in a healthy adoptive family that provided support (Jacob, 1987). One hundred twenty-six children born into families with schizophrenia were placed in adoptive families. Eight of these later developed a severe emotional disorder. Each of the eight had been reared in dysfunctional families.

We know there are many biological and social factors that affect mental health, from genetic material to extended family relationships. The power of the family unit cannot be underestimated in providing care to the developing individual. We will consider this further in the next chapter in the discussion on the emotional development of the infant and child.

Cognitive Development

Piaget's theory of development focused on the interaction of the child with its environment as the child explores and discovers objects and relationships and meaning (Piaget, 1985). Another psychologist, L.S. Vygotsky (1978), argued that development is understood only in terms of a social context. He suggested that as the child interacts with various aspects of the environment, it assigns meaning to events and things based upon the historical and cultural contexts, as well as the biological heritage and maturation brought to bear on the task. In many cultures, for example, competition is an important component of a child's learning experiences at home, in the class room, and on the playing field. But among several tribes of native North Americans competition is not a concept they understand, unless they have learned it from the 'immigrant' population. Self-improvement, cooperation and teamwork are the focus of interactions with peers.

Several systems within the human being are involved in providing the data from which meaning is derived. Data is brought into the central nervous system by way of all the sensory modalities, of vision, hearing, smell, taste, touch, and kinesthesia. What happens to it then is very much the subject of research, discussion, and debate. Several theories attempt to account for the transformation of light waves into an image of a tree, or sound waves into music of Mozart, or chemical esters to the smell of an orange. *Perception* is the process by which sensory information is organized into patterns. It includes the reception of the data by the sensory apparatus and transmission to particular parts of the brain, selection of particular aspects of the data to which to attend, and the assignment of meaning to it.

Over many years theories of perception have tried to explain what happens to the amazing number of stimuli that bombard our sensory apparatus. Only a small portion of these stimuli is taken in by the eye, the ear, and so on. Our nervous system has evolved from lower forms to develop mechanisms by which information is reduced and organized on its route to the brain as it moves from the sensory nerve cell along various pathways.

The sensory systems are part of our biological and genetic heritage. Given a set of equipment that is in normal condition, however, experience plays an important role in the development of those systems. For example, kittens reared in the dark do not develop binocular vision so are unable to integrate images from the two eyes. Research suggests there is a critical developmental period during which restricted experience will result in limited development for the sensory system involved. Extensive research focuses on the effects of practice on normal development and skill development of the sensory apparatus. Young adults raised in an urban community were compared with a group of Native Americans of the Cree tribe on ability to distinguish vertical, horizontal, and oblique outline. The Cree surpassed the urban dwellers on all parameters. The urban environment has an abundance of the vertical and horizontal, but few of the oblique. The homes of the Cree contain all three orientations. At one time, natives of the deep forests in the Congo seldom saw wide expanses of space or objects at a great distance. They had a poorly developed concept of the constancy of size in contrast to people of western nations. A buffalo was seen at close range in the forest; one could not see a long way off because of the foliage. When seen on the plain a long way off, a buffalo appeared as a speck or insect. This vision caused great concern to the pygmy guide of a cultural anthropologist who believed it was magic that the buffalo should get bigger and bigger as the jeep approached the herd (Turnbull, 1961). The sensory experience and perceptions of individuals who grow up in different cultures produce different schemata or cognitive maps. This concept is discussed in greater detail later in this chapter.

The form before us is more than brown hair, brown eyes, brown skin, several colors in fabric covering various shapes and forms of body and extremities. The brain organizes the millions of stimuli into a scheme that is a whole, that comes close to reality, but is not the reality, merely our construct of it. Perceptual organization is a process of the brain that brings together and coordinates many stimuli in some meaningful way. Assigning a meaning to this organized information is called interpretation. When we identify this form as a person dressed in traditional tribal fashion, we have simplified the complex and extensive information in order to deal with it in a timely manner. We have created an interpretation that is more than a sum of its parts, or a gestalt (Rock, 1985).

Our perceptual processes also allow us to derive meaning from incomplete information by completing that which is missing. We may observe a human form move out of our visual field around the corner of the building, but based upon the very limited data from body shape, clothing, and manner of stride, we can identify this form as someone we know. Based on the clues in the social context we draw conclusions and make judgments about the information that our senses have taken in. This process is discussed further in Chapter 13 in the context of an inference model that is applied to clinical judgment.

Learning and Learning Theory

Consciousness

Learning is a very complex operation that occurs whether we know it, or not, and whether we want to, or not. It depends to a considerable degree on the functions of conscious awareness. As you and I go about our daily tasks we function at several different levels of consciousness. Our mind operates at these levels to conserve energy and to optimize efficiency to arrive at decisions. Though there are many definitions, a general meaning of consciousness is that we are aware of mental processes in such a way that we can describe what is going on.

Through consciousness we construct our perception of the world around us. The process of attending limits the data that comes into awareness. For example, as we read these words we continue to breathe, move body parts, experience sensations from various internal organs and other parts of our bodies, and sounds in the space around us. But we are not aware of all of these simultaneously. We may not really be aware of the music on the radio until a special piece of music is played. Otherwise the sound recedes into a background to which we do not consciously attend. Our respiration goes on without notice, until a noxious odor causes a sneeze.

Automatic behavior

As we move the pen across the paper we do not consciously think about shaping each letter, or placing punctuation and capital letters, unless we are writing in a foreign language. We have learned through the development of skill, to automatize these activities. This automatic behavior occurs when we practice an activity to achieve a high level of skill that can be brought to bear without conscious thought. We are particularly aware of this as we observe others engaged in sport activity such as the Olympic games. The benefit of automatization is that we can engage in the activity, leaving our conscious processes available to process a multitude of other important data.

Consider the first few times you engaged in a new activity, whether threading a needle, playing tennis or golf, swimming, or parallel parking a car. Our attention is consumed by each small detail in the step by step process of accomplishing the task, doing each thing necessary to achieve our goal. We may be so focused on turning the wheel to avoid hitting the vehicle we are parking behind that we are unaware of the traffic approaching from behind. Within a relatively short period of time, with practice, we develop a level of skill that allows us to perform the task while attending to many other stimuli in the environment, the oncoming traffic, children playing nearby, and a pedestrian taking a short cut through the space into which we are backing. In the development of clinical skill, health professional students practice a great variety of activities with concentrated attention to the details of each component part. Within a short time much of this becomes automatic, allowing the professional to attend to other important aspects of the treatment situation, the patient's affect, the questions posed, and the performance today compared with that of yesterday.

Psychologists have described several levels of consciousness that have a bearing on perception and learning. We may become aware of data at a subconscious level when we are otherwise unaware, as in sleep. For example, mothers awaken at night to find themselves standing at the bedside of one of their children who has cried out or coughed in their sleep. Patients may be unconscious, unresponsive to stimuli in the environment, but nevertheless can report accurately the details of conversations that went on around them, once they regain consciousness. At some level, these people are aware of selected stimuli in their environments.

Theories of learning

Learning, fundamental to all human beings, is generally defined as a change in behavior as a result of experience. It is a process that continues throughout the lifetime. It allows us to adapt to our environment and the circumstances we find there. Learning may be good for us, leading to greater flexibility and responsiveness; or learning may impose restrictions on our behavior and lead to anxiety or unhealthy habits. The individual has a personality, which makes them distinguishable from others and that affects how learning takes place. The individual exists in a social context that also influences what and how learning takes place.

Psychologists have studied learning for many years. Here we will describe four theories that have been influential in our understanding of human development and inform us about this very human behavior: classical conditioning, operant conditioning, cognitive learning, and social cognitive learning. We learn in different ways and we learn different things in different ways. As we will soon discover, each of these theories is an attempt to describe the phenomenon of learning. Each has its own cultural context and time in history. Each contributes to our understanding of learning and explains a portion of the reality. We'll begin first with the work of the Russian physiologist Pavlov, whose work on associations brought him more notice in psychology than this same work on the digestive system which won him the Nobel Prize. The process of association has been studied since the time of ancient Greek philosophers, and more recently in the seventeenth century by philosophers such as John Locke, David Hume, and John Stuart Mill.

Classical or respondent conditioning

In our daily experience of life we associate many events with a particular meaning or phenomenon. When the telephone rings, we pick up the receiver as we have learned to associate that sound with the fact that someone is trying to reach us from a distance. If, as we prepare to walk across the street, the signal light changes from green to red, we stop because we have associated the red light with the meaning 'stop'. These stimulus – response associations are conditioned through repetitive experience of the same events in juxtaposition. We also learn to associate some of our actions with particular rewards or punishments. Rewards are more pleasurable than punishments, so we tend to repeat those actions that are rewarded and avoid those that elicit punishment.

Pavlov worked with dogs to determine the amount of salivation that resulted when meat was placed in their mouth in order to study the role of salivation in digestion (Pavlov, 1927). The dogs soon began to salivate when the laboratory attendant who fed them entered the area. The dogs salivated when the food cans or food trays were rattled in advance of presenting the food. The dogs ruined the experiment. Pavlov recognized that the dogs associated the attendant and the cans and the trays with food, with the result that they salivated, whether or not the food itself arrived. As a research scientist of that time, he believed philosophy and psychology to be unscientific disciplines. But his ability to scientifically measure an associative response was exciting, and led to continued study of responses to associations. His research apparatus has become well known. The soundproofed environment allowed him to present the stimuli by remote control while viewing through one-way glass. For several trials a bell rang at the same time food was presented to the dog harnessed in the apparatus. The dog salivated each time. Then a time delay was built in between the bell ring and the food. Salivation occurred with the ringing of the bell. Later the dog would salivate when the bell rang, even if food was not presented at all. The association of a previously neutral stimulus (the ringing of the bell) with food was called conditioning.

This process of respondent conditioning, or classical conditioning is shown in Table 3.1.

People can learn to associate almost any two stimuli, which allows for flexibility and adapt-

Table 3.1
Respondent Conditioning or Classical Conditioning

Action	Behavior	Label
Food in dog's mouth	Salivation occurs	Unconditioned response (UCR)
Taste of food	Salivation	Unconditioned stimulus (UCS)
Bell paired with taste	Salivation	Conditioned stimulus (CS)
Bell alone	Salivation	Conditioned response (CR)

ability; this may occur at the conscious level or out of awareness. When a particular stimulus is paired with an emotional response or object or image, the stimulus takes on a new meaning. Consider the implications for health care practice. Young children associate white coats and uniforms with pain; patients associate a health professional carrying a small tray with getting an injection or medication. The accidental repeated pairing of one stimulus such as a stern tone of voice, with another such as a placement of hands for support, may be associated in the mind of the patient with criticism or rebuke. The process of stimulus – response conditioned behavior is potentially very powerful, and dangerous when we do not know what we are doing.

The conditions of when and how often a stimulus of neutral strength is paired with another unconditioned stimulus determines the development of a conditioned stimulus (CS). Five different relationships of CS and UCS are identified in the literature.

- *Simultaneous* – the CS and the UCS occur at the same time.
- *Delay* – the CS occurs and continues until the UCS is introduced.
- *Trace* – the CS occurs and then discontinues before the UCS is introduced.
- *Backward* – the CS occurs after the UCS.
- *Temporal* – the CS is the element of time such that the UCS occurs at regularly calibrated intervals.

Of these five, research has identified that *delay* is the most effective and *backward* is the least effective. The organism is presented with the CS which is followed shortly by the UCS. After a number of repetitions these two become associated and the organism has learned to expect the two. The number of repetitions required for the CS to be associated with UCS in order to produce a conditioned response to the CS alone varies with the nature of each of the conditions. For example, a young woman became violently sick to her stomach after drinking the soft drink root beer. That one occasion was enough to cause a strong dislike for root beer.

When the conditioned stimulus is paired repeatedly with the unconditioned stimulus the conditioned response is reinforced. Once the CR is established, if the conditioned stimulus occurs repeatedly without UCS, the CR will gradually reduce in strength and disappear. This is called *extinction*. After a time, if the two are paired again, spontaneous *recovery* may occur. It is easier to develop a CR than to get rid of it. We have all seen applications of this in our own bad habits which are more easily acquired than gotten rid of.

Two major classes of conditioning have been identified: *aversive* and *appetitive* conditioning. Aversive includes those stimuli that the organism will try to avoid instinctively such as pain and loud noises. Appetitive are those stimuli the organism will instinctively move toward including food when hungry, shelter when cold, and sex when aroused. It is not only logical, but instinctive as well, that patients would try to avoid pain.

The process of respondent conditioning occurs so frequently in our lives that we take it very much for granted. Our health and safety depends upon this kind of response behavior. All kinds of warning signals alert us to the presence of danger, to which we respond quickly to avoid harm. The sound of the ambulance, smoke alarm, or signal lights at the railroad crossing alert us to attention. Advertisements in the media use this respondent conditioning extensively to attract potential buyers to their products. Fears and anxieties may develop as a result of respondent conditioning. For example, the small child who forces the fluffy puppy to shake hands and receives a bite for his efforts, may associate dog with pain and fear all dogs as a consequence. Taken to the extreme, this fear of dogs may extend to include all furry objects, so that a fur coat elicits the fear response. We would call this extreme response a phobia to fur.

Operant or instrumental conditioning

Thorndike is responsible for the early work in operant conditioning that focuses on the consequences of behavior in learning (Thorndike, 1898). He worked with cats in a maze activity and described the trial and error learning that he observed as the cats made fewer random movements. Our behavior is shaped by the consequences after the action. The *law of effect*, a major principle of this kind of conditioning, states that we select behavior that will obtain pleasure and avoid pain. B.F. Skinner's work followed the general line begun by Thorndike as he focused on voluntary behavior and how to modify it through the consequences that resulted. Skinner (1935) explained simply how classical and operant conditioning differed (Table 3.2).

Reinforcement, a key concept in operant conditioning, may be defined operationally as any stimulus that is more likely to result in repetition of the desired behavior. Traditionally the researcher chooses the desired response in advance, waits for that response to occur, and then provides reinforcement to increase the likelihood that it will occur again. Both *positive* and *negative* reinforcers are available. Positive reinforcers increase the likelihood of a response recurring and increase the rate at which they recur. Negative reinforcers increase the rate of response when they are removed. The terminology may be confusing to some because of the common association of positive with good and negative with bad. The reference here is arithmetic. In positive rein-

Table 3.2
Differences in Classical and Operant Conditioning

Classical Conditioning	Operant Conditioning
Conditioned response may not be present at all initially	A response must be made in order to reinforce it
Response is controlled by the stimulus that came before it	Response is controlled by what comes after it
Most applicable to internal responses, as emotional and physiologic	Most applicable for external responses, as verbal and musculoskeletal

forcement, something is added; in negative reinforcement, something is taken away. So if we take medication, and the headache goes away, that is an example of negative reinforcement.

Punishment is the opposite of reinforcement in that it decreases the likelihood that a particular behavior will recur. Like reinforcement, it has positive and negative types, in the arithmetic sense. Positive punishment is an added element: take the forbidden candy and receive a slap on the hand. Negative punishment is an element removed: drive recklessly and have your licence suspended. Our common use of language does not easily accommodate to the idea of positive punishment. The arithmetic reference is helpful in developing the correct mindset. Reinforcement and punishment are relative. What for one person is reinforcement, for another may be punishment, a bit like one person's trash being another person's treasure. Careful analysis of the individual's reward system prior to selecting an appropriate reinforcer or punishment is essential when trying to change behavior using operant conditioning. We frequently have seen that a parent's scolding of a child's behavior does not change the naughty behavior. From the child's perspective, the scolding is attention, and the naughty behavior is a way to get it. The scolding acts as reinforcement.

A practical application developed from this theory, known as behavior modification, serves as a foundation for much of what happens in education today. Skinner made a distinction between responses that were *elicited*, resulting from known and definite stimuli, and responses that were *emitted*, not linked with a specific stimulus but a matter of choice. Pupil constriction in response to bright light is an elicit-ed response. The emitted response is of particular interest to health professionals and is the focus of an extensive system of behavior change using operant conditioning.

The behavior one selects produces some reaction in the physical or social environment. The kinds of reaction vary with potentially important consequences for the individual; the timing and frequency of occurrence of the consequences may vary also, leading to differing effects on the individual and differing likelihoods that a particular behavior will be repeated and how often. If the reactions are reinforcing, the behavior will tend to be maintained, or if aversive they will tend to be extinguished. The conditions of reinforcement will vary over time as the behavior is shaped. For example, when the child first learns to brush their teeth, just holding and getting the brush in the mouth will receive lavish praise from the parent. Shortly, more is expected, so lavish praise is reserved for a few strokes of the brush on the teeth or somewhere nearby. Gradually the expected level of performance is raised and praise is reserved for the highest level attained when a good job of cleaning occurs.

Operant conditioning with emitted responses involves feelings and motivation as well as learning. It is not passive manipulation of an organism to achieve a desired behavior. MacMillan suggests a hierarchy of reinforcers (Table 3.3) that follow a continuum that has an implied maturation (MacMillan, 1972).

MacMillan found that using a higher level reinforcer along with the one in place eventually allowed the withdrawal of the lower level reinforcer. He acknowledges that the scheme does not work equally well with all learners.

Table 3.3
Hierarchy of Reinforcers

Reward	Example
Primary	Food, water, shelter
Desirable object	Toy or trinket
Token with back-up desired object	Paper money with which to 'purchase' favored object for playtime
Visual token as evidence of progress	Graphs, gold star, letter grades, work on display
Social approval	Public praise, special treatment among peers, e.g, being first in line
Mastery	Learning for the fun of it

We have already discussed that the value of the reinforcer to the individual is of key importance.

The frequency and timing of the reinforcement is thought to be very important by behaviorist clinicians. This is called *scheduling*. Several patterns of scheduling used in research attempt to identify the most successful: continuous, intermittent, fixed ratio, and variable ratio are just a few. In general, researchers conclude that with newly established behavior, continuous or frequent reinforcement is most effective in the early stages. The new behavior can be maintained later with an intermittent schedule. Punishment tends to become ineffective if it is not applied each time undesirable behavior appears. The variable ratio, basically a random type of reinforcement, is very effective. The participant knows that any effort may be rewarded. The gamblers and slot machine players get 'hooked' by this type of reinforcement.

The elements of generalization, discrimination, and extinction apply in operant conditioning as in respondent conditioning. We can look at the language learning of the very young child as an example of the first two (Brown, 1965). The early productions of 'da da' receive massive reinforcement from parents. When that is produced in the presence of the father, the reinforcement increases, if possible. The same is true for 'ma ma'. Soon the child applies these sounds to all adult figures, but the reinforcement is greatly diminished or is missing altogether. Gradually the child learns to associate 'da da' with father, and 'ma ma' with mother and discriminate these adults from others who are not 'da da' or 'ma ma'. Sometimes an individual's behavior may be modified through extinction, by ignoring undesirable behavior so it does not receive the attention-getting reinforcers.

Cognitive learning

Learning is described as a change in individual behavior that results from responses to events in the environment. A regular criticism of classical and operant conditioning theories to explain learning is that they fail to account for the will or intent of the learner, events that take place in the mind. More recent theories take into consideration knowledge, attitudes, and beliefs, collectively referred to as *cognitive variables*. *Psychosocial variables* are those socially influenced factors that affect what happens inside the mind. Those factors within the person are *intrinsic*; those outside the person are *extrinsic*. Both intrinsic and extrinsic factors are interactive and competitive.

Cognitive theorists study the many mental functions that have an impact on learning and behavior. Mischel identifies six cognitive functions that must be understood in our attempt to understand behavior: *cognitive competencies, self encoding, expectancies, values, plans and goals,* and *strategies to effect self control* (Mischel, 1979). These become integrated in any given situation to effect a particular behavior. In this conceptualization, cognitive competencies refer to one's abilities, knowledge, and skills. Self-encoding is how one sees oneself and evaluates oneself, while expectancies refers to how we perceive our ability to perform a given task and the consequences of our behavior. Values has to do with the priorities and weight we place on the importance of certain outcomes. This concept appears again in more detail in the chapters that focus on childhood and adolescence. Plans and goals are our strategies for achieving personal targets of performance. Self-control strategies are our personalized techniques to regulate our behavior. This last dimension moves us out of the realm of the stimulus – response uncontrolled behavior pattern into the realm of planned behavior. As we become more aware of our responses to particular stimuli, the better we are able to control those responses and channel the energy into successful behavior with predictable ends. Of these six, the dimension that has received the most research attention is that of expectancies. It features heavily in the concept of self-efficacy which is the subject of Chapter 10.

Cognitive theorists suggest that there is a range of ways in which learning takes place which includes classical and operant conditioning, observational learning, as well as cognitive mechanisms that affect learning and performance (Figure 3.1). We utilize cognitive learning in the process of gathering information, solving problems, communicating with others about our ideas, and developing proficiency in some aspect of our goal directed behavior. The learner is actively engaged.

Cognitive maps, as conceived by Edward Tolman (1948), are an internal mental representation of the present learning environment. While attending to the specific task in any given situation, the learner nevertheless assimilates information about the setting and the spatial

Figure 3.1 Ways of learning.

Classical conditioning	Operant conditioning	Observational learning	Cognitive learning

relationships to the task of various features within that setting. In addition to the physical features of the environment, this map includes the expectations and rewards in the system, and the emotions that co-exist. Tolman maintained that the fact that people are able to respond to changes in their environment indicates that there is a complex mental image that is brought to bear on the new problem, in the form of a cognitive map. Using rats in his research, Tolman demonstrated that they had an ability to identify and locate the route out of a maze based on a set of expectations. They developed a sense of the 'lay of the land' based upon their experience of moving up and down the several possible paths. This relationship of the elements Tolman labeled a cognitive map.

Leon Festinger developed this concept in a somewhat different direction in his 1954 publication to suggest that new information in the environment is brought into the brain and compared with what is already there in order to attach some sort of meaning to it. If the new information closely approximates a stored map, the meaning may easily apply. If no map exists that really fits, a new map may be created, or as sometimes happens, the map that comes closest to fitting is applied and a meaning that may or may not be appropriate is assigned. This provides the ground upon which misperception develops, that leads to errors in judgment. The process of making judgments is discussed more fully in Chapter 13.

Some cognitive theorists talk about a concept called *insight*, which we use rather loosely in our casual speech. As early as 1925 the German psychologist Wolfgang Köhler described an experiment with a chimpanzee in which the animal demonstrated a behavior that indicated an assessment of relationships between two known facts. The behavior was not a specific response to a particular stimulus, but a new behavior that resulted from integrating two pieces of information, demonstrating what he called insight. Bruner (1960) suggests that insight is the result of intuitive thinking that requires a holistic view of the problem. The individual

'...may be unaware of just what aspects of the problem situation he was responding to ... the thinker [is able] to leap about, skipping steps and employing short cuts.'

Expert health professionals draw conclusions from limited data and a non-linear problem solving strategy using a process of insight. They are able to grasp the holistic perspective quickly based upon multiple cues in the environment that lead to linkages with cognitive maps that fit the problem. These people frequently are not able to identify the process they used to arrive at their conclusions.

A brief description follows of several other concepts that enter into discussions of cognitive learning. We usually determine that learning has taken place based upon an observation of a change in the behavior of the individual. But sometimes learning takes place without immediate evidence of such a change. Theorists speculate that a change in one's ability may occur as a result of learning, without an obvious change in performance. They call this *latent learning*. For example one may acquire more and more information about how to perform a particular treatment procedure yet be unable to administer that procedure until all the pieces 'fall into place', or not be called upon to perform the procedure until a level of practice has been reached.

Observational learning takes place as one acquires information through the experience of others. A young woman had watched cardio-pulmonary resuscitation (CPR) many times on various television programs but had not received training nor ever performed the procedure. She had not 'learned' how to do it in the traditional sense. Yet, in an emergency situation in which an older man experienced a respiratory arrest, she was able to administer CPR under very difficult conditions for several minutes until the rescue squad arrived. The man had stopped breathing. There was no one else to do it. The man survived without residual impairment. The young woman had experienced latent learning through observation of the modeling of the technique. The television performers that had been observed were engaged in *modeling*. As a group of student health professional students watch their mentor perform a treatment intervention with a patient, the students are engaged in learning through observation, and the mentor is modeling the desired behavior. When the student then does the procedure with a patient he or she will *imitate* what was observed. We see this behavior throughout the childhood years as children imitate the behavior of others in their environment through speech, movement patterns, and specific activities. Parents are frequently dismayed when some of that imitation is of undesirable behavior. Of course imitation does not stop when one reaches adulthood.

If we could only do those things we had learned to do and observed others doing, our repertoire of abilities would be quite limited. We seem to have the capacity to make observations and infer rules of order about the activity, and then use those rules to generate new learning and ability. This is called *abstract modeling*. The child's acquisition and use of language is an example. We do not teach the young child about nouns, pronouns, verbs, adjectives, and adverbs, but the child acquires a vocabulary and uses the words appropriately by applying the 'implicit' rules that govern speech. If the child uses language incorrectly, they have learned to do so from the models in the environment. This abstract modeling is important in the more complex and sophisticated forms of cognitive activity and is considered the highest form of human intellectual behavior. Creativity, for example, may be the result of observing several models and deriving something new from them. When we are exposed to others who use creativity we are more likely ourselves to be creative (Belcher, 1975). Figure 3.2 identifies and organizes the several components of cognitive learning discussed above, as an extension of Figure 3.1.

With the technology available to us today, it is possible to study learning and psychological processes by observing behavior in minute detail. Through the use of video recording, and simultaneous collection of physiologic information on blood pressure, heart rate, temperature, and perspiration, brainwave activity in

Figure 3.2 Varieties of cognitive learning.

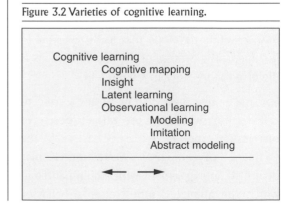

Cognitive learning
  Cognitive mapping
  Insight
  Latent learning
  Observational learning
    Modeling
    Imitation
    Abstract modeling

the form of electroencephalograms (EEGs), and activity in specific areas of the brain through position emission tomography (PET), we may piece together some of the critical ingredients of learning.

Cognitive and affective aspects of learning

The concept of cognitive learning may be used in a restricted way to refer to knowledge of facts alone, or it may include beliefs, values skills, and attitudes as well. These components of learning have both cognitive and affective aspects. For example, one may know facts and concepts that are in the cognitive domain, but have feelings associated with that knowledge. A young woman may know a great deal about mathematics, but have strong negative feelings when engaged in 'doing' math problems as a result of early learning experiences in which she felt discriminated against and thought the male students were favored in the class. We may hold strong beliefs and feel very positively about certain alternative health care practices, based upon limited facts and our feelings about using natural means and products in healing whenever possible. It is difficult or impossible to separate the cognitive and affective dimensions of learning. Researchers have found in addition that humans have a particular preparedness to learn some associations more than others. We have individualized ability to respond to the learning environment, and highly variable responsiveness to

different kinds of stimuli, dependent upon our genetic resources and maturation.

As we take all these factors into consideration in treatment planning for our client and patient, we also place them in the time continuum of the life cycle, and the cultural context of the society in which one matures. The *social cognitive theory* explains human functioning in terms of the three factors of cognitive, social, and environmental influences in one's life (Bandura, 1986). Bandura is one of several psychologists working in the area of social learning theory who was disenchanted with the limitations of earlier theories to explain human behavior and learning. These psychologists believed that the exercise of 'free will' had important implications for general personality development and learning in particular. The concept of expectations and expectancies grew out of this work, along with the important concept of self-efficacy that has particular relevance for learning and health care. This concept is the focus of discussion in Chapter 10. Figure 3.3 combines the segments represented in Figures 3.1 and 3.2, adding in the final component of social cognitive theory.

In the clinical setting we see an interesting application of learning theory in the behavior people learn to adopt when they become patients. Most quickly learn that the health care staff respond more quickly and effectively when the patient is perceived as 'good'. They also learn that there are few ways in which they are able to exert control over their

Figure 3.3 Ways of learning.

| Classical conditioning | Operant conditioning | Observational learning | Cognitive learning | Social cognitive |

environment. For many, this is an exceptional set of circumstances, very different from their existence in the 'real world'.

When these patients are in a situation in which they experience unpredictable and uncontrollable events, such as food arriving late or cold, or not of their choosing, uncomfortable tests, pain from their illness or procedures, administration of medication or reactions to it, and bad news, they learn that there is nothing they can do to improve, avoid, or escape these stressful circumstances. The initial frustration and anger leads to apathy, and finally 'learned helplessness' (Seligman, 1975). The patient is unwilling to initiate activity without permission, finds it difficult to concentrate and think logically, and lacks normal reactions to events in the environment. The physiologic correlates are similar to those found in people who experience post-traumatic stress disorder (PTSD). When these patients become involved in rehabilitation, the role of the health professional is to guide the process of recovery with the expectation that the patient will learn to help themselves. This is perhaps an unrealistic expectation, at least initially, if the patient has acquired a learned helplessness.

Memory

Memory is such an integral component of our cognitive processing and our daily lives that we take it very much for granted. We are hardly aware of 'using' it until we encounter a problem. Memory is fundamental to learning. Here we discuss a few of the basic principles of memory and how it operates. On the one hand, we have learned a great deal about how memory works in the past few years with the advent of certain new technologies such as PET scans and EEG. On the other hand, memory continues to pose mysteries yet to be solved.

The memory functions to maintain and update the record of accumulated data in order to deal with our day to day experience. It maintains files of specific episodes in our life, referred to as *episodic memory*; it stores the symbols we use to represent our thoughts and language, called *semantic memory*; and our memory holds and organizes the wide variety of rules that make it possible to function in our world, called *procedural memory*. Two major varieties of memory have been identified: *declarative* and *procedural*. Declarative memory is our representation of stored information that we use to think and to communicate. It contains information that allows us to know whether something is true or false (Tulving, 1984). For example, if someone asked whether you learned to swim by the time you were ten years old, you would be able to know whether you did or did not. How would you remember? Two types of declarative memory might have guided you to the response: *episodic* and *semantic*. Episodic memory stores specific experiences and may be very precise about some of these events. Semantic memory involves knowledge of language including the sounds, called phonemes, the shapes of the characters, and the meanings of words, known as semantic content.

So how did you remember whether you had learned to swim by age ten? You may have had an internal dialogue with yourself to the effect that if you don't know how to swim now, you didn't then. Semantic memory may have been sufficient to produce the response. If you know how to swim now, you may have had to go back in time to find what you were doing at age ten in terms of time and place and activity. You might use a process that included thoughts such as: where was I then, what was I doing that year or summer, when I was in the water did I know what to do, in order to remember whether you had learned the skill by that time. You would rely on both episodic and semantic memory.

The procedural memory is the repository for automatized schemata that were discussed earlier in learning theory. The millions of activities that become routine which no longer require attention to each detail in order to accomplish fall into this category, such as brushing your teeth, driving a car, dressing oneself, or riding a bicycle. Perhaps you remember when you first learned to tie your shoes and the difficulty you had with the task, or riding a bicycle. Now if you try to explain that task in words to another you will find that words do not represent the task very well. The psychomotor aspects are difficult to represent in words.

Our memory serves to organize and associate events in the past and make them accessible for use in the future. The more features or items associated with a memory, the more readily it can be accessed. The organization is a key aspect. Consider entering a library with the intent of finding a specific book and discovering that books are not organized in any particular manner. To find your book, you will have to begin on one shelf and work your way through all the books until you find the one you are after. Even in a small collection this would be a daunting task. So also with your memory, small items do not exist in isolation but are organized by association with other items. It would be a daunting task to search through billions of isolated bits of memory to find the one that fits the current need.

Consider the circumstances of a 76 year old woman who experienced a right cerebral vascular accident that affected her capacity to organize or sequence tasks. She had been a very active professional woman throughout her adult years. Now she cannot dress herself, or hang a shirt on a hanger to place in the closet. She asked her daughter what she could do to help with dinner preparations. The daughter understood her problem and suggested that she just sit and keep her company. Not to feel useless the woman said that she would set the table. She opened the drawer where the silver was kept and removed several items, put them down on the table, and then stood not remembering how to proceed. Her semantic memory had the information and 'knew' that she knew what to do, her episodic memory had all kinds of images of past table setting events, but her procedural memory had lost the sequence of the almost automatic behavior.

Watch a young child of five to six months of age involved in the task of moving an object from one hand to another. Just a few days ago the object was held in one hand, dropped and retrieved by either hand. At about this time the child also brings both hands together at the midline of the body so they touch. In a few days the child will bring the object held in one hand to the midline so the other hand can touch it, and then transfer it to the other hand. The infant does not have semantic representation for the object, her hands, nor the actions, as far as we know at this time. But the child learns from the psychomotor activity what works, is rewarded for the effort, and stores in memory the actions that lead to success for reaching, touching, grasping, holding the object in the hand, dropping and retrieving it, and finally moving it from one hand to the other. Within a few days the complex task of moving an object from one hand to another has been mastered, with the memories associated and stored for future use in similar tasks. With practice, this activity will become automatic.

Memory is an essential ingredient in the work of health professionals in health education, health promotion, and treatment of all kinds, whether for the client and patient, or for the family and caregiver. We will go into more detail on the processes of memory and factors that influence memory later in the discussion of making judgments in Chapter 13.

In this chapter we have looked at several conceptual tools and a few of the processes that relate to human development throughout the life cycle. We began with the biological and intellectual ability of the human organism to adapt to constantly changing circumstances that are essential to survival. The cultural context was identified as a critical factor in how these processes evolved and how they may be interpreted by those outside the culture. Cognitive development and learning theory occupied the remainder of the chapter with explanations of several different theories. We suggest that no one of them stands alone, but each contributes in particular ways to our understanding of this very human ability. Finally the capacity to remember things was introduced as an aspect of cognitive functioning, and will be continued in a later segment of the book.

References

Bandura, A (1986) *Social Foundations of Thought and Action: A Social Cognitive Theory*. Englewood Cliffs, NJ: Prentice-Hall.

Basic Behavioral Science Task Force of the National Advisory Mental Health Council (1996) Basic behavioral science research for mental health: family processes and social networks. *American Psychologist* 51(6): 622–630.

Belcher, TL (1975) Effect of different testing situations on creativity scores. *Psychological Reports* 36(2): 511–514.

Bruner, JS (1960) *The Process of Education*. New York: Random House.

Festinger, L (1954) A theory of social comparison processes. *Human Relations*. 7: 117–140.

Jacob, T (ed) (1987) *Family Interaction and Psychopathology*. New York: Plenum.

MacMillan, DL (1973) *Behavior Modification in Education*. New York: Macmillan.

Mischel, W (1979) On the interface of cognition and personality: beyond the person – situation debate. *American Psychologist* 34: 740–754.

Nsamenang, AB (1992) *Human Development in Cultural Context: A Third World Perspective*. Cross-cultural Research and Methodology Series, Vol 16. Newbury Park, CA: Sage.

Pavlov, IP (1927) *Lectures on Conditioned Reflexes*. New York: International Publishers.

Piaget, J (1936, 1952) *The Origins of Intelligence in Children*. New York: Humanities Press.

Piaget, J (1985) *The Equilibration of Cognitive Structures*. Chicago: University of Chicago Press.

Rock, I (1985) *Perception*. New York: Scientific American.

Seligman, M (1975) *Helplessness*. San Francisco: W.H. Freeman and Company.

Skinner, BF (1935) The generic nature of the concepts of stimulus and response. *Journal of Genetic Psychology* 12: 40–65.

Thorndike, EL (1898) Animal intelligence: an experimental study of the associative processes in animals. *Psychological Review* 2: Monograph Supplement 8.

Tolman, EC (1932) *Purposive Behavior in Rats and Men*. New York: Appleton-Century-Crofts.

Tolman, EC (1948) Cognitive maps in rats and men. *Psychological Review* 55: 189–208.

Tulving, E (1984) Precis of elements of episodic memory. *The Behavioral and Brain Sciences* 7, 223–228.

Turnbull, C (1961) Some observations regarding the experiences and behavior of the Bambuti pygmies. *American Journal of Psychology* 74, 304–308.

Vygotsky, LS (1978) *Mind in Society*. Cambridge: Harvard University Press.

4

Normal Growth and Development in the Infant and Young Child

Elsa Ramsden

Introduction
•
Normal Fetal Development
•
Developmental Tasks in the Young Child
•
Sensory, Perceptual, and Motor Functions
•
Psychosocial Agenda
•
Case I: Cindy Smith – Cerebral Palsy

Introduction

Getting to be me – genetic foundations

Each one of us at birth has a complex complement of genetic material with coded instructions for the developing human brain and body. The genes we received, half each from the male and female that produced us, are the basic components of heredity in all living things, made up of deoxyribonucleic acid or DNA. Every living cell contains DNA in its nucleus. The molecule of DNA looks like a twisted ladder with beads along its spirals. A specific gene pool has contributed to our genetic make-up, contributed by generations of those who have come before us. How those genes are expressed in our personhood is at least in part a function of the environment in which we live and grow.

The arrangement of the four chemical bases that make up the DNA molecule along its twisted ladder-like structure determines what and who we become. A gene is a piece of DNA that encodes a particular characteristic for the evolving individual. Twenty-three pairs of chromosomes together make up approximately fifty thousand genes that determine everything from skin and eye color to sex, bone structure, and certain aspects of temperament. How different are we from one another? Only six percent difference exists between us and a rhesus monkey; only two percent differentiates us from the chimpanzee; and between you and me, perhaps a tenth of one percent (Ornstein, 1993). In our everyday life we tend to exaggerate the differences that exist between us. 'I am entirely different from anyone else' is commonly heard from naive students.

We are more similar than we would like to believe. The children within a family inherit a complex set of physical characteristics and a variety of abilities that become expressed differently among them, except in the case of identical twins who develop from the same fertilized egg. How the genetic potential is expressed in the developing individual depends upon environmental and social circumstances and opportunity. Natives of South-east Asia tend to have shorter stature than do Caucasians in northern Europe and North America. However, Japanese and Koreans raised in North America grow to be taller than their family members living in their native land, largely due to improved nutrition. With increasing westernization and change of diet in Japan, there is an accompanying steady increase in stature. This has an interesting impact on the market place as well; for example, their automobiles have also increased in size.

In this chapter we will consider genetic inheritance, social and cultural values, and environmental circumstances which influence the development of the infant and child. Our objective is to increase understanding of human behavior so we can build that understanding into effective strategies in health care interventions. In our role as health professionals, we need to know and understand human behavior and individual differences in order to be intentional in our work with clients and patients, to plan intervention strategies that meet the particular needs of the particular person.

Normal Fetal Development

The developing fetus carries the genetic determinants that contribute to the individuality of that human being throughout life. Four governing principles operate for each of us: the rate of our development, abnormal features of development, individual traits, and the evolution of psychosocial development. While environment and experience certainly have an effect, genetic research has revealed the crucial role of the genetic inheritance on a wide variety of behavior and abilities.

Genetic technology has identified the location of the genes responsible for specific abnormalities such as Tay-Sachs disease, and cystic fibrosis. Currently and in the years ahead this technology will take us further, to enable us to modify directly the genetic structure, effectively eliminating many problems. The Human Genome Project initiated by the National Institutes of Health (NIH) in 1989 has set about to map the three billion base pairs of chromosomes that carry all the inherited traits of the individual. It is conceivable that in the near future scientists will be able to predict the vulnerability of an individual to certain diseases and malformations, and to treat diseases caused genetically through gene modification. The development of therapeutic interventions of this nature raise a new order of ethical issues that has an impact on the way we deal with these problems and the way we consider the meaning of life.

The course of prenatal development and the pattern it follows are guided by genetic information with strong influences imposed by the maternal environment and the psychosocial processes of the mother. The health and growth of the fetus are directly affected by all three of these sets of factors. Some of the maternal environmental factors include the age of the mother, use of medications and chemical dependency, diet, and the toxins in the environment to which she is exposed. Poverty is perhaps the most powerful of the psychosocial factors to have an impact on the developing fetus. Poor women are less well educated, know less about the risks of tobacco, alcohol, and drugs to the unborn fetus, are less likely to have been vaccinated against the infectious diseases that are harmful to the fetus, and are less likely to receive prenatal care in the early stages of pregnancy. Poverty is associated with malnutrition and increased instances of infection, diabetes, and cardiovascular disease, which in turn are linked to low birth weight and other physical and mental problems in the newborn (Cassady and Strange, 1987).

Developmental Tasks in the Young Child

In the first year of life the weight of the infant can triple; in any given week the infant may grow two inches in length. The rate of growth is dramatic. By two years of age, the basic ground work has been laid for voluntary movement, language development, and formation of concepts; these can be observed and recorded systematically.

The developmental tasks in infancy and early childhood may be categorized into five areas: *social attachments, sensory–perceptual–motor functions* used to achieve one's goals, *association of one's actions with their consequences* in behavioral terms, the *organization into categories of objects and events* that link people and events, and the *development of emotional responses* to people and events. The maturation of these developmental tasks leads to continuing growth in social relationships, intellectual pursuits, understanding of self, and meeting the challenges posed by the environment with physical strength and coordination that will lead to autonomous functioning in one's society.

Social attachment

The patterns of social attachment evolve through a process of building emotional bonds with a significant other, the mother or primary caregiver initially, and others later. The infant displays a behavior and receives immediate feedback from the mother that is associated with the behavior. This continuous signal and response activity leads to the development of an organized pattern that may be very positive, or very negative (Basic Behavioral Science Task Force, 1996). Ultimately patterns of social attachment develop that reflect distinctly different coping strategies in response to the stress induced by novel circumstances.

Four different patterns have been identified based upon research over the past two decades (Ainsworth *et al.*, 1978; Main and Solomon, 1986; Carlson *et al.*, 1989; van Ljzendoorn *et al.*, 1992). The infant who has developed a *secure attachment,* in the presence of the mother will actively explore the environment and interact with strangers. If separated from the mother, separation anxiety may be evident, but quickly disappears upon her return and the child will resume exploration of the surroundings. The *anxious–avoidant attachment* pattern is characterized by avoiding contact with the mother upon her return after separation, or ignoring her efforts to reestablish an interaction. The infant with an *anxious–resistant attachment* pattern is cautious when a stranger is present, and exploratory behavior ceases or is markedly diminished when the mother leaves the area. When the mother returns, the child seems to want to be near but is also angry, so is difficult to placate.

Most recently the pattern of *disorganized attachment* has been described by Main and Solomon (1986) as a combination of avoidant and resistant patterns (Radke-Yarrow *et al.*, 1985). These studies looked at children of mothers who were depressed, and children who had been abused. Later studies identified that the rate of disorganized pattern behavior increased as the social risk factors increased in severity (Lyons-Ruth *et al.*, 1993). An analysis of 32 research reports focusing on social attachment across eight countries found comparable results for China, Israel, Germany, Great Britain, Japan, Netherlands, and the United States. Within each country there was more variation in the distribution of the patterns across the population than there was between countries, with the secure attachment pattern as the modal pattern overall (van Ljzendoorn and Kroonenberg, 1988).

Several studies in the United States have examined cultural and subcultural differences in social attachment. They suggest that members of the several ethnic groups possess different mental representations of the parental role, which is reflected in their behavior toward infants. As one experiences parenting behaviors as a child, one tends to express that pattern later in life when in the role of parent. In addition, cultural beliefs about childhood convey information about the meaning of the child's behavior and how to respond to the signals. The world view of the culture contains coding that sets expectations for maternal sensitivity to the child's distress and responsiveness to it, length of dependency of the child, acceptable age for walking, toilet training, control of emotions, and manner of expression of feelings.

The quality of social attachment in the young child is a function of several factors as depicted in Figure 4.1 below. The personal factors inherent in the caregiver, along with the social environment, interact with the adult's own ability to provide a stable base of support.

Figure 4.1 Factors that contribute to the quality of social attachment.

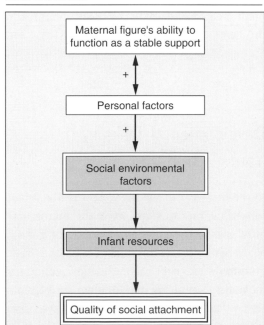

These work together with the malleable material provided by the resources the infant brings to the equation.

We infer an internal representation of how a child characterizes a particular relationship by observing the behavior (Main *et al.*, 1985). A set of implicit rules within this representation provides the child with guidelines for organizing information and experiences about that relationship. The kind of attachment pattern that is developed influences the way the maternal figure is perceived and interpreted, and affects the kinds of responses the infant and young child makes to that behavior. Later in the child's life, these representations may be altered as the child becomes capable of reflection and deeper understanding, and is able to reinterpret the maternal behavior based upon this new understanding.

Consider the infant who is cared for by a nanny or in day care during the day. At the end of the day until bedtime the mother is available to attend to the child. The mother's behavior displays interest in all the infant and child does. The child's behavior is rewarded with smiles, hugs, and gentle affection. Each new activity is greeted with praise and delight by mother and child. The child organizes all this experience into his understanding of what mother is all about in the mutually satisfying secure relationship. Later in his life the child may realize that not all mothers leave for the day, and are at home when the child returns from school. His friends seem to have something special that he does not have. How is this new information integrated into the child's understanding of mother's behavior? Given the confidence that has grown out of the early secure attachment, one might speculate that this child could create an understanding consistent with the love and affection experienced earlier in life.

When we consider the implications of the quality of social attachment during the infant's first months of life for relationships over the lifespan, we can appreciate that they are formative. Those children who have developed secure attachments are more likely to develop close relationships with peers and enjoy friendships throughout life. In many respects the relationships in adulthood may be characterized in a similar manner as those in early childhood, including physical closeness, sharing emotionally and intellectually, and being sensitive and responsive to another. In adulthood, those who formed secure attachments as infants are more likely to do so with their own children. Though many of life's experiences intervene to alter one's representation of social attachment, the concept is useful to describe and understand behavior at the individual level, in the dyad, and in larger systems. The person we see in the health care setting as patient and client is the product of many influences; one of these is the social attachment pattern that developed in infancy and was modified over the span of life.

Sensory, Perceptual, and Motor Functions

Maturity of newborn infants varies widely and influences their ability to sustain the essential functions of breathing, eating, and sleeping independently. The genetic coding has guided the process of development *in utero* so that most newborn infants have intact sensory systems and a well-formed brain. This brain has between 100 billion and 300 billion neurons, already linked through pathways to permit certain functions. Though the brain does not seem to change in terms of basic organization after birth, some details of its structure demonstrate plasticity for a period of time, especially in the cerebral cortex (Diamond *et al.*, 1985). Many human behaviors that are of particular interest to behavioral neurologists cannot be studied directly in the human brain. Experimental evidence is gathered from subhuman primates to enhance our understanding of some of the structural analogs that exist between the species (Mesulam, 1986).

An imbalance in the use of a receptor organ in the early period of life seems to result in a non-use or disuse retardation in development of that organ system. It seems that the neural networks of the brain are designed in such a way that those that are not used are abandoned, those that are used extensively are broadened, and in some cases enhanced where needed (Aoki and Siekevitz, 1988). Early patterns of association between object and response and familiarity with those patterns evolve through the child's interaction with the stimuli in the environment. This process shapes how the neural connections are organized and how they develop.

Interconnectedness

The sensory and perceptual capacities develop separately but function together in an interconnected system; they almost stimultaneously bring information into the central nervous system and provide interpretation about that information. Consider the first time the new born infant is put to the mother's breast to nurse shortly after birth. The stimuli include the visual data of the face, breast, and nipple, the olfactory data of body and milk, the kinesthetic data of mother's hands on body and face guiding the mouth to the nipple, and the data from the infant's mouth on the nipple with cheek against the breast, the gustatory data of the milk on the taste buds in the mouth, and the auditory data of mother's voice. This amazing amount of data is brought into the cerebral cortex where it is integrated and stored, to be reinforced with each repetition of the activity. Within a short time these stimuli are associated with satiation of hunger and comfort in the arms of the mother, so that simply seeing the breast or nipple brings about the open mouth and head-turning response.

The integration of the sensory information going in, and the perception of what that data means in terms of satisfying hunger is in place. These two functions together bring the outside world into contact with our brain in such a way that permits the formation of mental representations of reality in this case unrelated to words. The recognition of patterns is critical for identifying objects or places in the environment. The number of patterns an individual recognizes contributes to the development of expertise. Novices are different from experts in any field based upon the number of patterns they are able to recognize and respond to in a short period of time. As mentioned earlier in the discussion on learning, some of the 'recognition' may be out of conscious awareness.

The lives of infants and young children born with faulty sensory mechanisms are markedly different because the data brought into the central nervous system is different from that of other children. Therefore the perception and representation of reality is different. Young Bobby was a child described as awkward by his mother. He regularly bumped into door frames and knocked his glass of milk over at meal times. By age four the opthamologist thought surgery was indicated to correct a visual problem. When he regained consciousness after surgery, he saw his mother standing at the bedside and said, 'But mommy, there's only one of you now'. This child never really knew where the 'real' door frame was, or where the 'real' glass was placed on the table. His representation of reality had two images for everything along with the uncertainty about its placement in space. Consider the long-term implications for development of gross motor control, fine motor coordination, and eye–hand coordination when the data from the environment taken in by the visual system is faulty.

Motor development

Normal motor development proceeds in two ways: from the head, neck, and shoulders to the feet in what is called the cephalocaudal direction; and from the center of the body to the distal ends of the extremities in the proximo distal direction. This development results from the changes in the brain and spinal cord that evolve in the first few years of life. Dramatic changes occur from birth, when the infant has little strength or coordination, to a very few months later when they sit upright, creep, pull to stand, and move objects from one hand to another with accuracy. The increasing mobility allows the infant to explore the environment, testing and training new abilities, and encounter novel experiences for all the sensory modalities.

Motor skill develops in concert with maturation of bone growth and muscle development, coincident with maturation of the nervous system. For the achievement of competence to occur in the development of sensory-perceptual and motor tasks three factors interact in a synchronous manner: maturation, the circumstances in the environment, and the will or desire of the child to reach a goal.

The eight month old may have a strong desire to climb the stairs, and the environment may be supportive and protective, but if the maturation of the musculoskeletal structures involved in the activity are not sufficiently mature, the goal cannot be attained – yet. The three year old who goes shopping may want to imitate and 'help' his mother, who takes articles off the shelf and puts them into the basket, or may put them back on the shelf after looking at it carefully. He has the maturation level to do this, and the desire. The mother may perceive the behavior as disruptive or naughty rather than imitation and a learning experience. She will discourage the activity in a variety of ways, with the result that the social environment restricts, so is not conducive to accomplishing the task.

Sensorimotor schemes and early associations

The growth and development of intelligence was thought to evolve from elemental sensorimotor experience and adaptation by Piaget (1970). He suggests that the early reflex activity gives way to more sophisticated behavior, and that simple schemes develop into more complex schemes based upon increased exploration of the environment using the newly evolving sensorimotor resources. Patterns of movement become associated with particular events in the environment. At a very early age the infant learns to adapt the sucking activity from breast to bottle. Or if breast fed only, when the first teeth break through the lower gum, and the mother pulls away quickly during the nursing, the infant adapts and moves the tongue into a new position to prevent the pulling away. A new pattern develops from the sensorimotor experience. One could not explain in words to the infant how to do this.

This sensorimotor 'intelligence' is fundamental to the development of a sense of causality, that one action leads to a particular result. When the baby cries, mother will come and soothe or pick her up, or mother will ignore or hit her. Piaget and Inhelder (1966, 1969) presented a model to describe the evolution of these causal schemes from simple to complex in six phases. Researchers have recently con-

firmed these results since that earlier time (Fischer and Silvern, 1985). Table 4.1 displays the six phases in outline form.

Reflexes in the first phase affect the initial cause and effect scheme. The involuntary reflexive response to stimulation brings about particular associations such as sucking from the rooting reflex, grasping objects in response to pressure in the palmar surface of the hand, and leg extension in response to pressure on the plantar surface of the feet.

During the second phase from the second week to the fourth month the reflexive behavior is modified and expanded as the child explores a broader range of the environment. Increased musculoskeletal strength and coordination brings more objects within reach to investigate. Many are tested in the mouth, grasped, and dropped. Putting an object into

Table 4.1
Development of Causal Schemes: Six Phases

Approximate age	Behavior observed	Period
From birth	Specific stimuli elicit reflex responses	Reflexes
From the second week	Explore new stimuli using relexive responses	Initial habits
From the fourth month	Familiar action is used to achieve a familiar result	Circular reactions
From the eighth month	Use of a deliberate action to achieve a new goal	Coordination of means and ends
From the eleventh month	Actions are modified to reach goals	Experimentation with new means
From the eighteenth month	Recombining means and ends mentally	Insight

the mouth is a purposeful act that produces pleasure and can be repeated, an early form of causal behavior.

During the third and fourth phases occupying the fourth month to the eighth, and the eighth to the eleventh month, the child begins to connect cause and effect relationships, and learns to expect certain results from specific actions. They may express surprise if the expected outcome does not occur. Researchers believe that the child does not understand 'why' the one leads to the other, but does associate a cause and effect relationship.

In the course of the fourth phase also, the infant will use customary action to achieve new ends. They may shake the rattle to produce the noise, and then use the rattle to reach toward an object beyond their grasp in a purposeful manner. This is referred to as instrumental learning in the earlier discussion of learning theory.

During the fifth phase from the eleventh to the eighteenth month the child engages in more complex sensorimotor problem solving by modifying the means to achieve different outcomes. When unable to reach an object on a table, the child will employ a stool or box to stand on to reach the goal.

The last and sixth phase of sensorimotor causality evolves from the eighteenth month to produce mental representations of problem-solving activities to reach a goal without having to try each option separately. The child is able to think about a physical activity and decide whether it will work or not to reach the objective, and then move on to another possible alternative. This is the beginning of insight.

This ability to know that one is able to bring about a predictable change in the environment is basic to all future mastery and to the development of a sense of competence. The process includes investigating the circumstances in the environment, thinking about solving the problem, and expending effort to reach a goal (Yarrow et al., 1983; MacTurk et al., 1987). These same abilities in the adult depend on the early development of the sensorimotor capability.

Clinical application

Consider the infant born with cerebral palsy whose reflex activity is abnormal and whose sensorimotor development is impeded by the interference in the reception of the data from the environment and transmission of information from the brain to the muscles. The early development of sensorimotor causality described above will be severely disrupted. Because of the disturbed motor control more effort will need to be invested in the developmental tasks for each of the six phases, and each phase will take longer to master to a sufficient degree to move on to the next phase. The desire to accomplish the task may not be any less, but the sensorimotor resources to bring to the task will prevent accomplishment in the normal time frame, if at all. One would expect to see frustration and anger in a child who is not able to achieve their goals, even at this early age.

Object form and function and categories

When one watches the young infant move about in its environment, first lying and watching, then creeping, crawling, and then cruising upright by holding on to furniture or a hand, it is immediately apparent that exploration is a compelling need. First the eyes track moving people and objects, then the hand grasps, slaps, pushes, and pulls objects that come within reach. The object is felt, prodded, lifted, moved if possible, and perhaps tasted. Everything from toys and pets to tables and dirt are experienced in this exploration. The baby is an active investigator of its surroundings, not a passive recipient of it stimulation (Rochat, 1989; Ruff et al., 1992). In this process the child experiences the different properties of color, size, weight, shape, sound, texture, and boundaries.

In time, the objects take on two additional features of permanence and category. Piaget (1954) maintained that logical thought was founded on the understanding of the properties of objects. The child learns that when the object is out of sight it does not disappear from existence. When the toy rolls under the drapery hidden from view, the child can reach under or behind the place where he saw the toy roll from view and find it there (Wellman et al., 1986). The six month old will not pursue an object removed from view; the nine month old will watch the removal and go and search for it; the seventeen month old can pursue a hidden object even when they did not see it taken away. This progression in object permanence is apparent in the game of peek-a-boo. Initially the young child is delighted by the appearance of the smiling face, but loses interest when it is no longer in view. A few months later, the child waits with delight for the face to reappear when it disappears. And later still, the ambulatory child will go in search of the person hidden from them behind the chair or sofa.

It appears the development of object permanence and social attachment are interrelated and mutually enhancing. The young child of six months commonly experiences separation anxiety when its mother, with whom it has developed social attachment, is out of sight. It is not sure that the mother will return. As object permanence evolves, the separation anxiety gradually diminishes and disappears. It seems that object permanence applies to people as well as to inanimate objects.

The process of categorization has been studied by observing infants of three months respond to faces and objects. They smile at faces but not at objects. Researchers believe this finding emphasizes the importance of relationships in social development and growth. By the age of 12 months the child is able to sort objects upon request. For example, in helping to clean up the play area it can distinguish wooden blocks from soft toys, blue colored objects from others. By 18 months the complexity of this activity has increased so the child can sort into two groups a mixed assortment of objects such as colored blocks and human-shaped figures. Naming seems to be related to categorizing as the comprehension vocabulary develops from birth onward.

The young child whose movements are restricted by physical limitations or environmental constraints experiences retardation in the development of these abilities. For example, consider the circumstances of infants abandoned in war time and 'housed' in orphanages in light of the information discussed above. They were maintained in cribs with netting over the top, which kept them safe from falling out and injuring themselves. Their social attachments were seriously disrupted, and their learning environment so bleakly limited that they suffer irreparable developmental delay and emotional starvation.

Development of emotion

The expression of feeling in the infant is critical to receiving appropriate care. Caregivers watch for the emotional display, which represents some inner state of being, in order to respond to the need that produces that expression of feeling. The new born infant demonstrates distress by crying, interest through alert inactivity, and excitement through general body movement. These earliest expressions are soon increased to include the endogenous smile – turning toward the face of the care-giver and a moving object, the startle, and distress resulting from restraint of movement, discomfort, or covering the face. Within three months the infant displays pleasure which combines the smile with a generalized wiggle that consumes the entire body. These early states are accompanied by a distinctive pattern of motor activity, respiration, and muscle tone (Wolf, 1966).

The changes in the emotional state of the infant provide the stimulus to which the care-giver responds. The caring adult seeks to comfort the distressed infant and rectify the problem causing the distress, such as feeding when hungry or changing a wet or dirty diaper. When the child is alert parents try to make eye contact and use non-verbal behavior to elicit a 'happy' response behavior on the part of the child. The repertoire of emotional behavior displayed by the child expands rapidly in the first year of life, and continues throughout the first three years. Table 4.2 outlines this expansion in expressiveness over the first three years of life. The ages identified in the left column are those the literature suggests are the time the behavior is commonly seen.

When the infant is distressed and receives no soothing intervention it learns to cope with this situation by developing strategies to reduce the degree of distress (Dodge, 1989). The earliest forms seen in the youngest infants include turning their head away, sucking their hand or an object, and closing their eyes. When motor control is more under control the child can remove themselves from the environment, find distraction in the objects around them, or find solace through rocking movements, stroking, and sucking (Kopp, 1989). In extreme circumstances the child is not able to gain control of emotions and intervention by the parent does not help. These periods of high emotional intensity that cannot be controlled are referred to as tantrums.

The range of expression of emotion is culturally determined. In Japan, for example, the expression of emotion is generally considered inappropriate; to do so one loses 'face' or respect. Mothers restrict the opportunities for their children to experience frustration that would lead to anger. Parents seldom express anger to their young children, certainly not in public. The Japanese try to minimize the experience of anger in their attempt to regulate its expression (Miyake *et al.*, 1986).

In a study by Harwood (1992), Anglo and Puerto Rican mothers were studied to determine the boundaries of acceptable and negative behavior for their infants. Generally, the Anglo mothers preferred that their children control negative emotions and explore their environment while the mother was absent, but return to affirm the mother upon her return to the room. The Puerto Rican mothers found it more acceptable for the baby to cling to them when distressed, and

Table 4.2
Evolution and Expansion in the Repertoire of Three Qualities of Emotion

Month	Pleasure → Joy	Caution → Fearful	Distress → Anger
0 to 3	Endogenous smile; turning toward face of parent or moving object	Startle and pain; seeks attention	Irritation or anger when face is covered, with physical restraint, and physical discomfort
3	Pleasure		Anger and rage when thwarted
4 to 5	Pleasure and delight with active laughter	Caution and wariness	
7	Joy		Anger with increasing intensity
9		Fearfulness and aversion to strangers	
12	Increasing expression of elation	Fear and early signs of anxiety	
18	Views oneself in a positive way	Shame	Defiance
24	Affection		Intentionally hurts another person or animal
36	Proud of actions, love		Guilt

After Sroufe et al (1984).

preferred that the baby remain quiet and loving and stay close to them. Children learn to regulate their emotions through experiencing them and the reactions to them. They observe the range of emotional behavior of their parents and assimilate their parent's responses to their own emotional expressions, gradually learning what is acceptable and not acceptable. This is useful information that the child can apply to gain attention, or to control or disguise emotions in order to minimize pain or rejection.

Developing mutuality with the care-giver

As the infant matures, the state of tension develops between trust and confidence in the caregiver and mistrust accompanied by caution or fearfulness. In Chapter 2 this was discussed in the context of Erik Erikson's model of psychosocial development and outlined in Table 2.1 of Chapter 2. Trust is the result of an appraisal of another that they are reliable, honest, and caring, and that one may be confident to expect continued behavior of this variety. The infant does not have the language to put it quite that way, but the feeling of trust evolves based upon consistency in the relationship the child experiences and learns to expect in the future. Erikson (1978) associated trust with the concept of hope. He maintained that hope developed in infancy and provided the optimism that enabled one to continue through life to pursue new challenges and solutions to problems.

The key concept at this point in development is *mutuality* with the caregiver, a relationship within which each of the two individuals is responsive to the behavior of the other and regulates his own behavior in accordance with that of the other. Initially the caregiver responds to the signals of the infant. As trust develops the infant responds in kind. The early cries of the child are interpreted by the parent and the need is addressed. The child learns to expect that its needs will be met. Trust develops. Very soon the infant rewards the parent with smiles and wiggles of delight when they approach, and elicits more affectionate behavior from the parent. In normal development, as the child matures these exchanges become more sophisticated, increase in *coordination*, and become more subtle. Coordination refers to the ability of each to match the behavior of the other and the capacity to flow from one emotional state to another easily. This process contributes to the developing trust in the relationship.

Studies suggest that when parents were abused or neglected as children, are depressed, or are in a dysfunctional marital relationship, the parent–child relationship frequently lacks coordination, trust fails to develop, and there is less involvement with their children (Rutter, 1990; Alessandri, 1992). The first year of life is formative for the infant. The development of trust and mutuality have a strong bearing on the evolution of trust, building relationships, and intimacy with others throughout life.

Development through childhood

The developmental tasks throughout childhood follow a course of continuing complexity and elaboration at all levels. The one year old may be able to stand unsupported, take a few tentative steps, and manipulate objects with either or both hands. As strength, coordination, and endurance increases in the two to four year old, the tentative steps become secure and firm, with balance well under control to allow running, jumping, and climbing; eye–hand coordination allows the skilled manipulation of taking apart and putting together complex objects. These new abilities permit access to a wider environment with more stimuli to investigate, deeper investigation of objects, challenges to pursue and problems to solve and more risks. Fantasy enters into the play with increasing capacity for pretense with elaborate schemes to be acted out. Imaginary companions are a common feature of this age.

A central process in the development of the child is imitation. The child observes significant others in their setting, and plans their own behavior after that model. The imitation exists for its own sake, not because the child understands the underlying rules that govern the behavior being imitated. The eight month old will make faces to mimic the funny faces made by a parent; later words are repeated without knowing their meaning, but because they sound good or funny. The drive seems to be mastery of new skills. As the child matures they are more selective in the behaviors modeled and imitated, choosing those that serve their own particular objectives. Between the ages of three and six playing 'house' with peers involves an imitation of adults in real-life situations: setting the table, feeding the baby, house work, going to work, driving the car, scolding a naughty child. Playing 'school' allows the young child to imitate older siblings as they pretend to read, write on the board, and play at sports activities. These imitation activities enable children to develop links with other children in coordinated play when their social language skills do not permit skilled social interaction.

At the end of this chapter Cindy is introduced to us, a six year old who experienced a high fever with subsequent convulsions resulting in cerebral palsy at age two. She has difficulty in moving from place to place, and is delayed in skill development in many areas that require musculoskeletal coordination and controlled movement. As a consequence she is limited in her ability to explore her environment and interact with peers. Her conversation with the therapist illustrates several points discussed above: mutuality with the caregiver, sensorimotor schemes, object manipulation, and imitation.

Language development

The newborn infant is without language or the coding system to interpret the sounds of words that come to him from the immediate environment. Within a very short period of time they develop communicative competence that allows transcribing sound waves into meaningful symbols we call words. The *phonology*, or sound system, has a system of meanings we call *semantics*, and rules that govern how words are formed that we call *morphology*. Eventually the child learns the rules of sentence structure that we call *syntax*. The form of the words (morphology), and the rules of the sentence structure (syntax) form the grammar of the language being learned. All of this takes place without formal training in language, but through experience and the inductive and deductive processes of cognition.

The newborn infant is responsive to tone of voice. Gradually they associate particular words with particular meanings, though they are still unable to reproduce any words. The first to be associated in what might be called a comprehension vocabulary are the commonly used and functional words such as 'ma', 'da da'., hungry, food, milk, juice, cookie, dog, cat, and the special names of the family pets. The early sounds the child produces as babble are the precursors to intentional speech. Those sounds the child hears in the language around him are part of the babble; sounds that are not part of the language disappear from the babble.

Language production begins with naming objects. In English and American English, 'ba' represents ball, 'bb' represents bye, and 'baw' means bottle; these grow with an increasing number of partial pronunciations. Eventually the words take on more complete form and two word combinations develop in what is called telegraphic speech. The child links two words that are key to conveying the meaning, leaving out the non-essential verbs, articles, and so forth. 'More milk', 'no peas', and 'up now' convey the meaning without the burden of full sentences, and reduces the necessity for elaborate gestures. The evidence of increased language skill and the expanded comprehension vocabulary lead one to infer considerably greater cognitive ability than really exists for the child. Complex sentences can be repeated, for example, but the activity requested may not be completed. 'Go upstairs and get the sweater off mommy's bed please' Is understood in its component parts, can be repeated, but the cognitive ability and memory may not exist for execution of the task. When we consider the language skills and cognitive ability described in the introductory information in the case of Cindy we might question the phrase '… mild mental retardation'.

The interaction between parent and child is critical to the development of the child's language. That interaction, founded on effective social attachment, includes non-verbal and paralingual behavior (sounds that are not words), as well as the full range of words in the vocabulary. Talking, reading, singing, and playing activities contribute to the formation of language. Language is the medium through which the rules of the culture are transmitted informally and formally, and of course, the culture establishes the rules for language transmission. The culture determines who may speak to whom, in what manner, and under what conditions. Generally, children like the sounds of words and enjoy long and complicated words. They like to play with sounds and make up words, word games, and stories. Mastery of the production of sound that is meaningful to others is an important feature of the early years of development. Ron was a four-year-old boy who enjoyed telling stories to his mother, and she was delighted by their complexity and creativity. One day, part way through relaying the events of his experience at the house of a friend his mother interrupted him. "Ron, where in your story did it stop being 'real' and begin to be confabulation?" Ron said: "It was real up to the part about …, and the rest was confabulation." Ron knew what that big word meant, and the question had been asked before. It was a code that Ron and his mom shared. Story telling was fun and was all right to do under some circumstances, so long as each knew what was real and what was not real. He was demonstrating his delight in story telling, the sounds of words, and the attention from his mother.

As the child matures, language skills increase in complexity with a vocabulary that seems to explode in terms of number, from fifty at eighteen months to over 2000 by the age of three. Sentence structure becomes more complex, with correct use of irregular verbs and dependent clauses, descriptions expand, making language sound more as adult speech. Language allows one to engage in complex problem solving and reasoning, establish relationships and explore group memberships, gather new ideas and feelings and express them with others. The quality of one's spoken language leads toward the development of communication with another, which builds toward significant interpersonal relationships and intimacy. Language is the most commonly used channel to resolve interpersonal conflicts, develop group relations with family, friends, and others in the community.

Six year old Erika spoke English correctly and distinctly. Her parents were foreign born, had learned English in their native land, and expected Erika to speak as they did. They encouraged her to learn new words as something fun to do. She attended a school with a lunch program in the school cafeteria in which the children could buy their food. Erika brought her money to school each day, but soon decided the options did not suit her taste. She left the school quietly every day and went to a nearby family-owned and operated neighborhood grocery store. There she made her purchases of fruit and a piece of cheese, and sat on the counter to talk with the owner – at his invitation. After some time the teacher realized that Erika had not been in the cafeteria for several days. One day she followed her at some distance to the grocery store. She watched as the owner lifted Erika up on to the counter to eat her lunch and carry on a conversation with the owner and his wife. The teacher went in and joined the conversation. The owner said he was delighted just to listen to this little girl because she spoke so well and used so many big-people words. Of course Erika enjoyed their enjoyment.

Consider the restrictions imposed by physical limitations to explore the environment, as in the case of Cindy at the end of the chapter. The limitations impose difficulties in socialization when the muscles that control the prodcution of speech are involved. Daniel Day Lewis played the role of Christy Brown in the film *My Left Foot*, based on the book of the same title published in 1954. This young man had severe cerebral palsy that left him without intelligible speech and no productive movement for many years. His mother seemed to know that he was intelligent, though unable to let anyone know his thoughts and feelings. She talked to him, read to him, and ultimately provided a typewriter which he could bang away on with his left foot, over which he had developed some control. In fact, he began to bang out words, very laboriously, and produced a work of art. His mother's faith and insight provided an avenue to expression for this young man who had been locked inside his body.

Psychosocial Agenda

Autonomy versus shame and doubt

Psychosocial development for the two to four year old provides dramatic changes in physical and language abilities, the potential for increasing freedom from parents with commensurate decreasing dependency, and a growing sense of autonomy. We can refer again to Table 2.1 in Chapter 2, which outlines the psychosocial stages of Erik Erikson. This autonomy is gained through an extensive negotiation process between the young child and the caregiver, the one demanding to 'do it self mommy' and the other feeling the need to protect the child from harm. Persistence is a hallmark of this age, so the child will try again and again to accomplish the goal. When parents have been able to allow the growing competence to have expression without undue restraint, self-confidence emerges along with the new found independence. If, on the other hand, the child is not allowed to try, or experiences repeated failure at tasks attempted, and ridicule and discouragement from parents, a sense of shame and doubt develops instead. Shame is an extremely unpleasant feeling. When used as a method of control, the individual learns not to attempt 'risky' activities that might elicit the shaming response. Some cultures operate with conspicuous public shaming or humiliation as a method of social control. People grow up in this environment with a strong need to 'save face' in order to avoid public disgrace.

A classic arena for autonomy and shame to be negotiated is toilet training. It becomes clear to the child at an early age that he has the control to give or hold back, to produce or not, something that the parent thinks is important. The activity of control requires the association of internal sensory experience with the production of urine and feces, the language to signal the urgency, the muscular control to activate the anal and urethral sphincters, and the desire to please the parent. The neurologic mechanisms are not mature enough for control until the age of eighteen to twenty-four months. Control before that time is probably more a function of the mother's vigilance than the child's cooperation.

When physiologic readiness exists, and if the parents have not applied undue pressure to 'perform' ahead of this schedule, the child is likely to see toilet training as one more task over which to gain mastery and find pride in accomplishment. A struggle of wills leads to unsatisfactory experiences for both parent and child.

Gender-role identification

Many are confused about the appropriate use of the words sex and gender. In this discussion we refer to sex as a biologic description; gender has to do with how males and females are supposed to behave within a socio-cultural context. The fact that sports activities for male athletes are supported by the public in the United States, while female athletes struggle for public attention is a matter of cultural values, not a matter of sex or ability. In most professions and occupations, one's sexual identity is not a predictor of ability in job performance, or accomplishing goals or tasks. Sex is important most particularly in matters that are sexual.

Research results are mixed in reporting sex-based differences in abilities such as mathematics, spatial perception, verbal facility, music, and writing. If such differences really exist, they are very small (Ornstein, 1993). Important differences do exist in body size, weight, muscle mass, and distribution of adipose tissue, and significant differences exist in the way males and females are socialized in a society. The behavior sanctioned by a society for its members has evolved over a long period of time and is constantly tested by its members, which leads to further change. The rules that govern gender-based behavior are generally unwritten, and are part of the child's learning experience from the time of infancy. Each of us learns about how to behave as a boy or a girl first by observing our male and female adult caregivers, then imitating their role behavior in our relationships with them at home, and later in play activities with peers, and finally in particular roles as we move through adolescence toward adulthood.

Debate continues about the origins of gender, whether they are a function of biology or socialization, or an interaction of the two. Current research suggests the interaction theory has more merit as a resolution to this issue. Careful observation has also provided information about how the concept evolves in the mind of the child. Kohlberg (1966) suggests there are four stages in this developmental sequence:

1. Using the gender label correctly, as in 'Cindy is a girl, and Ron is a boy'

2. The gender is a stable condition, as in 'Erika is a girl, and when she grows up she will be a woman'.

3. Gender is constant, as in 'I'm a girl, and I like to wear jeans and play baseball with the guys'.

4. Gender has a genital basis, as in 'I'm a boy and I have a penis, and girls don't have one'.

The first stage is usually accomplished by 30 months, and the third between the ages of four and seven in Western societies.

Changing social circumstances may alter traditional gender roles in families. For example, in Mexican families that immigrated to the United States, the role of the wife and mother was initially passive and dependent. The husband was the wage earner and dominated the family with an absolute patriarchy called machismo. As the women obtained more and better education, and gained employment outside the home, they gained greater equality in decision making within the family (Ybarra-Soriano, 1977; Cromwell and Ruiz, 1979). Small children who observe the subtle shift in roles for their male and female adults in the environment might experience some confusion about the male and female roles; they also probably experience emotional distress from the conflict that normally accompanies such changes.

The culture establishes the standards for what is considered appropriate gender role behavior in any society, for the children and for adults. Those standards vary from one culture to another. Young children usually have greater latitude allowed for their behavior than do adolescents and adults. They learn the rules through behavior that is rewarded, and other behavior that is punished, and expectations expressed for future behavior. 'Nice little girls don't do that.' 'Boys don't cry.' 'If you want to be a good boy, you will do what daddy does.' 'Boys don't play with dolls.' The messages are endless. The pressure to identify with the same-sex parent is strong.

The manner in which parents manage the child's behavior may be identified as *authoritative*, or *authoritarian* (Basic Behavioral Science Task Force, 1996). Authoritative control provides a structure with reasonable limits and expectations for the child's behavior. This style of interaction also encourages the child to develop age-appropriate independence and control of their actions, social competence, and cooperation. An authoritarian style of control sets rigid rules with harsh enforcement in the face of irrational explanations: '... because I said so.' The dictatorial standards discourage independence and cooperation.

When the children reach school age they have experienced four to six years of a socialization process to role behavior for their gender, and experienced punishment for behavior that does not meet parental and societal expectations for that role. Punishment has many forms: it may be subtle, as in ignoring the child when they fail to 'perform' properly; active withdrawal of affection, as in 'I don't like that behavior'; angry expression of disaffection, as in 'I am angry with you for doing that'; and openly hostile, as when the parent shouts at or strikes the child. Fear of the loss of love is a powerful motivator.

The role definition includes words, expression of emotions, manner of dress, and body movement, as well as ritual acts. Recent research on the development of the concept of gender role in the mind of the child suggests that it is the result of a gender scheme. This scheme includes the cultural expectations and stereotypes related to gender, parental messages about their behavior, and information from their peers about how they 'should' behave. Children seem to focus their attention and organize their perceptions with reference to the scheme (Martin and Halverson, 1987; Levy and Carter, 1989). This concept of scheme is consistent with the earlier discussion on learning theory of cognitive maps. The role scheme is one kind of map that develops over time in the very young child, and is modified as the socialization experience includes others outside the family.

It is clear that many interacting factors enter the equation of the evolving person and personality. In this chapter we have considered the genetic heritage and fetal development as early conditions. Recent research suggests, for example, that language development begins in the womb, and math ability may be influenced by the kind of music the mother listens to during fetal development. The nature and course of sensory and motor development lay the groundwork for evolving skill. The character of the relationship between the infant and primary caregiver in the early months of life sets in motion patterns of social attachment that persist throughout life.

The emotional development of the child is a function of genetic predispositions and environmental factors expressed through enduring aspects of intelligence, personality, and temperament. The vulnerability and resilience of each individual in the presence of stress, and the styles of coping employed may be attrib-

uted to all those ingredients, set within the framework of social skills and self-esteem (Basic Behavioral Science Task Force, 1996). How is it that some people seem to succumb to stress with retreat and immobility, while others face the stress with competence and effective problem-solving skills? Recent investigations have pursued these questions through all the avenues identified in this chapter. We are coming closer to understanding how it is that our behavior is as it is.

Case 1: Cindy Smith – Cerebral Palsy

Cindy Smith is six years old, weighs 35 pounds and is 33 inches in height. Her diagnosis is cerebral palsy. Questions to keep in mind as you analyze this case are:

1. How has the normal developmental sequence been altered by the limitations imposed by physical disability?

2. What are the psychosocial needs of a child at this age. Do these needs change in the presence of physical disability?

3. If the health professional is a significant adult in the life of this child, what kind of relationship should be structured for the maximum benefit of the child?

General information

Cindy Smith is the third of five children in her family. The ages of her siblings are one, two, seven, and eight years old. At age two Cindy had a kidney disease accompanied by high fever and convulsions. This became prolonged, and the child was comatose for two weeks with resultant spasticity, mild seizures, and suspected mild mental retardation. Evaluation of intelligence has been difficult owing to her physical disability. She has mild slurring of speech.

Cindy has been maintained at home from that time to the present. There have been no formal treatment or education programs for the child until the current admission to a residential rehabilitation facility for children. At this time she is on a full program of daily therapy including physical, occupational, and speech therapies. Goals are aimed at independent ambulation and independence in activities of daily living (ADL).

The following conversations are excerpts from a treatment session in physical therapy between Cindy and her therapist on a Monday following a weekend visit home. Cindy enters the department in a wheelchair under her own power, slowly but steadily. She is dressed in a pretty red dress, white shoes attached to long leg braces, and a ribbon in her long blond hair. She has mild spasticity in both upper extremities, and moderate to severe spasticity in both lower extremities. At this time she is able to sit unsupported, stand in her braces between parallel bars or without braces with support. Her movements are slow and deliberate. At the time of this conversation she has been in the program for two months, working with the same therapist. It is anticipated that she will remain for the academic year and probably return for one additional year if she continues to demonstrate progress.

T = therapist (Mrs Hill)
C = Cindy
P = other patient

T Good morning Cindy. How are you today? My, but you surely look pretty this morning.

C Good morning Mrs Hill. Do you like my new dress?

T I sure do.

C You know what? [pause for the ritual 'what' from Mrs H] My mommy gave it to me when I was home this weekend. She said I was such a good girl that she would give me a present.

T And the dress was the present. What a nice present it is too. Are you ready to go to work now? We have a lot to do.

C Yes, I'm ready. Can I take off my shoes by myself? I know how. I'm a big girl.

T Yes Cindy you are a big girl. But I would like to help you off with the shoes and braces because they take such a long time to get off and on. When you are working with Miss Brown in O.T. this afternoon I know she will let you take them off all by yourself.

C OK. [the two proceed to work at taking off the shoes and braces] Did you see the pretty ribbon in my hair? You know what? My mommy says the ribbon matches my dress. [pause] What does 'matches' mean?

T 'Matches' means that the colors go together, that they are like each other so they look nicely together. The red ribbon looks especially nice in your pretty blond hair. Now, scoot over onto the mat so we can go to work.

C [makes transfer from chair to mat without assistance] There! What do we do first? I want to crawl. Can I crawl first?

T   You managed that transfer very nicely Cindy. Yes, you may crawl first if you like. That's a good place to begin. [Cindy proceeds to roll over into the hands and knees position and gets off to a bad start on the crawling activity] Whoa Cindy. I know you can do better than that. You had better stop and think about what you should be doing. When you move the right hand forward, what part moves next?

C   After the right hand comes the ... [long pause] ... You know what? My baby brother is learning how to walk but he's not very good at it. He keeps falling down. I can do better'n him 'cuz I don't fall down.

T   Cindy, you forgot what you were doing. Let's begin again with the right hand. What comes after that? Try to do it and maybe you'll remember which part moves next.

C   OK. [she tries and this time produces the proper sequence of movements] There! How was that? I went all the way across the mat before you could catch me. Did I do it right?

T   Yes, you did it OK. Now can you come all the way back without any mistakes? You try. This is the same set of movements we'll be using in the parallel bars soon, so it is important that you know how to do it well. [Cindy continues the activity, stopping often to look around the room and watch the activities of some of the other children] OK Cindy, as you come over here I'd like to have you walk your hands up the stall bars so you are in the kneeling position. Know what I mean?

C   Uh huh. I'm good at this aren't I? I can almost let go with my hands, but not quite. My baby brother can't do this at all,

'cuz I watched him and he kept on falling over and bumping his nose. I'm a big girl now aren't I Mrs Hill? I can do lots of things, can't I?

T   Yes dear, you can do lots of things. But there are lots of other things you'd like to be able to do aren't there?

C   Uh huh. [softly] My little sister can do some things that I can't do. You know what? In the dorm this morning, I was the first one to wake up and the first one to get out of the bed. Most of the time I'm a slow poke 'cuz I don't like to get out of bed. Most all the others are up ahead of me, but this morning I fooled 'em.

T   That must have been a surprise for them. Now, while you are kneeling there with your hands on the stall bars, I will give you some resistance here on your hips. And I want you to keep on kneeling just as tall and straight as you can. [Mrs H places her hands on Cindy's hip and applies small amounts of resistance, first in one direction and then in another] That's fine Cindy, kneel tall. Don't let me push you off balance.

C   Ooooh, that's hard. Don't push too hard! I might fall over. [pause] You know what? Jimmy, he's the boy in my class, was a bad boy. He was throwing spit balls at all the girls and one of them went onto the teacher's lap.

T   Uh oh. It sounds as if his aim wasn't very good. Did he get into trouble? [Cindy nods] What did the teacher do then? You may sit back down and rest for a minute now Cindy.

C   OK. The teacher made him come up to the front of the room and sit all by himself.

[she arranges herself, sitting tailor fashion, on the mat with elbows resting on knees for support]

T   What do you think he will learn from that?

C   I don't think he will learn anything from that. He doesn't like to sit so close to the teacher, but he does like to show off. When he sits up there everybody can see him, so he shows off all he can.

T   Maybe there is another way for the teacher to punish him, that he wouldn't enjoy so much?

C   Oh sure. She should put him at the back of the room where we can't see him, and where he can't reach us with the spit balls. Ha ha ha. [both join in a giggle over this suggestion]

T   Oh Cindy, that's good. I do enjoy your humor. Now sweetie, let's go back to work. This time I'd like you to walk your hands up the stall bars, all the way up, until you can get into a standing position. OK? You know what I mean? [Cindy nods and begins to move toward the stall bars. As Cindy manages to raise herself up, first to the kneeling and then to the standing positions, Mrs H kneels behind her with her hands in readiness, in case Cindy should fall] Cindy, you are doing very well on this today. And you haven't needed any help from me to do it.

C   Yeh, I dun good, huh. I didn't fool around either. [her balance starts to waver as her attention drifts from the activity]

T   Cindy, you better pay attention or you'll fall yet. When the job is as hard as this one is you really have to think hard about what you are doing. [pause, as Cindy gets herself straightened up again] There, that's better. It seems to me that you are getting tired. Would you like to sit down now? It's almost time to call it quits for today anyway.

C   Yes, I wan' to stop doing this. It's hard to do. My hand keeps coming off the bar [the spasticity causes the right upper extremity to pull into a flexion-adduction pattern] and my knees don't want to stay straight. [with this she lets go and plops down onto the mat into Mrs H's arms with much giggling] I fooled you. Ha ha ha!

T   Well, you surely surprised me. I didn't expect you to just let go and collapse in my arms, but now that you're here, I'll give you a squeeze. [gives Cindy a hug] There you go little minx. Time to get ready to go back to your classroom. You did quite well today, with the exception of that last falling performance.

C   You don't have to help me. I can get into my chair by myself. [she proceeds to scoot across the mat on her stomach, dragging her lower extremities behind her, transfers into the chair and begins to put on the braces. All this is accompanied by much chatter and gossip about doings in the dorm and her classroom]

T   I'll help you now Cindy. The shoes and braces are pretty hard to get on. And I don't want you to miss any more of your class. That's important too. [both work at this job together with Cindy teasing by putting hands in the way, unlacing or unbuckling what's been done and giggling all the while] Hey! you monkey! Are you trying to tell me something with that kind of behavior? You make me think you don't want to leave. Shall I put you to work scrubbing floors?

C [laughing] Oh, I don't want to scrub floors. But I like it here. I wish I could stay all day.

T That's sweet Cindy. I like to have you here too. But I have other children that I need to work with too. You all have to take turns with me. There, you are all put back together now [finishing the last buckle] And you still look very pretty in your new dress and the matching ribbon. You can go and show it off to your friends. Bye Bye. See you tomorrow.

C Bye bye Mrs Hill. See you tomorrow. [she turns the wheelchair slowly and pushes herself out of the department]

References

Ainsworth, MD, Blehar, MC, Waters, E, Wall S (1978) *Patterns of Attachment: A Psychological Study of the Strange Situation.* Hillsdale, NJ: Erlbaum.

Alessandri SM (1992) Mother–child interactional correlates of maltreated and nonmaltreated children's play behavior. *Development and Psychopathology* 4: 257–270.

Aoki, C, Siekevitz, P (1988) Plasticity in brain development. *Scientific American* 259: 56–64.

Basic Behavioral Science Task Force of the National Advisory Mental Health Council (1996a) Vulnerability and resilience. *American Psychologist* 51(1): 22–28.

Basic Behavioral Science Task Force of the National Advisory Mental Health Council (1996b) Perception, attention, learning, and memory. *American Psychologist* 51(2): 133–142.

Basic Behavioral Science Task Force of the National Advisory Mental Health Council (1996c) Family processes and social networks. *American Psychologist*, 51(6): 622–630.

Carlson, V, Cicchetti, D, Barnett, D, Braunwald, K (1989) Disorganized/disoriented attachment relationships in maltreated infants. *Developmental Psychology* 25: 525–531.

Cassady, G, Strange, M (1987) The small-for-gestational-age (SGA) infant. In: Avery, GB (ed), *Neonatology: Pathophysiology and Management of the Newborn* pp. 299–331. Philadelphia: Lippincott.

Cromwell, R, Ruiz, RA (1979) The myth of macho dominance in decision-making within Mexican and Chicano families. *Hispanic Journal of Behavioral Sciences* I: 355–373.

Diamond, MC, Johnson, RC, Protti, AM, Ott, C, Kajisa, L (1985) Plasticity in the 904 day old male rat cerebral cortex. *Experimental Neurology* 87: 309–317.

Dodge, KA (1989) Coordinating responses to aversive stimuli: introduction to a special section of the development of emotion regulation. *Developmental Psychology* 25: 339–342.

Erikson, EH (1978) Reflection on Dr. Borg's life cycle. In: Erikson, EJ, (ed), *Adulthood*, pp. 1–31. New York: Norton.

Fischer, KW, Silvern, L (1985) Stages and individual differences in cognitive development. *Annual Review of Psychology* 36: 613–648.

Harwood, RL (1992) The influence of culturally derived values on Anglo and Puerta Rica mothers' perceptions of attachment behavior. *Child Development* 63: 822–839.

Kohlberg, L (1966) A cognitive-developmental analysis of children's sex-role concepts and attitudes. In Maccoby, E.E (ed) *The Development of Sex Differences.* Stanford, CA: Stanford University Press.

Kopp, CB (1989) Regulation of distress and negative emotions: a developmental view. *Developmental Psychology* 25: 343–354.

Levy, GD, Carter, DB (1989) Gender schema, gender constancy, and gender-role knowledge: the roles of cognitive factors in preschoolers' gender-role stereotype attributions. *Developmental Psychology* 25: 444–449.

Lyons-Ruth, K, Alpern, L, Repacholi, B (1993) Disorganized infant attachment classification and maternal psychosocial problems as predictors of hostile-aggressive behavior in the preschool classroom. *Child Development* 64: 572–585.

MacTurk, RH, McCarthy, ME, Vietze, PM, Yarrow, LJ (1987) Sequential analysis of mastery behavior in 6- and 12-month-old infants. *Developmental Psychology* 23: 199–203.

Main, M, Solomon, J (1986) Discovery of insecure-disorganized/disoriented attachment pattern. In: Brazelton, TB, Yogman, MW, (eds) *Affective Development in Infancy,* pp. 95–124. Norwood, NJ: Ablex.

Main, M, Kaplan, N, Cassidy, J (1985) Security in infancy, childhood, and adulthood: a move to the level of representation. In: Bretherton, I, Everett, E (eds) *Growing points of attachment theory and research,* pp. 66–104. Monographs of the Society for Research in Child Development, 50 (1-2, Serial No. 209).

Martin, CL, Halverson, CF (1987) The roles of cognition in sex roles acquisition. In: Carter, DB (ed) *Current Conceptions of Sex Roles and Sex Typing: theory and research,* pp. 123–137. New York: Praeger.

Mesulam, M-M (1986) *Principles of Behavioral Neurology.* Philadelphia: FA Davis Co.

Miyake, K, Campos, J, Kagan, J, Bradshaw, D (1986) Issues in socioemotional development in Japan. In: Azuma, H, Hakuta, I , Stevenson, H (eds) *Kodomo: Child Development and Education in Japan,* pp. 239–261. New York: W. H. Freeman.

Ornstein, R (1993) *The Roots of the Self.* San Francisco: Harper Collins Publishers.

Piaget, J (1954) *The Construction of Reality in the Child.* New York: Basic Books.

Piaget, J (1970) Piaget's theory. In: Mussen, PH, (ed) *Carmichael's Manual of Child Psychology,* 3rd edn. New York: Wiley.

Piaget, J, Inhelder, B (1966, 1969), *The Psychology of the Child.* New York: Basic Books.

Rochat, P (1989) Object manipulation and exploration in 2- to 5-month-old infants. *Developmental Psychology* 25: 871–884.

Ruff, HA, Saltarelli, LM, Capozzoli, M, Dubiner K (1992) The differentiation of activity in infants' exploration of objects. *Developmental Psychology* 28: 851–861.

Rutter, M (1990) Commentary: some focus and process considerations regarding effects of parental depression on children. *Developmental Psychology* 26: 60–67.

Sroufe, LA, Schork, E, Motti, F, Lawrodki, N, LaFreniere, P (1984) The role of affect in social competence. In: Izard, CE, Kagan, J, Zajonc, RB (eds) *Emotions, Cognition, and Behavior*, pp. 38–72. Cambridge: Cambridge University Press.

Wellman, HM, Cross, D, Bartsch, K (1986) *Infant Search and Object Permanence: a meta-Analysis of the A–not–B Error.* Monographs of the Society for Research in Child Development, 51 (3, Whole No. 214).

Wolf, PH (1966) Causes, controls, and organization of behavior in the neonate. *Psychological Issues*, 5 (1, Whole No. 17).

Yarrow, LJ, McQuiston, S, MacTurk, RH, McCarthy, ME, Klein, RP, Vietze, PM (1983) The assessment of mastery motivation during the first year of life. *Developmental Psychology*, 19: 159–171.

Ybarra-Soriano L (1977) *Conjugal Role Relationships in the Chicano Family.* Unpublished doctoral dissertation, Department of Sociology, University of California, Berkeley.

van Ljzendoorn, MH, Kroonenberg, PM (1988) Cross-cultural patterns of attachment: a meta-analysis of the strange situation. *Child Development* 59: 147–156.

van Ljzendoorn, MH, Goldberg, S, Kroonenberg, PM, Frendel, OJ (1992) The relative effects of maternal and child problems on the quality of attachment: a meta-analysis of attachment in clinical samples. *Child Development* 63: 840–858.

5

The Adolescent Years

Pamela Hansford

Introduction
•
A Holistic Perspective
•
Universal Challenges of the Second Decade
•
Adolescents Talk About Their Experiences as Patients
•
Principles of Practice
•
Conclusion

'I'm Shelly McDonald. I'm very disabled. I can't talk or walk. I dribble a lot and some people really hate that. I think physio is very good for disabled people because they are not able to exercise their bodies themselves. When I sit all day I get stiff and it is so painful. I think physio could be improved if some therapists took more notice of what their people wanted, instead of making them so angry. I get angry when I'm treated by people like I'm stupid, not just disabled. Sometimes I think some therapists don't realise what it is like to be disabled. I can see some of them would prefer to ignore me just by their faces and some of the parents look at me as if I'm a freak.'

(Shelly, now nearly 14, p. 78)

'Looking at a baby photo of myself, I look extremely "normal". How I hate that word normal because in actual fact not one of us wonderful human beings are normal. We don't even know if God is normal so what right do these "normal" people have naming themselves with such superiority?

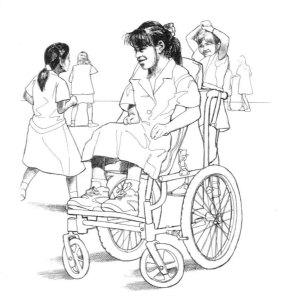

Figure 5.1 Shelley.

Figure 5.2 Theresa.

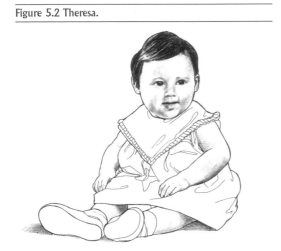

Anyway the photo, there I am sitting whether someone is holding me up I don't know but it looks pretty good to me, as good as my own "normal" children's photos. I personally don't think that I look very normal now. My right hand looks disabled and so do my legs.'

(Theresa had extensive surgery at 14, p. 78)

Figure 5.3 Sian (right).

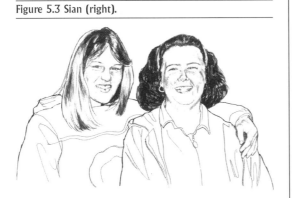

'I was angry at my friends for leaving me at a time in my life that I needed them most. My development as a teenager was reduced to an infant's status and I had to start my growing period all over again, but I had to grow up rather quickly. As a child I was not known for having patience and I had to learn to have patience while growing up again! Especially regarding losing all my friends who were young and not patient!'

(Sian was involved in a motor vehicle accident at 14, p. 79)

Introduction

The second decade is a period of rapid intense change, in which we face ongoing challenges, all offering opportunities for growth and mishap. If we see 'growth' as change occurring over time in all dimensions of the life cycle (physical, emotional, learning, social, creative, and spiritual), 'mishaps' are undesirable historical events which confront us with new issues and demand our attention. The voices of Shelley, Theresa, and Sian above testify to dealing with mishap in adolescence. Adolescence can be seen as a time of intensified risk for mishap, such as sport and traffic accidents and the results of experimentation with sex, alcohol or drugs. Leaving childhood behind, while moving towards adulthood may be perceived as being adrift in a sea of mishap, with the experience of dislocation being accentuated by the move from one school to another.

However, mishaps also offer opportunities for growth, even though this may only become apparent later in life. The urgent question leading us through this chapter is how as therapists we can best relate with our adolescent (and other) patients to take part in

- Helping them to deal ever more successfully with their challenges of daily living.
- Enabling them to take control of their own lives and responsibility for their own well-being.
- Empowering them to express their ideas at the level of their potential.

I have divided this chapter into four main sections. These are:

1. A holistic perspective A brief introduction to the theory of holism, the basis of this chapter.

2. Universal challenges of the second decade These include physical growth and development and taking responsibility for ourselves in relation to our worlds.

3. Adolescents talk about their experiences as patients We read verbatim comments on patient-identified issues such as respect and reciprocity in relationship, 'compliance' with the medical world and how adolescents perceive their own resources in the face of mishap.

4. Principles of practice These are offered as practical recommendations for health practitioners in relationship with patients in general, and adolescents in particular.

This chapter concludes with a discussion of the importance of relationships and the choices they require of us.

A Holistic Perspective

My goal in this chapter is to integrate theory and practice, and art and science, in therapy. I have adopted an experiential learning approach in a holistic framework. With a wide holistic perspective of human functioning, we can

- shift to new paradigms or ways of thinking about people through the contextualization process
- contribute towards the elimination of traditional opposites in human sciences, and
- explore new possibilities with regard to academic training, theory building, research, and practical application of knowledge (Jordaan and Jordaan, 1989:61).

The first person voice is used to shift our thinking from traditional healer–patient and adult–adolescent dichotomies, to interaction in a working partnership. Reflection on adolescent experience can be used to develop the empathy necessary for creating therapeutic relationships based on mutual respect and trust.

Holism – The whole is greater than the sum of its parts

South African statesman, Jan C. Smuts, introduced the concept of Holism as a fundamental factor in the universe in his book *Holism and Evolution* (Smuts, 1926:86). In a living whole, we notice a unity of parts which is so close and so intense as to be more than a sum of its parts. The whole and the parts reciprocally influence and determine each other, and appear to merge their individual characters: the whole is in the parts and the parts are in the whole. Holism is not only creative but self-creative, and its final structures are far more holistic than its initial structures (Smuts, 1926:85).

This concept about the integral relationship of the structure of the parts with the function of the whole illuminates our understanding of the second decade. Both structure and function change in relation to each other at an alarming rate, creating chaos in a previously well-ordered system. Body and mind are in turmoil much of the time, or need rest and recreation for recovery and reorganization at each new level. Our experience is largely fluid and plastic, with little that is rigid and much that is indefinite about it.

Holism and neuromuscular plasticity

Therapists have permission to work through touch. We hope to help people change the way they act and behave in space over time. Knowledge and experience teach us that change is possible. Our goal is to help people establish control of their immediate worlds through gaining a stable but dynamic base from which to reach out in all directions for easy, enjoyable interaction with the world. As therapists we take responsibility for directing change and need to identify basic principles to guide and direct our actions.

Sixty-six years after Smuts introduced his theory of Holism, Geoffrey Kidd, Nigel Lawes and Iris Musa in their aptly titled book, *Understanding Neuromuscular Plasticity* (Kidd et al., 1992), explain a holistic approach to therapy (based on potential for change of macromolecules) which utilizes plasticity in the sensor-neuro-motor skeletal system. An element of uncertainty of response is introduced into the central nervous system at the synapses (Kidd et al., 1992:xi). This principle of plastic adaptation is basic to our understanding of the possible effects of various clinical rehabilitation techniques, and operates throughout the lifespan in the 'timespace' framework (as conceptualized by Einstein). Form and function, like time and space, are 'wholes' and cannot exist independently of each other. The characteristics of form and function thus fuse into the concept of 'formfunction' (Kidd et al., 1992:xiv). Events, involving action in space and time, are real and form the units of reality (Smuts, 1926:22).

From a holistic perspective, effecting change in formfunction, in timespace, helps people achieve their goals and take responsibility for their own health and well-being by empowering them to develop more mature responses to daily challenges. We can improve quality of life through working in partnership in a goal directed, solution focused manner. Improving quality of movement in function will enhance the behavioral repertoire. As I move, others observe a change in my behavior. Because 'how I use my behavior' affects my interaction with the world, the quality of that interaction with the world and with people in that world, can be enhanced too (Milani-Comparetti, in Irwin Carruthers, 1984).

The focal concept for understanding the theories of holism and of neuromuscular plasticity is that change happens at the cellular level (where proteins are constantly broken down and reformed) and influences what happens to the function of the whole over time. The challenge lies in being able to initiate, support, and direct positive change to facilitate integrated, successful, experiential learning.

'It's the touching and the meaning of touching that matters. Touching is not only about hands or walking, it is also about eyes, ears and mind. Touch, in whatever form, sets up eddies in the flux of life, which can continue to effect responses through time and space far beyond the original contact' (Long, 1991:20).

The South African context

Although Smuts introduced his concept of Holism in South Africa 70 years ago, reductionism and fragmentation have been our experience, over the past half century. South Africa emerged as a 'new' nation in April 1994, but the legacy of apartheid remains. We are dealing with the consequences of adversity experienced as a result of years of legalized discrimination. Nearly half the population is under 19 years of age and 10% of the population controls more than 80% of the land. Being born 'black' predisposes children to experiencing a range of adverse life conditions which would not have arisen had the children's genes for skin colour been different.

In *Childhood and Adversity*, Dawes and Donald (1994) provide a psychosocial overview of the experience of childhood and adolescence in the context of adversity. In this book based on collaborative interdisciplinary research, all agree that most South African children and adolescents can be considered grossly disadvantaged and at risk for less than optimal psychological development owing to structurally generated conditions of disadvantage including poverty and political oppression.

In interpersonal contexts a range of major life struggles are generated in which individuals are subjected to abuse, experience the distress of divorce, or live with psychological illness or substance abuse of self or a family member. These adversities take place in the family or school, and it is clear that the risk of exposure is higher in poorer communities. In poor environments adult coping is frequently stretched to the limit, making it difficult for the adults to support their children and protect them from adversity.

Dawes and Donald therefore emphasize the concept of resilience as a research issue of major importance, as it changes the way we look at the relationship between adversity and development. Under what conditions, why and how are constructive coping strategies and resilience promoted in some children and adolescents, while vulnerability is reinforced in others? This has implications for research, intervention, and policy making (Dawes and Donald, 1994).

Developing constructive coping strategies under conditions of extreme adversity as reported in *Prospects for Africa's Children* (SCF, 1990) related to how people manage to survive protracted periods of drought. In Africa, although drought is common, famine that results in mass starvation is in fact surprisingly rare. Research revealed that in adverse conditions people planned ahead together, were able to preserve surplus from good years to build up stocks, and generated additional food from other sources in times of shortage, especially in poorer communities in more risky areas. This development of adaptive capabilities in response to real need, especially as part of the group, is basic to survival, growth, and development in all areas of life. This principle is highlighted throughout this chapter. Help is most valuable when it enables people to solve their own problems through developing creative solutions by building on and developing existing strengths.

Hope is the touchword in coping with adversity. South Africa and its children need a large dose of hope, together with the will to realize this hope, to face the future with greater confidence. Change is needed on all levels in policy making (at a national level, community, the organization, as well as at the individual level) to accommodate to the new health plan, and the reconstruction and development programs (ANC, 1994), to make the realization of hope possible. We must work towards greater understanding of childhood and adolescence in developing countries like South Africa, in order to contribute towards 'halting the historical theft of hope' which Monica Wilson refers to in her research (Dawes and Donald, 1994:vi). Adolescence is marked by a sense of idealism and omnipotence, which offers our society hope from an uncynical perspective (Elkind, 1991 in Santrock, 1992).

Universal Challenges of the Second Decade

From birth, we proceed stepwise through the process of life cycle development by dealing with the demands, tasks, and challenges of daily living. We meet these challenges through a process of survival, growth, and trial and error. We rise up against gravity, developing competence and confidence in our skills, knowledge, and attitudes and become independent and mature through learning to develop relationships in co-operation and collaboration with others.

The challenges of active engagement and conscious participation in our own development are very demanding in the second decade. During adolescence, we focus our energy on all aspects of becoming an adult person through dealing with the daily challenges of the present in the present as

'every dimension of the person undergoes qualitative and/or quantitative change' (Lerner, 1976: 205).

Erikson believed that optimal adolescent development is dependent on a balance between physical activity, the joy we derive from newly developed abilities, the social recognition we obtain and the status and approval it brings (Erikson, 1968). Bronfenbrenner (1986) has studied external influences that affect the capacity of families to foster the healthy development of their children through the research question 'How are intrafamilial processes affected by extrafamilial conditions?' and presents us with convincing reasons for looking both from within and from without as we examine relevant factors affecting the system. In this section, consideration is given to physical growth and development, self-creation with a focus on self-awareness and responsibility, and the social self in adolescence.

Physical growth and development

Bateson's example of presenting abstract thoughts in story form is followed in this chapter because it offers us a way of moving beyond logical thinking into the realm of interrelationships, enabling us to work on integrating physical and psychosocial aspects of the person. Since we communicate and connect through both touch and language in therapy, metaphor and humour are valuable in establishing ever more efficient and effective mind–body connections. After all,

'metaphor offers a way of holding the fabric of mental interconnections together' (Bateson according to Capra, 1989).

Eric Carle presents a vibrant metaphor for adolescent transformation through his simple, humorous story of change from birth and rebirth to metamorphosis into the adult form of *The Very Hungry Caterpillar* (Carle, 1969).

'In the light of the moon a little egg lay on a leaf'

sets the stage. In the passage of time the egg hatches. Maturation is facilitated by the warmth of the sun. He makes the most of his opportunities, applying himself proactively to growth from the moment of emerging from the egg. He naturally makes mistakes en route, but self corrects, as he benefits by learning through experience, and feels much better. He grounds himself by building a house around himself and enters the cocoon.

'He stayed inside for more than two weeks'

needing time to consolidate and prepare for proactive re-entry into the world. He

'nibbled a hole in the cocoon, pushed his way out'

and emerged as a beautiful butterfly. This adult form reaches out with vibrant wings which free it to explore space and deal with new, more varied challenges at higher levels. In this chapter, this metaphor for growth, development, maturation, and expansion of self is applied to the reality of the adolescent world.

For a child, the extraordinary level of growth and development at birth is revealed in the following responses to face, voice, and smile elicited when the newborn is in a state of peak alertness, as demonstrated in the course of performing Brazelton's Neonatal Assessment (Brazelton 1984). In the first year, 'touchpoints' are strikingly evident.

'Touchpoints, which are universal, are those predictable times which occur just before a surge in rapid growth in any line of development (motor, cognitive, or emotional) when for a short time the child's behaviour falls apart ... Predictable spurts raise equally predictable issues in virtually all families.'

The chaos necessary to create new order, precedes mastery of the next skill. The child appears to regress in several areas, but if seen as

'windows through which parents can view the great energy that fuels the child for learning,'

'touchpoints' become maximum growth points for both child and family.

'Rebirth' through adolescence into adulthood is a similar stormy process. We can use this concept to understand the process more clearly. Interaction within the family is frequently abrasive as the child struggles to gain sufficient control to achieve the next major milestone. The whole family needs to deal with the ensuing change, whether this is the achievement of crawling which enables the baby to leave the parent and explore, or whether it is our initial experiences with dating and experimentation with sex as adolescents. Exploration results in feelings of vulnerability and exposure, providing true 'touchpoints' for the introduction of new learning.

'When seen as normal and predictable, these periods of regressive behavior are opportunities to understand' individual teenagers and to support growth 'rather than become locked into a struggle.' (Brazelton, 1992: xvii–xviii).

After the dramatic changes that take place in the first year, the infant, then toddler, preschool, and primary school child grows consistently in reciprocal relationship to the environment. Periods of growth and development and periods of maturation, consolidation, and enrichment interchange in such a way that change is often only evident once it has happened and reintegration taken place. But rates of growth and change vary.

During the first decade, it is as if we are looking at a series of separate photographs taken over a long period of time. Not so in the second decade, when we see an often loud, action-packed, drama video, demanding recognition and response! The opposite state is much in evidence too – in adolescence we gain strength for growth through long periods of sleep at times of our choice! Physical growth demands that we deal with the physical task of redeveloping a sense of position in space and place, a task with a strong psychological component, which parallels a much earlier stage of development. With several extra inches suddenly attached to each of our

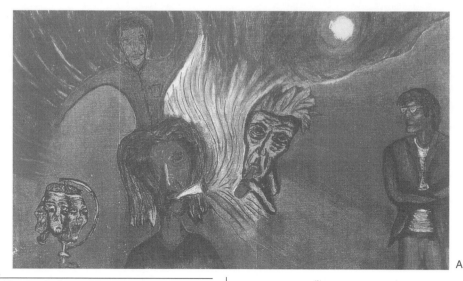

Figure 5.4 Liam's painting and later drawing.

extremities, even inanimate objects in our environment become aggressive and attack us in passing, bruising both body and ego! Even more demanding of our attention are the bodily changes and turmoil produced by the hormones, including the specific sex characteristics, hair growth, and skin changes.

Adolescence is a time of increased freedom and experimentation with all the attendant risks and there is therefore increased need for decision making. Choices cover a wide range from simple to complex and the mundane to the ridiculous, including what to eat and how much, what to wear, what hairstyle to risk, what face cream to try next, whom to be friends with, what subjects to take at school, what to do after school, whom to date, whether to have sex or not, whether to follow peers or adhere to family values, whether to take drugs, and even whether life is worth living. The choices we make during this second decade, and the lessons we learn from them, affect our paths into adulthood and influence our personal definitions of self in relation to

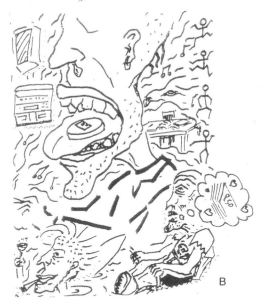

the world. As we emerge from a self-constructed cocoon of adolescence, we use our new knowledge, gained through reflection on experience, to develop decision-making abilities, widen our behavioral repertoires, and investigate new possibilities. Liam's story conveys these points. Liam, at 17, compared a current drawing of his experience of adolescence with the picture of 'Teenage Life' which he had painted the year before (Fig. 5.4). He commented on the fact that anything missing, like sex, was only absent because it wasn't important to him when he produced the pictures! In a year Liam had developed a greater sense of freedom. His drawing showed this as it pictured him abandoning his desk and dancing around, exploring possibilities with a sense of humor and light relief.

A family move from his home town to Cape Town, with the concomitant loss of close friends and a change to a more autocratic school, proved to be one stress too many. He was not coping in the context of family or of school. His first self-portrait reflected his unhappiness with his malaligned, vulnerable self. Eight physiotherapy sessions over eight months, helped him to begin to realign himself and to enjoy putting energy into physical activity again. His second self-portrait reflects his satisfaction at having been able to add layers to the self, an enjoyment of the filling out process, satisfaction with his change in 'form-function' in 'timespace' and particularly, his re-emerging sense of humor.

In retrospect, Liam intuitively understood our need as adolescents to develop the physical self first to center, stabilize, and give balance and focus to life. Adolescents need to throw their energy into something that has meaning for them, becoming totally and egocentrically involved, for example in a particular sport (and seemingly unaware of the needs of the rest of the world), particularly when struggling to deal with issues of loss like divorce and death. Elkind (1976) in Santrock (1992) speaks of this stage of apparent egocentrism as an explanation of our sense of recklessness and feelings of invulnerability as adolescents when the attitude of 'It could never happen to me'

leads us into experimentation with little sense of boundary or safety.

Self-creation

Growth, development, and maturation bring an increase in experience, a widening of the knowledge base, and an increase in speed of response and automaticity, first of the physical side, then in skill development and competency, and finally in the cognitive processes, in preparation for testing ideas in collaboration and co-operation with others. Through our learning experience, our ability to construct new knowledge is increased: we reflect on and learn from the old, and learn to make ever more complex connections as the basis for projecting into the future. Adolescence is a time of hypothesizing and theorizing, and of questioning, evaluating, and planning in an attempt to define a sense of self (Santrock, 1992). Mann (in Santrock, 1992) believes that adolescents with their increased cognitive abilities are more able to generate options, examine situations from a variety of perspectives, examine consequences of decision making, and consider the credibility of resources.

AJ Fernando focused on credibility in the context of society in his presidential address at the World Confederation for Physical Therapy Congress in Washington in 1995.

'Our patients will be the source of our credibility'

if we can predict the outcome of whatever intervention we discuss and account for the outcome by measuring it. It's time

'that credibility has to be in a valid context. It has to be in the context of the society we live in, the economics of our society, and the cultural influences that guide our society. And our education should prepare us to do the job in our society and in our economy. When we can achieve that, we have credibility within that context.'

Our capacity for self-awareness is the unique human attribute which allows us to accept the challenge to engage consciously in our own development. We are able to experience all aspects and attributes of our being from without and within, as individuals, and in relation to the world. Each person's self-image is a picture of what, whom, and where we are at that particular time.

'Every person forms a self-image on the basis of self-knowledge acquired through the act of self-evaluation'

which

'is carried out with a greater or lesser degree of awareness in various life contexts'

(Jordaan and Jordaan, 1989:683), thus giving us potential for enhancing the fluid, dynamic character of our own images in reciprocity with others in our world. This self-image, both internal and external, can be changed by choosing what is used to create it, just as a painter chooses each brush-stroke for its special effect, as well as the type of stroke, the direction in which it moves, the degree of pressure with which it is applied, and so on.

Conscious engagement in the process of becoming a person involves confronting of both positive and negative feelings about our behavior, and making choices accordingly based on current beliefs, values, and attitudes. In this way we can

'take responsibility for creating our own reality, moment by moment'

(Davis, 1994). A major challenge of maturation in the teenage years is the need to learn to take responsibility for ourselves, in preparation for behaving responsibly in relationship to others.

This central issue of rising above both nature and nurture and taking

'responsibility for creating our own reality, moment by moment'

is epitomized in the way in which Victor Frankl (1963) found meaning in life through choosing to create a lifeline of hope into the future. Covey (1992:69–71) describes how Frankl found meaning in the most inhuman and degrading circumstances imaginable while imprisoned in the death camps of Nazi Germany. Although he had no liberty,

'as a self aware being who could look as an observer at his very involvement'

he was still able to exert his freedom of internal power to choose his options.

'He could decide within himself how all of this was going to affect him.'

He understood one of life's basic principles, that between stimulus and response lies freedom of choice, regardless of instincts, training, and circumstance. He worked at choosing and developing his own coping skills. By working on what he was learning from the circumstances and focusing on the heroism and courage he saw around him, Frankl literally worked out what he would pass on to others and mentally prepared lectures for his future students based on what he was learning there at that time. Through the process he formed his own lifeline that sustained him.

Kwezi, a seventeen year old boy with athetoid cerebral palsy arrived at the same understanding of this crucial existential question through his own experience in Cape Town and presented his thoughts in a short paragraph entitled, 'What Its Like To Be Disabled'. Kwezi types with his right big toe.

When I was about four years old. I thought I was the only disabled child in Gugulethu, because I always only saw people that were able to walk and do things without any help. I started schooling at Thembalethu pre-school and only then did I see I was not the only one. I liked school so much and school helped me a lot. I used to watch my cousins and some children who were the same age as me play. They ran and chased girls, and played soccer, rugby and other games. I wished I could be like them. I got tired of sitting on the wheelchair. I wanted to be able to run like them, to do things for myself. I found this so unfair. I kept on asking myself why me, why me? There was no answer. The only person who knows the answer is God. I forgot about the world around me and found my own, the TV. The telebox became my world. It helped me with languages – Xhosa, English and Afrikaans. It answered questions clearly, like 'Where do babies come from'. At the age of seven years old, I knew all about babies and about maturity. It taught me that it doesn't matter if you can't be like the other people, you still can use your brain and you can do something wonderful by yourself. Don't let anyone tell you what you can't or can do. Don't let them make fun of you, because you ain't no punk. That is a rule you must always remember.

Kwezi takes responsibility for his health and well being by exercising his ability to choose his response. Covey (1992) suggests that the freedom to choose one's own response is based on the human endowments of self-awareness, imagination, conscience, and independent will.

The self in relation to the world

Cultural, psychosocial, and political influences shape the context for life cycle growth. As we grow, we come into contact with an ever widening social spectrum from which we derive our support networks, pleasure, variety in experience, and an increase in potential for mishap. We need to achieve independence en route to interdependence in adolescence. We need to learn to be able to stand on our own two feet figuratively, and derive enjoyment from challenge in order to learn from experience, derive meaning, arrive at understanding, take ownership of our own feelings, and take responsibility for ourselves in relation to the world.

'To become fulfilled members of their society, adolescents must understand when childhood ends, adulthood begins and what their culture expects of them'

(Cohen, 1991:45). Many traditional cultures mark and celebrate this transition to adult status with an initiation ceremony

'characterised by some form of ritual death and rebirth'

(Santrock, 1992:440) which serves to facilitate the passage.

'Separation from the normal life of society, the liminal state of betwixt and between and, finally, reincorporation into society with a new status'

form the

'classic tripartite structure of all rites of passage' (Cohen, 1991:70).

Aspects of initiation, such as what is considered proof of adulthood and how to adapt to changing lifestyles in practice, may change, though transfer of cultural values and behavioral expectations of young adults remain the same.

Ironically through the adolescent years young people remain dependent on parents and other significant adults, but in different ways. The process of evolution to adulthood requires that our parents be mature enough to let go consciously and free us as adolescents to experiment and explore and make our own mistakes, learn from them and develop constructive coping skills as we reach out to take our places in this world. We achieve this most successfully in our teens if our parents have been working on 'letting go' appropriately from the time when we were born. A loving, non-judgmental attitude on the adult's part offers psychological safety. The adult also needs to offer support and facilitate decision making in daily living, and in risk-taking behaviors. Our progress therefore requires continual change on the part of our parents. Shifting responses from holding and caring, to guiding and directing, followed by give and take, allows parents to step back and take on the role of consulting and advising as requested when their children become adults. Success in dealing with these developmental tasks leads the young person from the adolescent cocoon into adulthood as an adult capable of loving and of being loved.

The dialectic task of adolescence incorporates striving to be oneself and to share oneself, thus being able to accept and enjoy one's own individuality as one takes responsibility for oneself and for one's part in this world. Covey (1989) describes this constant dialectic between reaching in to deal with personal concerns and reaching out to have an influence on the world. Mastery of developmental tasks described by Erikson does not result in exclusion of one element and inclusion of the other. Both elements can and must be present when reflecting on the meaning of experience. What we have worked

through remains an integral part of ourselves, but may need to be reworked again in a later developmental stage.

Ramsden, in a summary of Erikson's epigenetic stages of development (Ramsden in Davis, 1994:20), gives prominence to an appropriate pace as an element of reciprocity in the process of transfer of responsibility and privilege. Time perspective versus time diffusion becomes the dilemma. Erikson describes the diffusion of time perspective as a

'disturbance in the experience of time'

or

'a decided disbelief in the possibility that time may bring change, and yet also of a violent fear that it might. This contradiction is often expressed in a general slowing up'

which makes the person behave

'as if he were moving in molasses' (Erikson, 1968:169).

Successful resolution of issues in the second decade with a sense of time perspective, enables us to experience a sense of achievement as we work through experimentation with different behaviors and roles, and learn to express initiative. By contrast, resolving the conflict between

'identity versus identity diffusion'

by choosing

'behavior and roles in conflict with parents or the community'

may result from the perception that a

'negative identity is preferable'

to experiencing ourselves

'as being nobody at all' (Ramsden in Davis, 1994:21).

Adolescents Talk About Their Experiences as Patients

The people whose voices you will hear in this section form a group of mainly middle class South Africans. They are not representative of the majority of South Africans who do not have access to individual therapy. However, the key issues of adversity and the experience of dealing with issues arising in our teenage years affect all of these people, as they do in any social class and culture.

Participants were invited to express their feelings about growth following mishap, using their own words and art forms. Some preferred to be interviewed rather than to write, some combined writing with interviews, while others presented art work or poetry. They were asked to contrast what was most beneficial and most detrimental in their experience of physiotherapy in particular and the medical world in general. They were invited to identify and discuss issues they would like health professional students to be aware of from the beginning of their careers. Responses are organized around key headings reflecting common issues to give structure and direction to the wonderful variety of material received:

1. *Respect and reciprocity.*
2. *Compliance* where there is an absence of respect and reciprocity.
3. Clients' perceptions of their own resources.
   - *A sense of humor.*
   - *Self–motivation, self–determination and assertive behavior.*
   - *Integration of therapy with daily living.*

Respect and reciprocity

The theme which runs through the responses, and enables all to speak with one voice is that all people are people first and foremost and share a basic need in relationship to one another. People need to be treated with respect and be in a position to reciprocate. In this section we hear from Theresa, Shelly, Sian, Peter, and Annalu.

Theresa, a married woman in her twenties with two young children who works in a property agency, feels relationships are all important. Theresa has cerebral palsy and had physiotherapy in special schools throughout her teenage years.

I think it's important that you have a good relationship with the person you are working with. You would not really be able to relax with someone whom you cannot get along with and at therapy you have to be able to relax to achieve what you are there for. After greeting, when I arrive, Annelore asks me what should we do, what do I feel I need to work on. We take it from there and as she works with me she asks if it is comfortable. We try to get the muscles relaxed to get movement. We work until we have achieved the goals for that session.

This theme of developing a good working relationship was repeated consistently by other respondents.

Shelly, a thirteen year old girl with cerebral palsy, is one of the first severely disabled children in this country attending a mainstream school. She was taught at home for a number of years after being deemed uneducable by 'medical experts' in the special school system. Shelly sits in a wheelchair and uses a computer to communicate, with her facilitator, Jan, supporting her arm. She had just started to communicate with her therapist between sessions via fax and was delighted both to be asked her opinion, and to link up with *Sian* in discussion. She was asked questions during her therapy session or via fax and she in turn would type her answers with Jan's help and these would be faxed back.

I'm Shelly McDonald. I'm very disabled. I can't talk or walk. I think physio is very good for disabled people because they are not able to exercise their bodies themselves. I come to physio to help me stay mobile. When I sit all day I get stiff and it is so painful. Physio feels sore when I go. When something is painful I shout and Caroline stops the therapy. She asks me what's sore and where it's sore and she doesn't do it again. Caroline always talks to me – she won't do anything until she has explained it all to me. The ball feels better to me than the floor because it is softer but yesterday it was so good to use the blocks and the ball together. I could feel all my spine stretching. I'm very happy working with Caroline. She makes me work hard but it is so good to be stretched out. I wish she did more. I feel comfortable working with Caroline because she thinks about what helps *me* Shelly no one else.

Sian, now 22, has just returned from an exciting two week tour of Europe with her friend, Claire, in the company of over 50 young adults. Stories, photographs, and farewell messages all emphasize Sian's contribution to the fun and humor they shared as a group. Sian was hit by a truck as she pushed her bicycle across an intersection at a designated crossing on her way home from school when she was 14. She sustained head injuries which resulted in the development of massive tension throughout her body (especially on the right). She lost her ability to speak, as well as her freedom of movement and ability to sustain an antigravity posture. Initially she wasn't expected to live and was told emphatically that she would never walk again. She did not

return to school and was wheelchair bound for many years.

It's important to form a good rapport with your therapist. It makes it so much easier when a patient is able to indicate they are in pain, or have discomfort in a particular place or position. It is a relief when a professional of some sort actually listens to you! I've been to many so called professionals to do with different parts of my broken body. Some talked down to me and some would talk right over me as if I wasn't there, or as if I was just a thing with no scruples. My physiotherapist is completely different. She really gets involved in your recovery process and just about throws a party when a muscle releases and I do something spontaneous. Before we start our session she always asks *me* what I think should be worked on. She is not like other therapists that work to time. Once she gets hold of you and she's on a roll you're there for the day, unless you open your 'trap' and tell her 'Time out!' The physiotherapists I had before would not really listen to me when I indicated to them that I was in pain. So I had to do my best to grin and bear it but in her case she encourages me to let her know about any pain or discomfort, or if I do not like a certain position.

Peter, highly motivated and determined, struggled scholastically all through primary school. He enjoyed a telephone interview and described his gains from therapy and how this affected his school work and all other aspects of his life, and elaborated on how his self-concept changed.

My name is Peter Statham and I am nearly 16. I came to physio to help me with my schoolwork two and a half years ago. My main problem was that I couldn't read at my age level when I started high school. Physio helped a great deal with my reading and my writing and with my spelling too.

Peter feels it was important for him to learn to be able to say

'I'm here to be treated like a human being like you'. In therapy I had the experience of being treated by adults as a fellow human being, whereas at school I always felt I was like a little person who could get walked all over. In therapy I learnt to be able to accept help. We made plans together, and I could take over as my confidence grew. I now use these skills every day. What I'd like to tell others who are struggling is 'Don't ever let anyone say you're stupid or can't do something because, with the right help, improvement is always possible'.

Annalu, an adult with athetoid cerebral palsy and a doctorate in computer science, has specialized in alternative and augmentative communication for non-speaking people. She lectures around the world, skis, and has a particular interest in learning through play.

When I look back on my school physio, I remember doing the same exercises day after day, week after week, and spending the whole session worrying about finishing the cycle of exercises so I could get dressed in time for the next period. The worst was having physio in the last period – I worried about missing the bus if I didn't finish in time to get dressed. Absurd things worry children. When I left school, my mother insisted I continue with physio. I met Joan and then Pam, people who interacted with me while we 'played' with my body. It was so exciting to discuss and analyze how my muscles were working and what we wanted to change. I began to view 'exciting' physiotherapists as fine tuning people mechanics who listened to what my needs were. Sessions are never exactly the same. Excitement comes from identifying a situation that can change and seeing, feeling and celebrating change together by the end of a session.

There are many funny examples of having physio with Pam. A classic was when she arrived at the flat I was looking after. I opened the door and collapsed in laughter as I greeted her. We spent the session working on my laughing without collapsing into a ball. What a change when I said goodbye – I was laughing but standing up straight! I also remember being nonplussed the day Pam put a ball of string in my one hand and the tail of the string in the other, and proceeded to work on ways I could relax while standing and talking. It slowly dawned on me that Pam had attended a lecture of mine and had seen potential for change. The ball of string represented the mike I had been holding during the lecture. As I write this, I can remember the sense of achievement, fulfilment and wonder as I felt my body reacting in a different, strange, and yet positive way.

But the best has still been playing ball! It took me into my twenties before a physio helped me to kick, bounce, throw and catch balls of all sizes and colors...

Unfortunately, many physiotherapists do not see the need for post-school physio. I once sought a physio in the city I had recently moved to, but was told that I should know the exercises I needed and be able to do them by myself. That was the point when Pam and I decided to make videos of our sessions when I was on holiday in Cape Town. I took these back to Scotland with me and we used them for distance training, first of a medical student friend of mine and later a physio who was keen to learn to help adults gain not only range but also increase balance, control and their repertoire of possibilities in daily function. This problem solving approach makes me a partner in a fun process.

In summary, all the participants feel mutual respect is essential to build trust in a working partnership. Respect is conveyed through one's attitude which is translated into touch and speech, but most importantly, in the way in which one person listens to another, and indicates that they have understood by the way they act. Follow through with action that can help the patient achieve short and long-term goals is essential so that the person can carry gains through into everyday life easily and automatically.

Compliance

The pervading theme regarding what was detrimental within the relationship was absence of reciprocity. People were expected to comply with whatever medical professionals deemed appropriate treatment and behavior, and were discouraged from voicing their feelings. The responses of Annalu, Theresa, and Jenny follow in order, with a focus on Theresa's dual mishap experience.

Annalu contrasts her experiences with medical professionals.

My first memories of physio are of discomfort, even pain, and embarrassment. I used to have to bear my hamstrings being stretched while standing astride a roller because 'it was good for me'! My mother knew when I was in pain as I collapsed in giggles (an effective cop out as I realized that therapists and my mother coped better with giggles than with screams). Physio was never fun, except on Fridays when the whole class played games. However, most of my classmates had good upper arms and better legs than mine, so ball games were frustrating. Looking back, the physio could have done more by helping me play the game.

I remember as a young child being made to walk up and down in front of a circle of strangers, mainly male orthopedic surgeons, other medical staff and therapists. My parents were not always present. As I grew older, these sessions became more embarrassing. I remember later being told to walk up and down in a huge gymnasium dressed only in my bra and panties while the surgeons constantly discussed 'cutting this and lengthening that' with no consideration for my growing fear and panic.

Shortly after this, I was flown to Cape Town. There we saw Mr. Goldschmidt, a wonderful white-haired

gentleman. I immediately took to him. He treated me with dignity and took time to talk, explain, and above all, get to know me. It transpired that my right hip was in danger of dislocation and I had an adductor release four days later. Mr. Goldschmidt was amazing! He even took time to play noughts and crosses with me. Years later he reminded me of all of the times I had beaten him. He remembered playing with a twelve year old all those years before – he saw me as a person.

Theresa describes the denigrating effect of the labeling process used by medical professionals which serves to reinforce inequalities in the patient–professional relationship.

Looking at a baby photo of myself, I look extremely 'normal'. How I hate that word normal. In actual fact not one of us wonderful human beings are normal. We don't even know if God is normal, so what right do these 'normal' people have naming themselves with superiority? In the photo there I am sitting whether someone is holding me I don't know but it looks pretty good to me, as good as my own 'normal' children's photos. I don't think that I look very normal now. My right hand looks disabled and so do my legs.

Theresa's experience of the medical world during her teens was traumatic – having to submit to authority, and even to accept pain and major disfigurement. I remember a conversation held in the passage outside an orthopedic clinic. Theresa, who had undergone the rhizotomy procedure, was discussing with a friend what the surgery meant. They felt hurt by the fact that the doctors claimed that surgery was their own choice, but implied at the same time that they would be stupid not to accept it. These wise teenagers knew that something else would again be offered the following year as the next new and best option.

I have had quite a few operations and personally I don't remember having a choice of whether to have them or not. Besides the rhizotomy having reduced the spasticity in my muscles, I now have a great big scar going down my back, numbness in my legs and feet and sharp pains which make my legs jump.

Theresa employs the sarcastic ridicule of 'gallows humor' (Robinson, 1991) to relieve the distress she still feels regarding this surgery.

I know I wanted this op. because boy, oh boy, there was a miraculous chance of recovery – 50/50 chance of coming out paralyzed or just dying. Well which one would you opt for if you were a 14 year old young girl? None of the damn irritating side effects were told to us. We certainly weren't prepared for the pain. Not that I think they knew about it themselves. Guinea pigs is what we liked to call ourselves. I feel, especially with kids, the person does not exist, only the body. They feel they have to sort out the problem with the body, but they forget about the mind, and the person inside, which I think is more important. They should have more respect for kids and give them a real choice.

The rhizotomy, the numbness, we were paralyzed from our waists down and those nurses would just fling you around, as if they just could not care. We had no clothes on, and there were many students around. We were young girls, teenagers at the time. And the doctors would just come and rip your bedclothes off you and start explaining to the students what was happening, telling them to look at this and that and not even bothering about the person lying in the bed and how we felt. That is just one of those things. If you are disabled you just shut up and let everyone walk all over you.

I remember going for physio – I'm sure their motto was 'No pain, no gain'. Well if only these people were taught that if you just guide the muscle and do some massaging what they could do. A friend of mine at school would have done anything not to go for physio – he no longer thinks he needs therapy. As for myself, I just look forward to my monthly massage, workout and problem-solving session.

Being treated as a non-person by the medical world, special schooling system and maybe the parents as well affected Theresa profoundly. As a teenager she internalized this dehumanizing attitude to such a degree that

I was under the impression I wouldn't be able to have children because I am disabled. I thought that until the day I found I was pregnant. Tyrone was born when I was 16 years old. People should be taught more about being adult and about having children – that was never explained to us. They should be told that they are just as human as everyone else and that those things can happen.

She felt that the protective attitude of those in authority was one of the biggest blocks to the disabled children's personal growth.

They shut you out from everybody else because they are scared something is going to happen to you. They try and prevent it, but in the same instance, instead of informing you what to expect, they don't, and you are totally shut out from everything. Until it happens to you.

However, Theresa's turning point came when she brought her baby home.

The social worker said, 'I think you should give your child up, because he is going to be like your brother, not like your son.' She never gave me the choice whether I wanted to keep the child or not. It was just 'You should give it up because you are not going to be capable of looking after this child.'

This, as Trevor says was *the kick start* they needed, which, combined with the couple's determination to work things out together, served as the starting point for building the firm foundation of a solid family unit.

All those who have described their experiences thus far have been able to contrast positive with negative ones. For some people, experience with the medical world is only negative. Jenny, now 26, contracted myalgic encephalomyelitis (ME) in her mid teens.

At that stage ME was not well-known and certainly not well accepted by medical professionals, who were quick to label an illness they did not understand as psychosomatic. It is difficult enough coping with an ongoing illness and all it entails without having to continually fight to have people even accept that one is ill … We wanted them to listen to what we were saying and recognize that since they had no experience with this illness, they needed to investigate the things we were telling them were problems, accept that what we were saying could be accurate despite their own theories and work with us to find the answers.

Going to a doctor or physio appointment takes an enormous amount of effort and when I get there I am faced with criticism, disbelief and being told time after time that I am wrong. I have lived with this illness all this time and have had to accept, however reluctantly, the changes it has made in my life. I have remained positive and hopeful in spite of it and learnt a lot about myself and others. In the beginning I was in my teens, facing experienced professionals and having to say that I was right. I know it is impossible for anyone who has not suffered this illness to understand what it is like but I wish health professionals would come to realise that too, and learn from and work with their patients.

In summary, they felt that they were not being treated as people and that their feelings, especially those related to pain, were discredited and ignored or judged inappropriate. Any judgmental attitude of the medical professionals was experienced as dehumanizing and aroused frustration, resentment, embarrassment and hurt which often aggravated their physical problems. However the participants ability to analyze the situation and put it into words, provides us all with great learning opportunities!

Clients' perceptions of their own resources

A sense of humor   Sian informs us about her use of humor as a major coping mechanism when dealing with adversity.

In the beginning I was extremely angry, at life basically. I used to take most of my anger out on my parents which I am really ashamed and embarrassed about. Especially since I know now that they are doing everything they can to speed up my recovery. I am very grateful to them for not just tossing me aside and forgetting that there is a person in this rigid lump of a body. I was a real '—up' (sic) physically. My parents were told to find an institution as I would be a total VEGETABLE.

She picks up on the humor of stereotypes, having previously been the butt of redhead jokes but now uses it to her advantage.

Being a redhead really helped because everyone expects you to be stroppy and to fight for things. Little did they know just how determined this little (at the time) redhead or her parents would be! My present physiotherapist encourages me to be my own person. There is no pussy-footing around at her practice. Thankfully I had not lost my sense of humor, and I think my wit has improved somewhat – I always manage to make my therapists laugh … Physical torture does help! At least you get to sleep like a baby, however old you are!

Sian elected to convey her thoughts via the computer which allowed her to proceed at her own speed, and her thoughts to flow most easily. Much to her therapist's delight she also produced a full hand written page entitled *'You, your therapist and pain'*. She feels her strength lies in her family, her sense of humor, her determination and their ability to find the right people with whom to work. Her sense of humor is also evident in understatement. Her response to the question 'How do you feel about having had a major car accident when you were fourteen?' was *It set me back a bit in terms of my growth and development.* When asked what she had lost, she succinctly replied that *everything came to a full stop.* By contrast to her previous lifestyle, when as a gregarious and outgoing teenager she was *quite active in spite of being a bit plump* and played tennis and enjoyed modern dancing, she was *suddenly stuck in one place, not able to do anything,* for herself. Movement returned gradually *but only with much effort.*

Sian uses humor consciously to reduce tension because she has learnt that 'Less pain, less strain, more gain' keeps dynamic stabilization at its optimum level, and frees her for more efficient function in all activities. She concluded her piece written on the computer with a list of a dozen abilities, finishing off with '*I am also able to play the fool*' in a position of importance at the end of this list.

She also uses humor, including irony, to deal with issues of loss of her previous lifestyle including loss of body image, loss of sense of self, loss of freedom and particularly, loss of friends.

I was angry at my friends for leaving me at a time in my life that I needed them most. My development as a teenager was reduced to an infant's status and I had to start my growing period all over again, but I had to grow up rather quickly. As a child I was not known for having patience and I had to learn to have patience while growing up again! Especially regarding losing all my friends who were young and not patient!

Sian lost confidence in meeting people and talking to strangers because of her speech difficulties. She can produce each sound, but coordination of breathing, voicing and articulation in an upright posture takes time and effort, is slow and can't be maintained long. She recognizes that loss of speed in speech impedes the flow of meaningful content, so she asked her aunt to read the moving speech she wrote on the occasion of her twenty-first birthday. However, she has now learned to compress a wealth of meaning into a few words and has refined her sense of humor, which she uses proactively to reduce tension for herself and others. She thus enables others to be comfortable with her and invites them to seek out her company, a most constructive coping skill for someone who had lost all of her friends after her accident. Occasionally unintentional humor creeps in! To our collective amusement Theresa did use the word abnormal once! She said, when discussing her relationship with Trevor.

We have been through a lot of difficult patches and some of them have been more difficult than others. One thing I must say about the two of us is we have a very close relationship, which sometimes seems a bit *abnormal* (sic) compared to other people. We can discuss anything and everything. Whereas when I speak to friends of ours they won't speak to each other about certain things but we don't have a problem with that.

Theresa laughed as she said that there is

Definitely room for laughter, room for lots of fun as well. I think physio should be serious to a point that you get out of it what you need to cope with, but at the same time *you need a bit of humor, because that is what life is about.* Imagine if we did not have humor to restore our balance.

As they said, they can both laugh together because they can both laugh at themselves, an important element in the closeness of their relationship.

Trevor emphasized the reciprocity in their relationship:

'It's very much give and take, it can't be one sided.'

He said that sharing and responsibility

were not just the kids, it's the household, everything that you basically go through you have got to share. She does her share just as well as any 'normal' person would do, it might be a bit slower, but it is there. She is just as good as the next person.

Theresa recognizes that for Trevor '*it has not been easy married to me with my disability. There are times when things get tough, when he gets a bit frustrated.*' They haven't been able to take things for granted. They have had to think things through more carefully and make conscious commitments. They negotiate and agree on what they are going to put into something and aren't able to be spontaneous. In fact the outstanding feature of the interview was that although the disability issue had divided them initially, over the years they had worked through the issues in such a way that they had strengthened their relationship and now spoke with one voice on the subject, supporting each other constantly!

Self-motivation, self-determination, and assertive behavior Reality-based self-motivation and goal oriented determination were vital themes for all and formed the basis for the development of assertive behavior. Here is an example from Sian:

I had to endure an unbearable amount of pain, but it eased a bit at times. My feet were going every which way but straight and were blue most of the time too. My right arm was virtually under my chin. My speech was incomprehensible and inaudible. That made me feel inadequate. My confidence started withering away. Also, my breathing was not in control. My hands were tight fists, so tight my nails were growing into my skin. My left knee would not bend. My biggest goal was to get out of

the wheelchair. I gave myself time, saying I would walk on my 21st. I really wanted to be up for my 21st birthday, so I kicked butt, preferably mine and much to some people's astonishment I was up and walking well before my 21st. I celebrated my 21st itself by walking down the passage from my room to the bathroom alone without any aid or assistance whatsoever! All of these successes result from a combination of going to my physiotherapist, my determination and my family support.

Sian's mother Pat added to this in her interview.

After hearing the initial diagnosis (she'll be a total vegetable, put her in an institution, forget about her) I just had to be there. People told us to surround her with what was familiar – people, smells, perfumes I wear, voices, sounds, music, read her things she most enjoyed. It was just keeping us connected, probably on a subconscious level. It was a case of getting stuck into this situation and dealing with it and getting it out of the way as quickly as possible. I did not know that this would take as long as it did. Anyhow eight years is not too bad. Her dad and I were both prepared to put in whatever it took. It was just one of those things and it's paid off.

Carson, a 15 year old who applies himself assiduously to realizing his goals, demonstrates that determination is the driving force behind success. Through application and practice he increases his competence. Nemaline rod myopathy resulted in his muscles having exceptionally low tone. Eventually that became his spur to more and more skill development.

Many different things helped me with my physiotherapy. But to me the thing that helped me most was Exercise. Since I have low muscle tone it was important to get exercise regularly. I have always worked hard to be able to do things for myself, so that I would feel more certain about myself. Once I learned to play certain sports such as roller blading and skate boarding I was more confident about myself. Finally, I was able to roller blade and skateboard just like the people you see skating on the beach front. I admit I took longer than most people to learn, but I was able to do so and that's what's important.

My parents always encouraged me to make my own decisions and treated me with respect as a growing person. I have problems when people don't give me a chance to say what I feel. People judge by appearances and then tell me to be careful in some exercise situation – but not my younger brother! They don't stop to find out how I feel and then they make decisions for me as to what I can or can't do. They treat me as a helpless little child. It really gets down on your self confidence being treated like a much younger child. I've seen it happen to other people in the same situation as me – these people are voicing their opinions, but those in authority don't listen, don't give them a chance to speak, and speak for them instead. Sometimes you think that what you're saying is just going in one ear and out the other! I guess they think they're helping but we need to remember that our self-concept can go from positive to negative. For some people it takes a lot to get back to positive.

Therapy at its best is an assertiveness training program. Carson now perseveres, and sticks to his guns when he feels its necessary to protect his sense of self. When he went to a special school for his initial interview, the doctor wanted him to run down the passage in his underpants. Carson couldn't run and was very conscious of the fact that he didn't have much muscle, but he had learned to state his needs in therapy previously. He refused to walk down the passage unless he was allowed to keep his T-shirt on, and he explained that he would be walking, not running. He won his point!

Integration of therapy with daily living Jacques, an Afrikaans speaking young man in his early twenties, is at university doing his masters degree in English. He is blind and was referred for physiotherapy in his final year at school. His body was very tense, he lacked confidence to explore the space around himself, and literally waited to be led everywhere – even to the bathroom in his sister's flat. He was already an accomplished writer and poet and had won the National English Olympiad competition that year. His postural control and ability to move changed to such a degree in six sessions that several people who saw the televized prize-giving ceremony said he looked more confident going onto the stage, than the person leading him up the steps!

The first thing that struck me when I met my physiotherapist was the ease with which our sessions got under way, but I only realised later on why this was so important. The moment I walked into her office she started analyzing my posture, and before I knew it, we had joyously launched into one of our therapy sessions. I suddenly realised how thin the boundary between therapy and non-therapy had always been. My point is simply this: she was able to make me feel that what I was learning from the sessions was somehow intimately connected with the rest of my life and interests, as I watched her use whatever I happened to be doing at the time in order to teach me something. Not for a single moment did I feel that I had to enter an alternative, therapeutic universe in order to understand what she was saying.

Maybe this idea of life being integrated was the most valuable thing I learned during my time with her. Once, when I was fifteen, I overheard someone saying that I sometimes acted like a five-year-old, sometimes like a twenty-five-year-old, but never my age. I was disconcerted and hurt, but understood what he meant. At that time my life seemed hopelessly fragmented, and I hoped to hide my confusion by concentrating on aspects of my life with which I felt confident, trusting other people to look after the rest. She suggested links between these parts, so body posture became important while having a philosophical conversation, and stretching the muscles in my fingers a metaphor for redefining my personal space in the broadest sense.

On a practical level, I had to learn how to move my body in new and adventurous ways, to express myself with it. Blind people are naturally less confident expressing themselves through body language. My strategy for coping with this was to compensate by concentrating on my verbal abilities. Through her suggestion of links between seemingly unrelated things, she taught me how to use new strategies to achieve new goals. I still often need to be reminded by friends to loosen up. I remember one of my first experiments in loosening up outside of sessions. Standing in a crowded bus, clinging to a railing for all I was worth in order not to be pushed over by the crowd, I realised I simply had to lean forward and shift my weight to be comfortable. It felt like a major discovery, and it was. I had begun to see my body as a tool with which I could extend my personal space, rather than an inconvenient package other people had to lug around.

This theme of connection between what one learns in the therapy sessions with one's life and interests (for the purpose of freeing oneself up on a day-to-day basis) was echoed by others. Like Jacques, and Carson, all indicate a growth in self-confidence as they apply the principles of what they have learnt in their own environments, and learn to deal more successfully with daily personal challenges.

Theresa describes how her therapy is linked to her everyday life and how she practices conscious carryover of what she has learnt to reinforce the gains in her daily life.

When I have been to physio I have to think a lot between that session and the next about what I can accomplish with what I got out of that day. When my shoulders get stiff, it is difficult to answer the phone and take messages fast enough at the same time. I need freedom in my shoulders to do a lot of typing and to work fast.

Peter explains how physiotherapy helped his schoolwork. Determination alone is not enough because effort produces tension which blocks success. In physiotherapy he gained the ability to free up on physical and psychological levels simultaneously by building confidence through experience of success. He was able to carry his gains over into everyday life, consciously at first and later on an automatic level.

In my first session I improved my writing speed by 30% and started to read more easily. I left feeling pleased with myself. My hands were able to relax so I wasn't holding my pen so tightly. I could write faster and stay neat. Before, the harder I tried to write fast or neatly, the more tense I became and the more I cramped up. So much so that I used to get spasms in my hands and couldn't write, especially if I was trying to get a lot of notes down fast.

Peter had difficulty reading for comprehension because he was trying so hard to read for accuracy.

My reading improved because my whole body was lifted up out of my hips. I had a lot more freedom instead of being so cramped up over my work. My chest was opened up. When I had to read out aloud in class, I was able to read out and up to the teacher. Previously I was so tense and hunched up that I was reading into my book. In this way I was able to project what I was reading and I wasn't worried any more about what others would think about me. Previously they couldn't hear me and so my friends would have to listen very intently and would then find all my mistakes.

My comfort has improved when I sit and work. I used to get pain at the top of my spine. Now my muscles are relaxed, I don't get tired, I don't feel pain and I finish my work quickly. My hands feel more comfortable because they are freer and I write a lot easier and faster because I don't have to stop to relax my hands and warm them up. I'm pleased physiotherapy helped me grow a lot too. As I relaxed, I could feel my whole body lengthening out. Improvement in my spelling was a bonus. Physio relaxed me so I wasn't so intent on having to get it right. Without the struggle it came right naturally.

I have more time to finish my examinations so I now have time to check my work and go back and find my mistakes. My Science mark is now close to 80% and my Maths mark (the first to improve) was 90% at the end of last year, having been around 60% when I came to physio. This year it also helped having a change in the Maths teacher who is good at taking time to explain the work.

Peter has done well in public speaking. Once his self-confidence started to improve, he took part in a Toastmaster's course at school.

My self confidence grew because the more effort I put in, the better I did. Before I came to physio the harder I tried, the more tense I became, and I became frustrated and 'aggro' because even when I tried my best at something new, it wasn't good enough. My friends were getting higher marks, but now I'm up there with them too. Although I was nearly ready to give up, my own determination and my mother and father and all those who were helping me, kept me going.

Scouts has always been very important to me. I've always felt valued as a person and my effort has been recognized. Physio taught me to say what I feel and also improved my physical ability. My running speed has improved incredibly too. I was always very slow (no push off in tense muscles). Last year I started cross country running. I improved quickly and now I am the fastest cross country runner in the school, captain of the team and I still have three years to go before I finish school.

In summary, these accounts of emerging from adversity are exciting. With one exception, all reflect on harnessing innate resources and strengthening of people and relationships in this often painful process. As they used mishaps as growth opportunities, families, friends and health practitioners helped them deal more effectively with the challenges of daily living. They felt empowered to take responsibility for their own attitudes, health and well-being. Their positive coping skills were used to build confidence through experience of success. After the interviews, we realized that organizing and exploring their ideas in this way with others has been the logical next step in helping them work towards realizing their goals.

Principles of practice

The people whose words are used in this discussion are privileged to have received therapy adapted to their needs. Therapy at all in South Africa is a privilege. Study of and reflection on the richness of their experience, enables us to explore psychosocial issues together, and to abstract key principles regarding health and well-being in the family. We can also examine empowerment of people in the context of their own environments, and apply what we learn to our own practice, regardless of where and how we work.

In South Africa, a land of contrast and great diversity, therapists, like the adolescents, are experiencing the need to deal with massive change quickly and on many levels. The alternative is not whether to engage in the process or not, but how best to plan to deal with the current and future challenges. There are now over 40 million people in the country with fewer than 4000 practicing physiotherapists, whereas in highly developed countries in Europe like Holland, the ratio is 1: 1000. In South Africa, therefore, we need to develop creative problem solving and planning skills to find ways of meeting the basic needs of the largest possible number of people. Creating opportunities to demystify our expertise and place practical skills in the hands of the people working with the children and adolescents of this country, especially those with special education needs, becomes a supremely important challenge and the basis for introducing and developing problem-solving consultancy models.

Are we doing therapy or working together as agents of change?

We have established that successful therapy starts with an invitation to work together in a partnership based on mutual respect and trust. Our goals as therapists are:

- to enable people to deal ever more successfully with their challenges of daily living,
- to empower them to take control of their own lives and responsibility for their health and well-being,
- to help them achieve a position in life to express their ideas at the level of their potential.

What principles can we apply to help us relate successfully to the adolescent? What are the aspects of the therapeutic relationship that are mutually beneficial as we create a framework of interdependence? How can this relationship benefit us as well as our patients in terms of growth, development, and maturation? People

entrust themselves to us as patient teachers. Their mishaps become opportunities for growth for therapists too as we follow the patients' lead in working for change to develop strength from adversity. How can we learn to follow, in order to learn to lead more successfully?

Establish the starting point for success from the outset

Young adults in their late teens and early twenties form the main body of the therapy student population. Physiotherapy students need to learn to enjoy putting fun into function. One way to accomplish this goal is to learn with the patients to find new ways of using mishaps as growth opportunities. Willingness to engage actively in the process of learning leads to change which leads to excitement and fun.

Barry, who was having therapy after a subdural haemorrhage and several weeks in a coma, was invited to help teach a group of physiotherapy students about the importance of fun in learning, even for an adult. Barry happened to be an educational psychologist who was keen to get back to work. A basic principle in building confidence through experience of success, is that of offering the person a choice between two elements. This gives the opportunity to practice being right by paying attention, listening, selecting an appropriate answer, putting it into words and following it through into action with help. The choice between engaging in group discussion and delivering a lecture was designed to enable him to take a first step back into teaching and begin to rebuild confidence in his own decision-making ability. Barry was brave enough to choose to answer questions, although this choice was influenced (as most are) by the fact that the alternative was worse. He knew he was not yet in a position to be able to prepare and present a lecture, but was nevertheless keen to undertake the challenge of helping others learn.

The first question invited mishap by giving Barry the opportunity to demonstrate his inadequacies. The second question enabled him to move immediately to a position of strength, to engage in discussion and establish a flow and a rapport with the group. How do we encourage the latter type of response?

The first question from a student therapist was 'Can you tell us about your accident and what happened afterwards?'. His answer appeared brief, disconnected and incomplete and he seemed to be struggling with ordering and sequencing. Barry couldn't respond in the informed, accurate way that he as a psychologist would expect to answer that question. He was being asked for facts about a period of his life that was full of gaps. Information was stored in fragmented form, out of sequence and not readily accessible. As a teacher-psychologist, he couldn't readily admit to his lack of information either, even to himself. He felt most inadequate, and the situation created a feeling of discomfort for all.

The second question from the student group was: 'What do you feel is the main problem in your life?'. This gave Barry the opportunity to demonstrate his articulate command of language and answer logically and coherently as he expressed his frustration and distress about trying to come to terms with this huge gap in his life. *Imagine going back to the hospital and being greeted by the staff, fellow professionals, as a long lost friend and having no idea who any of them were!* His focus on feeling enabled him to let the words flow so the entire group sat up and

took notice, literally and figuratively.

Later Barry's wife Cathy joined us and was able to fill in specific details. Barry indicated that asking her first would have reinforced his feelings of being out of control of his own life. On reflection, we understood that a basic component of empowerment was to enable people to act from a position of strength, knowing that what they say will be heard and acted on as this is an integral part of the process. We observed that opportunities for growth and mishap occur each time we interact with one another.

The first question we ask the patient is especially significant, as it carries messages about our attitudes, both in general regarding life and people, and in particular regarding this person at this time in therapy. The presentation of this question indicates where our starting point will be, and has profound implications regarding the therapeutic relationship. We choose whether to recognize the patient as a person, focusing on their feelings and strengths first and foremost, or to operate in a medical mode concerned primarily with 'what happened?' and 'what's wrong?'. Do we choose to engage by offering the patient the opportunity to present themselves in the best possible light or ask the patient to struggle with a question or task that demonstrates his or her inadequacies?

When we regard the patient as a person, it's vital that the person themselves has the opportunity to take the initial step in making contact with each new therapist (or someone else in the family only if they themselves are not in a position to do so.) The first question becomes 'What are your strengths – what do you enjoy?'. This is followed by 'Where do you struggle – what are your difficulties?' so a basis has been formed for the next question: 'What are your needs?'. Having identified needs together, we formulate an answer to 'What's the way forward?' and create a mutually acceptable plan of action.

Practice makes perfect – or does it?

The old adage 'practice makes perfect' is based on two assumptions, namely that each time an action is repeated it will improve, and that perfection is a desirable goal. Further implications are that the more repetitions and the more effort one puts into the process, the better. We can challenge the notion that practice makes perfect by examining these underlying assumptions, and see what happens with practice in the neurological system. Do we become proficient with practice, or merely proficient at what we practice? Can we become perfect – and would we want to? What are the implications for therapy?

Repetition merely reinforces what's already happening
Plastic adaptation is

'the ability of cells to alter any aspect of their phenotype, at any stage in their development, in response to ... changes in their state or environment' (Brown and Hardman, 1987).

At the synaptic junction, a threshold has to be reached before the message can initially cross the synapse. With each successive passage, less neurotransmitter is required, and both the number and complexity of arrangement of the 'knobs' on the dendrites increases. 'Formfunction' is thus affected in 'timespace' (Kidd *et al.*, 1991). So 'practice makes perfect' is a fallacy because it's actually only the message which passes more easily, merely reinforcing established patterns. More repetitions then lead to more reinforcement – unless natural variation and elaboration takes place or change is consciously and purposefully introduced into the system.

One's self-esteem may well remain low when the focus in treatment is on doing more and trying harder. Feeling a failure can be reinforced by not quite satisfying our own standards of perfection and the expectations of others, however hard we try. We need to switch to a model of behavior in which we can congratulate ourselves each step of the way for specific improvements and for reaching each successive goal. In an 'excellence model' we feel good about ourselves as we learn from our mistakes.

'Pay attention to the tension and ease it away' or *'Try softer, not harder – or hardly at all!'* 'Freeing up' is the starting point of the process of change, regardless of whether we focus on the physical, emotional, behavioral, social, or spiritual level. Therapy has many unchallenged traditional injunctions, all demanding compliance and effort such as 'grit your teeth' and 'grin and bear it'. Trying harder calls for maximal concentration and effort and builds the tonic component in the phasic muscles, thus increasing tension and distorting alignment and body–space relationships throughout the entire neuro–myofascial–skeletal system. By contrast, optimum function on a daily basis involves a much lower level of effort for maximum efficiency in the tonic muscles, as this supports effective automatic antigravity responses and control of movement and posture. This allows the system to vary speed and degree of response, gain the ability to start, change direction and stop, and also to devel-

op stamina, endurance, and the ability to produce bursts or periods of maximal effort as appropriate. We can now begin to understand the value of 'less strain, less pain, more gain'.

Improvement requires the introduction of change – only specific change produces specific results Therapists are responsible for introducing change and directing change. We choose patterns we want to introduce and establish them through practice. When we initiate and reinforce change, we can learn to risk and learn from our mistakes, so we can 'free-up' and improve with practice. We need to help people move beyond stereotypical, repetitive actions practiced through conscious effort and reach out with responses which can vary, elaborate, and adapt, according to the needs of the situation. The goal is to release tension in all soft tissues, realize range as we re-form the body, activate muscles (particularly the slings of support of the dynamic stabilizers of the trunk and limb girdles – Vleeming, 1997), warm people up from the inside out (Dorko, 1996:43) and establish a relaxed response to movement.

As agents of change we learn that we can best help others by first changing what we ourselves are doing. We need to pay attention to the tension in ourselves (Edgelow, 1997) and cut our efforts by half, and half again, so we can ease it away by lightening up, and trying softer, not harder – or hardly at all.

Specific changes can be introduced if we ensure that we:

- *Recognize the individual's worth* by the way we meet, greet, introduce, interact and work together.
- *Focus on experiential learning to integrate gains.* Invite whole person participation in a fun environment; promote learning through exploration and discovery; develop thinking skills; encourage perception of contrast and offer assertiveness training choices to develop self-confidence.
- *Guarantee success* by following their lead and promoting, recognizing and celebrating success. When someone falls do we say 'Ooops!' or 'Well done, you caught yourself!'? And do we give them time and space to recover themselves, thus preserving integrity and supporting self-concept?
- *Introduce and establish efficient dynamic stabilization to support all functional activities* by creating arches of support and using novel sequences of movement in real function. For example, establish light active support (not propping) through the shoulder girdle to activate the shoulder girdle stabilizers, thus reversing the origins and insertions of the trunk muscles and promoting the passage of new and more efficient pathways in which trunk stabilizers support the body actively and more automatically against gravity. This allows for more spontaneous adaptive responses in function and easier more natural give and take in interaction.

In favor of excellence

Perfection can only be discarded as an inappropriate and unattainable goal when we realize that in fact perfection and humanity are mutually exclusive. Perfectionism offers a reductionistic and restrictive, but therefore predictable framework, because if

'something that is perfect is completely correct or accurate, or is done so well that it could not be any better' (Collins, 1987), then process is obliterated. Options are reduced to polarized opposites of perfect or not perfect, i.e. right or wrong. If we choose an attitude of perfection, we set ourselves up for failure by ensuring that the goal is unreachable (in spite of, and perhaps because of, our best intentions and efforts!). By definition, one only has one opportunity to make the 'right' choice, with elimination of all other influences and no room for improvement. The definition of 'the perfection of something' as 'the act or process of improving it' thus becomes a contradiction in terms. On the whole, we are all schooled and conditioned to the ideal of perfection – and then spend the rest of our lives trying to move past this block to progress!

A switch to excellence is a decision-making process which allows the possibility of improvement with each practice, as opposed to setting oneself up for failure. Decisions are made, revised, and adapted as necessary as the plan of action is explored. If we apply the principle of regeneration through rest and relaxation too, we ensure that planned rest is included from the beginning, giving opportunities to celebrate task completion, recover, and optimize the starting points in preparation for each successive phase.

Timing Timing is possibly the most crucial dimension of excellence. Since

'time perspective versus time diffusion becomes the dilemma'

in adolescence, Ramsden (in Davis, 1994) reminds us of the importance of an appropriate pace as an element of reciprocity in the process of transfer of responsibility and privilege.

'Successful resolution of issues with a sense of time perspective enables us to experience a sense of achievement.'

Sian's mother, Pat focuses on the need to follow the patient's timing.

I think Sian can still achieve a lot more than she has to date. We tried to force things such as eating, using a spoon, putting it in the mouth, closing the mouth, things that we do in seconds. She was just not ready for it when we wanted it, so we had to leave it. Then two or three weeks later she would just pick up the spoon and do it automatically in her own time. We learnt a lesson from that so when it came to walking, I was keen to encourage her but I had to wait until she was ready. Right through the whole process we had to wait until Sian was physically, mentally and emotionally ready, where she had reached the point and felt right about it. Even today, eight years after the big bang, if she decides its time to walk with a single stick we have to go with the flow, whether she falls, breaks teeth, collects a few bruises, it is her choice because she feels that the time is right. The accident changed our lives totally and drastically, from having a daughter going towards independence and then having almost a brand new baby, where almost 100% everything had to be done for her. That was time consuming, energy consuming, everything consuming – no time for anything. There was not much time for sleep or rest, friends, visitors, social life. Even meals were reduced to sandwiches at around ten o'clock at night, when we had just brought her home from hospital ... Now we all have time to develop our other interests!

A further point on the subject of excellence is that of being able to get appropriate therapy at the appropriate time if there is to be maturation in the rehabilitative process itself. This aspect of excellence is especially vital for the adolescent in linking mind and body to integrate therapy with daily living. Sian's family described how they expanded their horizons by expanding their team from the confines of the multidisciplinary unit, to a group of separate therapy practices, each of which offered an exciting range of new challenges in terms of locations, relationships, learning, and development of thinking skills. As therapists we tend to claim excellence by virtue of offering all of the services in one location such as a special school or rehabilitation unit, but we need to understand that the perceptions of patients and their parents are not only valid but all important. Sian stayed with the multidisciplinary approach until she and her family perceived it no longer adequate or challenging. They sought more change faster for their money.

Things were starting to happen, but not fast enough for us. She got bored with some of the stuff. I needed to know that change was a continuous thing and be able to continue with simple easy exercises, without causing pain or problems or putting her back, to use all the time between sessions.

Shelly's mom, Shona points out that *time frames differ* and asks us to focus on response time. She draws attention to the way in which we want to

step in to fill gaps or initiate movement because of our own discomfort with empty silences and need for closure when communicating with someone who has no speech. Our thoughts and predicted replies long to burst out and fill this 'vacuum', which draws us, as social creatures, conditioned by a speaking society, to respond, affording us reward for our communicative intent, satisfying and reaffirming our mere existence. We instinctively expect the response to bounce back with the rhythm and casual ease of our own spoken words. Eliciting a communicative response from Shelly can

take upwards of a minute (count 60 slowly). It's tempting to overlook her reply and pre-empt it, and in so doing, rob her of her initiative, self worth and independence. How can we become comfortable with these spaces in time? How can we change our own time frame and use these opportunities to observe carefully and quietly *so that we learn to* pick up subtle cues and unspoken messages which often shout out their responses in a most direct manner.

Moral and ethical behavior   Children are often principal victims of war, violence, and abuse. We have a moral and ethical obligation as therapists to recognize signs and symptoms of torture and violence, within the framework of timing and social context. The psychological effects on a teenager of being lashed in a riot crowd will be very different from the psychological effects inflicted on that same child or teenager by subjecting them to ongoing, institutionalized violence specifically for the purpose of breaking down their spirit and defenses. We need to understand that in the case of abuse, signs may be masked or hidden. We must respect the person's reluctance to discuss their situation, but be prepared to take responsibility for dealing with what we can, and to refer appropriately for counseling and support as necessary.

Health as a key to development   Poor health leads to uneconomic performance, especially in poor countries in which infectious diseases, malnutrition, and accidents are the most serious threats to the child's survival. We all need to be aware of the priorities of basic health care needs such as adequate nutritious food and clean drinking water. We need to participate actively in promotion of health and well-being on all levels, realizing that sustainable health care requires action against poverty within the framework of primary health care. What does primary health care mean for us as therapists? In order to assure accessible, affordable, appropriate health care we must use our time and other resources efficiently and effectively to reach and meet identified health needs of as large a proportion of the population as possible. In a balanced ecosystem, promotion of health and well-being includes assisting the adolescent to meet the challenges in function of the evolving changes that occur as a natural part of development and as a result of disability. The larger community may either support or undermine the adolescent's efforts to work through the tasks and challenges of this demanding period of their lives.

Therapists must be able to identify needs and offer solution focused brief intervention. This important goal requires a basic understanding of the wider socio-economic context for health and well-being. Some of us will focus on community-based work with the aid of community initiative, but participation becomes a challenge for all of us as we attend to individuals in the context of their own environment! Development of communication skills becomes a primary responsibility, especially in terms of adult education.

Linking needs and resources reciprocally in an integrated framework becomes essential. We need to link self-resources and other resources, remembering that our primary resource is our discussion with the other person with whom we work. In all challenging environments, students, therapists, assistants, and community-based rehabilitation workers will gain by working in partnership in pairs or threes.

The paradigm shift

If we are to abandon the perfectionistic approach of Western medicine, we must shift our attitude to a model of excellence. When the patient is examined out of their social context based upon their level of impairment, in doctor's rooms and hospital settings, they are judged to be sick or well, normal or abnormal, and treated accordingly. In the medical model the procedure is one of problem identification and diagnosis. Injury or illness is labeled according to the level of bodily impairment. The need for therapy is presumed to be directly related to the degree of severity. The polarization of opposites which occurs in this deficit model is at odds with a holistic approach of working together with a person for constructive change within the context of their environment.

In a dynamic biopsychosocial model of wellness and well-being, we describe observable, measurable, behavioral patterns which change over time in relation to relevant environmental and personal factors. We adopt a solution-focused approach to functional efficiency. At the same time we recognize that even the most subtle problems of posture and movement may compromise function by disrupting the muscle balance so necessary at the centre to support efficient distal function.

This paradigm shift enables us to develop a co-operative partnership based on mutual respect and trust. We start with abilities, and with what the person enjoys, and work for change in pursuit of excellence, promoting, recognizing, and celebrating success along the way. This is true at any age but vital in work with adolescents undergoing intense change, especially in their relationships with adults.

The basic prerequisite for an attitude of self-direction is the development of self-confidence in our own ability to deal with the tasks and challenges of daily life, and confidence to carry them through to completion.

Conclusion

- Change happens in the organism at the level of the cells, in all of the cells, where proteins are constantly broken down and reformed (Kidd *et al.*, 1992).
- The only real choices are therefore related to direction, timing, and quality of change, and to whether we as therapists assume responsibility for what happens in therapy.
- The choices we make will be directed by our attitudes, values, and belief systems.
- As we deal with the challenges of daily life and engage in the process of a search for self-identity in adolescence, *change is the route for learning*. The map is not the territory but merely a two dimensional representation of it. Negotiating individual passages through this potentially dangerous territory requires engagement in a complex decision-making process. Many alternatives must be considered on which to base 'life and death choices' moment by moment.

Relationships are all important as we consider adolescents as changing beings in the broader context of which they are a part. Relationships define the context of interaction by providing 'the pattern which connects' as described by Bateson (1972). Duality not only exists within a dynamic relationship, but is necessary to the relationship. Relationships contextualize opportunities, and lead to a reciprocal dance of choice and decision making, resulting in change which precedes the next opportunity.

The adolescent is part of a family, which is in turn part of an extended family, which is part of a community with its own particular culture and place in society. She or he cannot be considered as an isolated being, however much they may experience their life as being isolated. If the family is the natural environment for growth and well-being of its members, economic pressures can and will disrupt family life and render the children more vulnerable. When children become separated from their parents and are cared for by others, disabled children are seen as a particular drain on inadequate resources. Therapists need to work with a person in the context of the family. A better understanding of each person's situation is possible once we meet in their own environment. It is not only the adolescent who experiences change through disability. The family too is influenced by the disability, and has an influence on the effect of the disability. Each family unit is different and has unique ways of coping with change. These coping strategies will also both influence and be influenced by the adolescent. When we meet the person on home ground, we have the opportunity to convey respect, and to begin with what that person enjoys. We observe and celebrate achievements, abilities, and strengths and show willingness to learn together. We can enable the person and their family to take the initiative in identifying needs and encourage them to participate in creative planning, organizing and problem-solving skills. One of our goals is to help the people with whom we work deal ever more efficiently with the challenges and demands of everyday living. To accomplish this we foster automatic carry-over into everyday functions with elaboration of pattern, and generalization from the specific in order to deal with new and different situations when we invite participation of the wider family.

References

African National Congress (ANC) (1994) *The Reconstruction and Development Programme – A Policy Framework.* Johannesburg: Umanyano Publications.

Bateson, G (1972) *Steps to an Ecology of the Mind.* Nortvalwe, New Jersey: Jason Aronson Inc.

Brazelton, TB (1984) *Neonatal Behavioural Assessment Scale, 2nd ed.* Philadelphia: Lippincott.

Brazelton, TB (1992) *Touchpoints – Your Child's Emotional and Behavioural Development.* A Merloyd Lawrence Book. Reading, Mass: Addison Wesley

Bronfenbrenner, U (1986) Ecology of the family as a context for human development. *Developmental Psychology* 22: 723–742.

Brown, MC, Hardman, VJ (1987) Plasticity of vertebrae motoneurons. In: Winlow, W, McCrohan, CR (eds) *Growth and Plasticity of Nerve Connection.* Manchester: Manchester University Press

Carle, E (1970) *The Very Hungry Caterpillar.* London: Hamish Hamilton.

Capra, F (1989) *Uncommon Wisdom: Conversations with Remarkable People.* London: HarperCollins.

Cohen, D (ed) (1991) *The Circle of Life.* London: HarperCollins.

Collins (1987) *Cobuild English Language Dictionary.* London: William Collins.

Covey, SR (1992) *Seven Habits of Highly Effective People.* London: Simon & Schuster.

Davis, CM (1994) *Patient Practitioner Interaction: An Experimental Manual for Developing the Art of Health Care.* Thorofare NJ: Slack Inc.

Dawes, A, Donald, D (1994) *Childhood & Adversity: Psychological Perspectives from South African Research.* Cape Town: David Philip.

De Bono, E (1978) *Opportunities.* London: Penguin.

Dorko, BL (1996) *Shallow Dive: Essays on the Craft of Manual Care.* Thorofare, New Jersey: Slack Inc.

Edgelow, PI (1997) Neurovascular consequences of cumulative trauma disorders affecting the thoracic outlet: a patient-centered treatment approach. In: Donatelli, RA (ed) *Physical Therapy of the Shoulder,* 3rd ed. New York: Churchill Livingstone

Eliot, TS (1963) *Collected Poems 1909–1962.* London: Faber and Faber.

Erikson, EH (1968) *Identity: Youth and Crisis.* London: Faber and Faber.

Fernando, AJ (1995) Presidential addrress. World Confederation for Physical Therapy (WCPT) International Meeting, Washington.

Frankl, VE (1963) *Man's Search for Meaning: An Introduction to Logotherapy.* New York: Washington Square Press

Hanford, PK (1987) Motoric competence, behavioural confidence and classroom function. *Physiotherapy* 43(4): 111-115

Irwin-Carruthers, SH (1984) Extract from Milani-Comparetti, A (1983) A theoretical model for developmental neurology. Symposium International Paralysie Cerebrale, Toulouse, France, 1983. *SA Journal NDT* 7(3): 9-12

Jordaan, JJ, Jordaan, WJ (1989) *Man in Context.* Isando: Lexicon Publishers.

Kidd, G, Lawes, N, Musa, I (1992) *Understanding Neuromuscular Plasticity: A Basis for Clinical Rehabilitation.* London: Edward Arnold

Lerner, RM (1976) *Concepts and Theories of Human Development.* United States: Addison Wesley

Long, R (1991) *Walking in Circles: Exhibition at the Hayward Gallery.* London: Thames and Hudson

Robinson, VM (1991) *Humour and the Health Professions.* Thorofare, NJ: Slack Inc.

Santrock, JW (1992) *Life–span Development,* 4th edn. USA: Wm C Brown

Save the Children Fund (SCF) (1990) *Prospects for Africa's Children.* Sevenoaks: Hodder and Stoughton

Smuts, JC (1926) *Holism and Evolution.* London: Macmillan

Stewart, I (1990) *Does God Play Dice?* London: Penguin

Vleeming, A, Snijders, CJ, Stoeckart, R, Mens, JMA (1997) The role of the sacroiliac joints in coupling between spine, pelvis, legs and arms. In: Vleeming, A, Mooney, V, Dorman, T, Snijders, C, Stoeckart, R (eds) *Movement, Stability and Low Back Pain.* Edinburgh: Churchill Livingstone

6

The Adult Years

Lena Nordholm

Introduction
•
Theories of Adult Development
•
Developmental Tasks of Adulthood
•
Life Patterns of Men and Women
•
Mid-Life Crisis
•
Health Problems in Adulthood
•
Activating Psychological Resources in Patients
•
Summary

Introduction

In a conversation with two children I happened to ask them what they thought it meant to be an adult. The boy (age 9) did not hesitate: 'It means to have a job and support yourself.' The girl (age 11) gave a more elaborate answer: 'To be adult means that you must take on a lot of responsibility — you have to look after your children — it is very hard work to be an adult.'

These answers reflect traditional sex roles of adults, emphasizing important tasks in adulthood: work and love. Most developmental psychology textbooks ignore adult development. It is as if nothing of interest happens to the development of the person beyond the age of

20. Even though several researchers (e.g. Havighurst, 1972; Neugarten, 1973; Vaillant, 1977; Levinson, 1978; Erikson, 1982) have studied adult development, their findings and theories rarely make it into developmental textbooks. There are at least two explanations for this. First, it may be that because adult development has been studied in the context of aging, it has been associated with aging rather than with development. Secondly, it could be that the physical model of development, which describes a growth in functions for the young person, a plateau for the adult, and a decline for the old person, has also influenced thinking about psychological development. Yet, nothing could be further from the truth than to describe adult devel-

opment as a plateau. During the adult years major psychological development takes place. The adult continually faces new developmental tasks; new challenges to his/her psychological growth, which he/she must cope with.

This chapter will describe adult development. Coupled with this description will be the theme of the adult as patient. It is the major thesis of this chapter that illness and disability heighten the experience of predictable crises in adult life, or passages as Sheehy (1976) calls them. At the same time, the experience of a psychological crisis may heighten already existing physical symptoms or bring out latent illness. Insights about this interdependence may increase the health professional's understanding of the patient. For example, the apparent overreaction in the patient with a 'trivial' complaint may be better understood with reference to the existential crisis of mid-life.

Another theme which will be highlighted in this chapter is the importance of interpersonal relationships. Psychological health, and thus by implication physical health also, is dependent on satisfying, warm, respectful, and life-giving human relationships. If only health professionals knew how much of their beneficial effect is due to this kind of relationship.

Theories of Adult Development

In his book 'The Life Cycle Completed', Erikson (1982) outlines a theory of psychosocial development in eight stages. One of these stages, 'adulthood', the seventh stage, is relevant to this chapter. Erikson has assigned this stage the critical antithesis of *generativity versus self-absorption and stagnation*.

Generativity includes procreativity, productivity, and creativity. It involves 'generating' new human beings, new ideas, new products as well as a new identity. Stagnation, on the other hand, is failing to be involved in generative activities. Erikson suggests that a sense of stagnation may overcome even very creative and productive people at times. This psychosocial crisis of generativity versus stagnation is resolved in a positive way through *care*,

'...a widening commitment to *take care* of the persons, the products, and the ideas one has learned to *care for*' (Erikson, 1982, p. 67).

Thus, care is the characteristic virtue of adulthood, the essential generational task. As adults we must care for our children, our parents, our societal institutions, the environment, our cultural heritage, our humanistic values, the world, so that we have something of value to pass on to our children. However, generativity implies more than productivity and care. Implied in the concept is the notion of social responsibility. The generative adult is a socially responsible adult, who assumes the responsibility for the continued existence of his/her 'products', be these the children, the inventions, the works of art, or whatever. The adults (parents, teachers, inventors, artists, workers) are only generative if they acknowledge their social responsibility for the consequences of their productivity.

Erikson (1982) describes care and *rejectivity* as two opposites of a contrast. While care is the sympathetic side of the contrast, rejectivity is the unwillingness to include certain people, certain groups in our caring, i.e. one does not care to care for these people.

'In fact, one cannot ever be generative and care-ful without being selective to some point of some distinct rejectivity. It is for this very reason that ethics, law, and insight must define the bearable measures of rejecitvity in any given group, even as religious and ideological belief systems must continue to advocate a more universal principle of care for specified wider units of communities. It is here in fact, where such spiritual concepts as universal caritas give their ultimate support to an extending application of developmentally given care' (Erikson, 1982, p. 68).

Erikson suggests that rejectivity may express itself as

'...suppression of what does not seem to fit some set goals of survival and perfection' (p. 69)

and gives examples of cruelty against children or prejudice against certain segments of the community as well as against large groups of foreign people. The ultimate expression of rejectivity is in wars against those nations (or ethnic groups within a nation) that threaten one's own kind.

The conflict between generativity and rejectivity can bring out the best in man in expressions of loyalty, heroism, and cooperation while at the same time making people wage wars and bring death and destruction to those who are different. Erikson (1982) also states that where rejectivity is merely inhibited, a form of self-rejection may develop. Thus, the concept of rejectivity has far-reaching implications for the psychosocial development of the individual.

Levinson's (1978) conception of adult development is based on the idea of pursuit of 'the Dream', a vision of glorious achievement. To help the man realize his dream (Levinson studied men!) there are two significant other people: 'the mentor' and 'the special woman'. For Levinson the developmental process is defined as 'individuation', which refers to 'the change in a person's relationship to himself and to the external world' (p. 195). Levinson discusses three different developmental tasks of adulthood: building and modifying the life structure, working on single components of the life structure, and becoming more individuated. Among the men Levinson studied, achievement and success, the struggle toward recognition and glory, take priority and human relationships play a relatively subordinate role. Vaillant's (1977) account of adult life also emphasizes work. Based on interview data, Vaillant suggests the thirties as an era of 'career consolidation', which will bring societal recognition. Vaillant emphasizes the relationship of self to society and minimizes relationships to other people.

In discussing the various male models of adult development, Gilligan (1982) concludes:

'Thus, there are studies, on the one hand, that convey a view of adulthood where relationships are subordinated to the ongoing process of individuation and achievement, whose progress, however, is predicated on prior attachments and thought to enhance the capacity for intimacy. On the other hand, there is the observation that among those men whose lives have served as the model for adult development, the capacity for relationships is in some sense diminished and the men are constricted in their emotional expression. Relationships often are cast in the language of achievement, characterized by their success or failure, and impoverished in their affective range' (p. 154).

Gilligan's own contribution is to note that in the various studies

'... the women are silent' (p. 155),

and bring forth the missing line of development. She argues that development toward maturity is not only a question of achievement and individuation, but also

'a progression of relationships toward a maturity of interdependence' (p. 155).

Gilligan has been influential in bringing in the voices of women, correcting the one-sided view, which equated adult development with male development. According to Gilligan, women identify themselves in terms of their relationships, as mother, wife, mistress, child, friend, etc. They also assess themselves by a moral standard of relationships

'an ethic of nurturance, responsibility and care' (p. 159).

The women in Gilligan's study, despite their professional and academic achievements, did not define themselves in terms of such achievements.

In her studies of moral development, Gilligan (1982) found that men and women use different points of departure, different ideologies: justice and care. This is a parallell to the emphasis placed on achievement among men and on human relationships among women. Gilligan concludes her insightful discussion in the following way:

'To understand how the tension between responsibilities and rights sustains the dialectic of human development is to see the integrity of two disparate modes of experience that are in the end connected. While an ethic of justice proceeds from the premise of equality – that everyone should be treated the same – an ethic of care rests on the premise of non-violence – that no one should be hurt. In the representation of maturity, both perspectives converge in the realization that just as inequality adversely affects both parties in an unequal relationship, so too violence is destructive for everyone involved. This dialogue between fairness and care not only provides a better understanding of relations between the sexes but also gives rise to a more comprehensive portrayal of adult work and family relationships' (p. 174).

Developmental Tasks of Adulthood

The notion of developmental tasks is an appealing one. It suggests tasks, problems, to be mastered at different stages of development, and it suggests an expectation of achievement. Havighurst (1972) describes a developmental task as

'…a task which arises at or about a certain period in the life of the individual, successful achievement of which leads to happiness and to success with later tasks, while failure leads to unhappiness in the individual, disapproval by the society, and difficulty with later tasks' (p. 2).

Developmental tasks vary for different ages and to some extent for different cultures. However, the notion of a development task has an implicit universal meaning. Therefore, although there may be some cultural variation with respect to its expression, a developmental task is basically universal, applicable to all mankind. When we consider early child development many of the developmental tasks are related to physical and cognitive growth such as learning to walk, learning to talk, etc., and these show great regularity and universality. The older the individual gets the more influenced by culture will the developmental tasks be. Thus, finding a mate may involve different rituals, different tasks to be mastered in a village in Africa compared to a village in Sweden. Marriage and childbearing may occur at different ages and with different rituals, but they *do* occur in all cultures, testifying to the universality of these developmental tasks.

Havighurst (1972) lists the developmental tasks associated with adulthood as: selecting a mate, starting a family, rearing children, holding a job, establishing and maintaining a home, participating in civic affairs. Later in adulthood come the tasks of: preparing older children to make the transition into adulthood, adjusting to physical changes associated with aging, developing leisure time skills.

Task development is a major focus in clinical practice for occupational and physical therapists, who guide their patients to master skills in habilitation and rehabilitation. Banus (1979) discusses the concepts of task, activity, and occupation, and the relevance of the developmental perspective to occupational therapy. One may easily apply this perspective to physical therapy and other rehabilitation disciplines.

We will now turn our attention to the two major developmental tasks of adulthood in Erikson's (1982) seventh stage of psychosocial development: parenthood and work.

Parenthood

Finding a mate is usually associated with the age range of the twenties, so this task will not be discussed here. However, parenthood, although it starts for some in the twenties or even before, is viewed as the foremost developmental task of adulthood. It is the essence of generativity, according to Erikson (1982). What could be more productive than creating new human beings? Furthermore, this kind of productivity is very important for the psychological development of the adult.

The role of mother is traditionaly the most important function for women. Women today are expected to fit motherhood in with career, no matter what type of work they are involved with. Motherhood is a lifelong occupation, which once entered into cannot be resigned easily. Every woman must decide about this issue of motherhood, whether she has children of her own, or whether she adopts a child, or decides against it. Eliasson and Carlsson (1989) wrote that the idea of motherhood is more sacred to men than to women, to the low-income person than to the high-income person, to younger than to older people, and to married than to unmarried people.

The motivation to become a parent seems to be different among males and females. Women are less hesitant to become parents than men, and answer 'yes' more often than men to the question of whether children are the meaning of life. However, 35-year-old women without children perceive meaning in life despite being childless, and have a less positive attitude toward parenthood than their male counterparts (Swedish Bureau of Statistics, cited in Eliasson and Carlsson, 1989).

No doubt becoming a parent means different things to men and women. Motherhood brings status and social identity to the woman. These reasons are less prominent among men. However, for the woman, motherhood is associated with both internal conflicts as well as conflicts at the societal level. The conflicts concern women's right to have autonomy and control over their own lives and the children's rights to a harmonious psychological development. It is extremely important for the child to have a good mother. Good mothers traditionally put their children's welfare before their own. This may mean that many women subordinate their own lives and interests to the children's. The long-range implication of this is that their own adult development may be put off until the time when the children are grown up. Women who do not become mothers may experience both disappointment over not fulfilling expectations, and anger that they are not allowed to choose for themselves. In some societies it is considered 'unnatural' not to have or want children if you are a woman, and such women may be regarded as maladjusted (Eliasson & Carlsson, 1989).

Becoming a parent is an overwhelming experience in many ways. Your whole outlook on life changes. Suddenly you are not the center of your world – the child is. Without the parent's (or substitute parent's) attention to the needs of the child, the child will not survive. The realization of the utter dependence of the child brings an end to the egocentrism of the young parent, who must subordinate his/her life to the needs of the child – day and night.

At the same time that the child brings immense pride and happiness to the couple, an enormous psychological adjustment to the new roles of mother and father must occur. Many new emotions are aroused by these role responsibilities. The mother may grieve over her lost career opportunities. She may find little satisfaction in much of the tedious child-caring chores, and she may feel guilty about each of those emotional experiences. On the other hand, she may feel relieved to have left a job that wasn't satisfying, and flourish in her new role as mother and home-maker. The father may find it difficult to adopt to and accept his responsibility to this new family, and continue to put first priority on his work. He may not understand the impact of lack of sleep and lack of stimulation, and may not be sensitive to his wife's complaints about boredom.

Although it would today appear that the sex roles are more fuzzy at the edges, these roles are basically intact, as they always have been. For example, when the Swedish government introduced paid paternity leave in addition to maternity leave, very few males used this benefit. Many males claim that they cannot afford to take time out for childcare because of their careers. The ones who do are younger, and are occupied in service professions such as teaching.

Ideally couples need to negotiate a satisfactory solution to their new circumstances as parents. If the wife takes the major child care responsibility during the first years, it is often with the understanding that she will return to her work and career in the near future. The husband may be willing to assume his part of the responsibility for the home and child care to facilitate his wife's return to the work force. However, the demands can be overwhelming at times for both the man and the woman, and put severe strain on the relationship.

Through the adult years the roles as parents require constant adjustment to new demands, and mastery of new tasks. Not only do young children depend on their parents, but teenagers may revolt against them, young adults learn from them, and old people frequently require assistance from them. The adults are seen as all-powerful protecters by their young children, as stuffy conservatives by their teenage children, as influential maintainers of society by the young adults. It is no wonder that the adult years constitute a period of responsibility, authority, and influence. Adults are those who teach, guide, influence, change, reform, protect, and carry on.

Work

In the Erikson (1982) model of psychosocial development, the concept of generativity is also expressed in work. Early in adulthood the person decides on a career to pursue which will bring fulfillment of his/her lifegoals (compare Levinson's (1978) concept of 'the Dream', referred to previously in this chapter). During the adult years the work role is established. Work is an enormously important factor in providing structure for the life of the person. Work occupies many of our waking hours for a large part of our lives. No wonder young adults agonize over the choice of occupation to pursue.

To achieve a professional training, to master work skills, to develop an occupational role and an occupational identity are the kinds of developmental tasks associated with work. For many people the work experience brings endless opportunities for generativity, for example the teacher, academic, health professional, engineer, priest, social worker, scientist, artist, etc. However, the work one undertakes is very much a function of what one brings to it. In many work places there are opportunities to effect change through creative effort. For example, in human organizations one may come up with good ideas and suggestions that lead to improvement of the social climate of the work group. The value of *care* in Erikson's

(1982) theory about the adult years embodies a key concept for this age. There should be numerous opportunities for 'care' in our daily lives, whatever work we may be doing. When adults assume the responsibility to care, they achieve psychological growth.

During this agespan (30–50), many adults reach leadership positions in their chosen fields of work. Clearly there are important aspects of generativity possible for the person in a leadership position. Through leadership in one's chosen profession one will be able to influence goals and has the legitimate power to affect developments in the field. The aspects of generativity are inherent in that one turns not inward but outward with the ambition to do something for others, for one's patients, colleagues, and fellow workers, for mankind even. Social psychologists have studied leadership both in terms of leader characteristics and leader functions. During the era from the 1940s to the 1970s, many attempts to identify leader characteristics were made. It was found that personality traits such as responsibility, will-power, endurance, ability to take initiative and be goal directed could be attributed to effective leaders, but correlations were generally rather low. For most researchers today, leadership is seen as a social psychological process, an interactional process, whereby effective leadership depends on the situation, the task, the leader, and the followers. More attention is focused on the behaviour of leaders and followers, their communication and interaction, rather than on personality traits. Still, the leader is attributed to have a key role in this interaction (Malten, 1992).

A leader should help his/her group with two major tasks: to reach the group goal and to maintain good relationships in the group.

These two general tasks hold for all types of group and at all levels of good leadership, be it the local Red Cross society, the soccer team, the health team, the gym group, the 'back-school' therapy group or whatever. Health professionals have an extremely important function to lead various groups, both patient groups and groups of colleagues. The implication is that with good leadership the therapeutic goals may be more successfully reached, and good leadership requires insight into the social psychology of group interaction.

Many of the physical problems adults experience, such as back and neck pain, repetitive strain injury, headaches, and ulcers, are associated with unsatisfactory work situations. It may be that the actual physical conditions of the work place are detrimental to the employee through the provision of poor work positions, poor light, high noise levels, and poor ventilation. It is also possible that the psycho-social climate is destructive to one's self-concept. The individual may lack autonomy, receive little or no respect or appreciation, fail to experience success or opportunities for advancement, and may feel oppressed by authoritarian leadership. The working conditions at one's place of work not only affect the individual in that environment, but have an impact on his/her whole life situation, including physical and mental health. One can easily see that there is an impact on the family too.

For some people illness may be a way to escape an unbearable life situation such as conditions at work. To receive a pension and to be excused from work legitimately can give a new lease on life. For others, there is an opposite reaction. They refuse to admit to ill-ness and cling to their work. For them it seems the way of survival. The following case stories illustrate that work can have very different meaning for chronically ill people. The stories are excerpts from interviews with individuals having chronic illness (Blomdahl-Frej, 1988).

'Mrs C is 37 years old, married without children. She lives in the countryside with her husband in a house they own. Mrs C married when she was 19 and has been a housewife most of the time. She has also held part-time jobs as cleaner and textile worker. She has no occupational training. In 1973, Mrs C was afflicted by an acute neurological illness and in 1982 one of her lungs collapsed. She has been treated at a lung clinic. Mrs C does not miss her part-time jobs. With the help of her husband she can do the housework. Although her life is restricted, she has accepted her illness and the fact that she can't have children' (pp. 205–207).

'Mr E is 41 and has a wife and teenage son. His wife works part-time. Mr E has a small business. They live in a house of their own. Mr E has suffered from asthma the last seven years. He has been a frequent patient at the lung clinic and was once hospitalized for four months. Despite his illness it is possible for Mr E to run his business relatively well. Work is terribly important to him. He would never consider receiving an illness pension. He enjoys meeting people and finds achievement stimulating. He would not want to be considered useless, and says that he would feel worse if he was home. He says that the days he can work he feels a lot better. It is clear that he is trying to avoid a sick role and that he has learnt strategies to live with his disease' (pp. 108–209).

Mr E's way of coping with his asthma illustrates a relationship to the illness which was found characteristic among patients with asthma in the study by Hansson-Scherman (1994). She entitled her study: 'Refusing to be Ill', since this was the dominant pattern among the chronically ill patients with asthma/allergy. The findings indicated that chronic illness and medication threaten one's identity. Patients developed various strategies to maintain their identity as healthy persons, by distancing themselves from prescribed medications, without any detriment to their state of health, as studied over 8 years.

Life Patterns of Men and Women

Since love and work are the two major tasks of adulthood, according to Erikson (1982), it is useful to look at the various ways in which men and women go about building their adult life structures with respect to love (marriage, children) and work (career). The following model and descriptions of life patterns are based on Sheehy's (1976) analysis, that continues to be relevant today. The frequencies of people in each of the categories may have changed in this decade, however. Sheehy (1976) describes five different patterns for men: the locked-in; the wunderkind; integrators; never-married men, paranurturers, latency boys; transients. She also describes six different patterns for women: the care-giver; the nurturer who defers achievement, the achiever who defers nurturing; late-baby superachievers; integrators; never-married women; transients. Note that some of the category names are identical for men and women such as integrator, never-married, transient. Though the name is the same, it does not necessarily mean that the patterns for the males and females in that category are identical, but they do share

important features. In the discussion of the categories that follows, similarities and differences for males and females are contrasted.

Locked-in/care-giver I see great similarities in the patterns described as *locked-in* for men and *care-giver* for women. Men who follow this pattern have as their goal to get settled early, often without much reflection. Many follow in their fathers' footsteps in terms of career choice. They are the conformists who do what is expected of them. They avoid risk taking, play safe, do not want to be different as they start climbing the career ladder in their chosen field of work. Many men in the longitudinal Harvard study of adult development were locked in (Vaillant and McArthur, 1972).

The care-givers also want to get settled. They want to marry and have a family and do this early in their twenties, without any intention of going beyond the roles of wife and mother. They too do what is expected in terms of traditional sex roles. I believe that this pattern for women is less common in Western societies today. As I reflect upon events in my own country, Sweden, where few families any longer can be supported on one salary alone, and 80% of women of working age are in the work force, I am forced to conclude that the sole role of care-giver is probably less valid today.

Nurturer who defers achievement/achiever who defers nurturing These two patterns characterize women. They represent an either/or pattern. Either you have a family first and then go back to school/work, or you try to get established in a career first and then have children. These patterns are probably exclusively female patterns. Few men would reason like this, not even today in more egalitarian societies. The men prepared to commit themselves to nurturing will probably be included among the integrators (see below), those wanting to combine it all at the same time: career, marriage, and family. One effect of the women's movement may be that we see less young women today in the *nurturer who defers achievement* pattern than in the *achiever who defers nurturing*. The astonishing fact is that so many of the women who are middle-aged today and who had excellent school achievements made the choice to become a nurturer who deferred occupational achievement.

Wunderkind / late–baby superachiever According to Sheehy (1976) the wunderkind is the man who plays to win, not the one who plays to avoid loss. In other words, the wunderkind is the risk-taker who enjoys career success early. He is competitive, absorbed by his work, pursuing his dream. He has high visibility in sports, show business, arts, science, politics, or business. Of the women's patterns described by Sheehy, the late-baby superachiever seems to me to have similarities with the wunderkind. The female superachievers also have high visibility and spectacular accomplishments in show business, arts, science, or business. Moreover, many of these women do not become mothers until they are 35 or over. Some well-known examples are Margaret Mead, Barbara Walters, and Sophia Loren. Having a child so relatively late in one's childbearing life puts one in a special situation. Some women have been perceived as grandmothers to their children, and some children have lied about the 'ancient' age of their mother. When the young girl's puberty coincides with the mother's menopause, it is bound to affect the mother's self-concept. This is a different experience from that of her contemporaries, who are living through the empty nest syndrome at this age.

Never–married Western culture has tolerated unmarried men more than unmarried women as we see in the favourable connotations of 'the eligible bachelor' and the unfavourable ones of 'wallflower spinster'. In a hisorical perspective, marriage and children have defined womanhood and given women status in most cultures. The unmarried woman often had a marginal position although she may have had important work such as teaching, or nursing. Sheehy (1976) writes that

'Our society is stingy about acknowledging this [being unmarried] as a legimate pattern for women' (p. 343).

But the evidence is that single men and women below 35 are very similar in terms of education, occupation and income (p.287). As time goes by the distance between them widens. By the time they reach middle age, single women are more educated, have higher average income and work in more prestigious occupations compared to unmarried men. The unmarried woman appears to bring stronger psychological reserves to bear on the challenges of her position in comparison with unmarried men. It has been found that single women experience greater happiness and less discomforts than single men, who suffer more depression, neurosis, and antisocial tendencies (Gurin *et al.*, 1960).

Many unmarried persons of both sexes become *paranurturers*. They involve themselves in nurturing tasks either through their work (e.g. as teacher, clergyman, nurse, social worker) or volunteer work involving nurturing. Another category of unmarried men is also described by Sheehy as the *latency boys*. For these men the life cycle never gets under way. They remain bound to their mothers and are underachievers in their careers.

Transients The transients are the men and women who keep their options open. They do not commit themselves either emotionally or careerwise. In a way they are prolonging their youth, trying out courses, jobs, places, lovers in a prolonged wandering. This could occur in a positive way whereby the try-outs and wanderings become a basis for self-knowledge and a serious commitment later. It may also occur in a negative way through drifting and self-destructive behavior, whereby the individual ends up isolated from human relationships. The positive aspect of the transient pattern is often seen as acceptable, maybe even desirable, for people in their twenties to prevent too early a locked-in pattern.

Integrators Integrators are the people who try to do it all: career, marriage, and children *at the same time*. Sheehy (1976) wrote:

'Women like me were the mutants of our generation. Marriage did not stop us from working toward accomplishment, nor did childbirth, although it usually caused us to slow down. The guilty rub at the center of our twenties was, "How will I integrate the baby with my life so it won't cut me off from the world"' (p. 339).

Many integrators at this time paid a high price in either a wrecked marriage, a disrupted career, or neglected children. Sheehy suggested that the expectation to be able to integrate it all so early in life was unrealistic, and pre-dicted that integrators would be more successful at 30 or 35 years of age. Whether this prediction is true today, toward the turn of the new century, is a question for research.

The male integrators are the men who try to achieve a balance between their career commitments and a genuine commitment to family life. Here we find the husband who takes paternity leave and time off to be with sick children, and who supports his wife's career ambitions rather than just his own – not only in theory but also in practice. The integrator is a role model for a more involved father, not only one who brings in the financial support to the family, but one who resumes responsibility for the human support too. This is obviously not an easy pattern to follow in societies dominated by competitiveness, and where success in life is measured in accumulation of material rewards. For the man it may involve not accepting a job with hours that are too long or involving absences from the home that are too extensive. It may also involve having a part-time job to facilitate the wife's education or career ambitions.

A pattern which has become more prominant is the *one-parent family*. In Sweden today for example, approximately one marriage or de facto marriage in three ends in divorce/separation. In about 70% of the cases the woman has taken the initiative (Eliasson and Carlsson, 1989). In most cases the woman will have the major childcare responsibility. For the single parent, life may be a constant struggle against loneliness, poverty, and guilt over having split up the family.

It will be interesting to study the generation of young people now entering adulthood in terms of their solutions for combining work and family, and the new patterns that may evolve in the new century. After all, our world is constantly changing and when the premises change, so must the life structures which young people will build.

Mid-life Crisis

'When I was about 40 years old I was set in a life–pattern of work, home and family. My husband and I were both academics and did not see much of each other working at different universities in a big metropolitan area. Our two children – a boy of 10 and a girl of 8 (the perfect nuclear family) – were pretty much self–sufficient. They were outgoing, doing well at school, and able to take care of themselves. Since we were not living in our native country we had no family nearby, but we had a network of wonderful friends. We lacked nothing, yet I would wake up early in the morning around four o'clock, and think about my life. Was this to be my life from now on? Was this all there ever was going to be of my life? Would I ever live in my native country again? Would my children grow up not knowing their roots, their relatives, their place in the family history? I also remember feeling so utterly alone and afraid of old age. I knew I had a loving and caring husband, despite the fact that we did not spend as much time together as I would have liked. Why did I feel this awful sense of time running away, of time slipping by, half my life had gone now? Thinking back I realize it was my mid–life crisis I was experiencing. Three years later my situation had changed completely. We had moved back to our native country, we had new jobs and we had a new baby! The mid–life crisis resolved through new expressions of generativity!'

The mid-life crisis at about 40 years of age has been called 'the deadline decade' by Sheehy (1976). She refers to the decade between 35 and 45, when individuals suddenly realize that half their life is gone and they have to take stock of their situation. The realization that life is not endless strikes you as a thunderbolt: 'What am I doing with my life? I have only this one life – and half of it is gone.'

Sheehy (1976) describes the work of Elliot Jacque (1965) suggesting that Jacque may have coined the term 'mid-life crisis'. Jacque had observed that great artists (e.g. Beethoven, Goethe, Ibsen, Voltaire) had experienced a crisis in their creative work at mid-life. He went on to study his own patients' life stories and concluded that a mid-life crisis manifested itself not only in creative geniuses, but in everyone in some form.

The creative crisis described by Jacque (1965) may express itself in three different ways. For some people the creative capacity may now emerge for the first time. The most famous example is Gauguin who after having left his job in banking became a famous post-impressionist painter by the age of 41. Another way in which the creative crisis may express itself is that the person may burn out or actually die. In his study, Jacque found a sudden jump in the death rate between 35 and 39. Yet another way is a smooth transition, that is the work of the artist does not change decisively. Sheehy (1976) suggests that Jacque's analysis of the creative crisis is

'a strong metaphor for the change in quality and content we can all begin to feel in our chosen enterprise at this time' (p. 370).

It may be comforting to know that great men before us have suffered through the mid-life crisis and come out ahead, such as, for example, Dante and Shakespeare.

In her interviews with men and women in mid-life, Sheehy (1976) discovered a consistent pattern of: (1) a sense of time urgency (How much time do I have left? Will it be enough to do the things I dreamed of doing? If I want to change my life, I must do it now or it will be too late); (2) troubled thoughts over loss of youth, vitality, and diminishing physical prowess (Do young men still look at me or only old men? Why do I have this pain in my shoulder so often. Why can't it go away? Why do I get so tired?); and (3) the existential questions without answers (What is the meaning of life? Why do *I* live? What happens after death?)

The ways in which people experience the mid-life crisis depend on the life structures they have been building up to this point. For instance, there are both distinct differences due to gender, as well as overlap between the life patterns of men and women. Furthermore, the ways in which people experience the mid-life crisis is in a more general sense dependent upon all the various environmental factors, such as the family and work situation, the social, political, and economic situation of the society in which they live, and various personal resources such as genes, intellect, and personality.

Menopause

Miss G, 52 years old, never married, career in business, has of late experienced embarrassing symptoms. At inopportune moments she has felt a hot wave through her body and sweated profusely. At night she has woken up so wet from sweat that she has had to change her nightdress. She is well aware that these symptoms are connected to her menopause, but finds the inconvenience a nuisance. When discussing menopause with her friends at work she discovers that many of her contemporaries have these physical symptoms but at the same time feel relieved to be rid of 'the curse'.

Mid-life crisis in women is often associated with menopause. Many beliefs exist about both physical and psychological problems at the time of menopause. Some of these beliefs seem well founded in research. For example, the physical symptoms of hot flushes and sweating have been established in many studies of menopausal women (e.g. Collins and Landgren, 1994; Koster and Garde, 1994). However, the beliefs about psychological problems such as anxiety and depression, irritability, restlessness, lack of self-confidence, and poor self-image are much less substantiated in research (Richter, 1994). In clinical studies of menopausal women seeking medical assistance for physical problems, psychological problems may also be present, but several studies have failed to support the claim (e.g. Plesner, 1981; Collins and Landgren, 1994). It seems more likely that psychological problems at this age depend on the many changes in the life situation, rather than the lack of estrogen. Furthermore, it appears that the experience of menopause may reinforce already existing psychological problems or bring forth latent ones (Plesner, 1981).

The health survey by Collins and Landgren (1994) was answered by 1400 women born in 1942. The women from the district surrounding the Karolinska Hospital in Stockholm, Sweden, were surveyed by mail. This study showed that hot flushes and sweating were the only symptoms directly related to menopausal status. They were significantly more frequent among women who had stopped menstruating. However, psychological symptoms appeared to be secondary; they were more common among those who had hot flushes and sweating than among those who did not have these physical symptoms. Furthermore, the secondary symptoms were not directly related to the loss of menstruation, but correlated to several other variables such as earlier reproductive health, lifestyle, smoking, physical activity, etc. The results of the study indicated that active, independent, women with interests of their own had the least problems during menopause. Many of these women experienced this time as a stage in life that provided increased freedom, and improved self-image and self-confidence.

Health Problems in Adulthood

Lifestyle and health

Many of the health problems which affect people in adulthood are directly related to lifestyle. For example, the risk of suffering a heart attack or stroke is related to sex, age, blood pressure, cholesterol, cigarette smoking, and diet. In addition, workload, stress, and behavioral factors such as coping mechanisms have an impact on the known risk factors of blood pressure, smoking, cholesterol, etc. (Lundberg, 1994).

The belief in personal control over health has been suggested as a crucial variable in explaining health problems. Rotter (1966) first proposed the personality-like construct of internal/external control as the person's level of expectancy that outcomes depend on one's own actions. People high in internal control believe that they themselves can affect out-comes, while those high in external control believe that fate, luck, or powerful others affect the outcomes. Wallston and coworkers (1978) have developed a multidimensional instrument to measure internal/external beliefs about health with three dimensions: internal health locus of control (HLC), and external health locus of control divided into two: powerful others HLC and chance HLC. Wallston et al. (1983) have found that people with higher internal health beliefs also show preference for control of, and active involvement in, their own health care. On the other hand, patients who believe that their health is controlled by powerful others are less likely to endorse self-treatment or active involvement.

Another useful concept related to health beliefs and locus of control is 'self-efficacy', first introduced by Bandura (1986a) within the framework of social-cognitive theory. Perceived self-efficacy is defined as

'people's judgments of their capabilities to organize and execute courses of action required to attain designated types of performance' (Bandura, 1986b, p. 391).

His definition of self-efficacy is concerned with what the individual thinks he is capable of doing, not his actual ability. Bandura suggests that the self-efficacy theory may be useful in understanding the psychological and cognitive factors that mediate health outcomes. A growing body of research indicates that self-efficacy can have a significant impact on anxiety, stress reactions, and pain that affect the quality of life and development of chronic dysfunctions (e.g. Bandura, 1986a). Later studies indicate that self-efficacy can be modified through therapeutic interventions (Lomi et al., 1995).

The mechanisms that explain the cause and effect relationships between psychosocial factors and somatic illnesses are not clearly delineated nor understood. Several theoretical models have been described in a review by Melin (1992). The major feature of these models is an interactionistic and multifactorial way of approaching the problem. This approach holds that environmental and individual factors interact and result in different adaptation strategies. For instance, the balance between perceived demands from work, home, and family, and belief in one's own resources to meet these demands may be connected to different biological functions that affect the interaction. The area of type A personality and heart disease is one area of research where these relationships have been closely studied, but before we turn to this we must examine the major culprit – stress.

Stress

Stress is used by many lay people as the culprit that explains the contemporary ailments that afflict them. However, there is no single uniform definition of stress agreed upon by the scientific community. Stress can be viewed as a stimulus, a stressor such as heat. And stress can be viewed as a response, a stress reaction such as the physiological reaction to a noxious stimulus situation. A transactional view suggests stress is the interaction between the environment and the individual's experience of the situation (Bailey and Clarke, 1989).

Selye's (1936) classic study demonstrated the physiological effects of stressful situations as in stomach ulcers. Much research has followed this line of investigation, so it is now clear that stressors will affect the organism at the cellular and molecular level (Arnetz, 1995). In order to understand the illness – health continuum and its relation to stress, both physical and psychosocial stress must be considered.

Psychosocial stress can be experienced during major life events such as the loss of a loved one, loss of work, and other life changes that have great impact on the person's life situation. Unemployment is a major societal problem in most industrialized countries, which now witness structural changes in a transition into the Information Technology (IT) age. Many people have been forced out of employment situations, or live under the threat of losing their jobs. Some predict that not every able-bodied person will have employment in the future. Yet, the importance of work cannot be overemphasized, as we discussed earlier in this chapter under Theories of Adult Development, and unemployment can have serious consequences for health.

In an interdisciplinary study described by Arnetz (1995), several hundred individuals were studied on several variables over two years. One group was unemployed, one group lived under the threat of unemployment and the third group was securely employed. One of the major findings of this study was that unemployment and threat of unemployment was associated with strong physiological stress reactions affecting cholesterol level, blood pressure, immune function, and psychological reactions such as hopelessness and depression. Various coping strategies were also studied. It was found that people who used a coping strategy that focused on problem solving had more favorable outcomes than those who used coping strategies oriented to their emotions.

The advance of the IT society has spawned research interests related to occupational health hazards and computer work. One line of research has focused on factors that have detrimental effects on the skin. Berg *et al.* (1992) studied two groups of computer operators, one with skin problems and one without. They found that those with skin problems had a higher level of physiological stress reactions present at work but not at weekends. These reactions could not be explained by physical factors alone, such as electromagnetic fields, but included a poor work environment with dust, heat, or dry air as potential contributing factors to the skin problems. In addition, psychosocial stress in the form of powerlessness and individual coping strategies were related to the presence of skin reactions.

Psychosocial stress as experienced by people in their work situation is perceived as a growing problem in society. Stress leads to decreases in an individual's sense of well-being and lowered productivity. Stress results in a lot of human suffering and leads to increased health care consumption. Arnetz (1995) claims that stress is a major health problem. He suggests that every work place should survey the work situation and identify major problem areas. Programmes need to be developed and implemented to improve the work environment. These steps must be followed with evaluation studies to check on the effects. Arnetz (1995) suggests that a continous monitoring of the psychosocial work environment is as important as monitoring the productivity. These kinds of effort in program development and evaluation will lead to increased knowledge of stress-reducing techniques that can be applied to combat the illness produced by stress.

Type A personality and heart disease

Mr P, 53 years old, twice married with two families (four children), was burning his candle at both ends. He is hard driving, in a high administrative position, is a workaholic, slightly overweight and smokes. He felt constantly pressed for time. His greatest wish was that the day would have twice the number of hours in it. His friends had begged him to change his lifestyle for the sake of his health, but it took a heart attack before he listened.

This description is representative of a person with type A personality. In the original study by Friedman and Rosenman (1974) the patients who were impatient, aggressive, and perceived themselves to be under constant time pressure were called type A, while the patients who had a more relaxed attitude toward life were called type B. Later studies have used a variety of questionnaires to measure type A behavior. In general, the type A behavior is seen as a personality trait characterized by speed and impatience, job involvement, and a hard-driving attitude. This trait is approximately normally distributed in the population (Lundberg, 1994).

Large epidemiological studies (Jenkins *et al.*, 1971; Rosenman *et al.*, 1976) have documented that while controlling for other risk factors, the individuals with type A personality had twice the risk for heart attack. More recently Lundberg (1994) argued that the research conducted during the 1970s and 1980s is not convincing in implicating type A behavior. He postulates several explanations for this, such as a diversity of measurement instruments across the many studies, and instruments which have low correlations with each other. Another reason may be that type A behavior is becoming more common in our Western industrialized societies in general, which makes it difficult to find differences between type A and type B behaviors. Some research has pointed to hostility as a particularly significant aspect of type A behavior. This hostility is described as a hostile and aggressive attitude to the world, probably founded on lack of basic trust (Barefoot *et al.*, 1983).

Lundberg (1994) concludes, based on both American and Swedish studies of children as well as adults, that type A behavior begins early in life and is reinforced in the type of work these individuals seek. They select jobs with status, high salary, power, responsibility, and control, and work environments where their personality traits are reinforced through competition and time pressure. The research results on type A personality serve as good examples of the interaction between health and behavior.

Musculoskeletal problems

Mrs E (43 years old) is divorced with no children. Mrs E dropped out of high school and worked as a waitress until she developed problems in her upper right arm. She consulted several doctors and finally had surgery. However, the relief of pain was only marginal. The search for a cure continued over several years, with periods of sick leave interspersed with periods of work. Mrs E has now resigned herself to this chronic problem and works part-time as a receptionist.

Mrs T (38 years old) is married with two daughters. She works full-time as a dentist. Recently, she has started to experience pain in the thumb of her right hand. She has consulted a doctor and exercises have been recommended. She has begun to increase her general level of fitness in order to withstand the physical demands of her work.

Mrs M (41 years old) is divorced with two children who live with her. Mrs M works full-time in clerical work sitting 8 hours a day in front of a computer. Despite instructions to take minibreaks and follow the schedule of exercises, problems with her right wrist (repetitive strain injury) continue to bother her, sometimes worse than at other times. It seems to her that this vulnerability appears especially when the work conditions are stressful, e.g. when there is time pressure to get something finished.

Miss K (37 years old) is unmarried, smokes, and works as a nurse aid. Her job involves lifting many heavy patients so Miss K has experienced repeated back problems and associated periods of sick leave. She has received instruction in how to lift, and physical exercises have been recommended to strengthen her back muscles. She is a very dedicated and conscientious person and wants to continue her work.

What these four patients have in common is that they are all women, approximately 40 years of age, and suffer from various pain problems of the muskuloskeletal system. Psychosocial factors are often suspected in health problems relating to the musculoskeletal system. In addition to loss of income and intense suffering for the individual, these problems are very costly for society. Despite big investments to improve the ergonomics of many workplaces in Sweden, these problems have increased rather than decreased during the 1980s and are today the most common cause of sick leave and disability pensions (Sievers and Klaukka, 1991). Furthermore, pain problems are as common in light as in heavy work (Bammer, 1990). Many investigations into this problem area seem to indicate that a whole host of factors interact to increase the risk, such as work stress, work dissatisfaction, repetitive movements, static work load, physical condition, smoking, and diet (Holmström, 1992; Ohlsson, 1995).

Many people experience pain on a daily basis. Much research has focused attention on low back pain, an occupational hazard in many jobs, not only the ones involving heavy lifting. Research includes epidemiological investigations of the prevalence of pain as well as clinical studies examining treatment effects (Kvarnström, 1983; Nachemsson, 1991). Some have tried to unravel the origins of low back pain through the study of the different risk factors such as work-related factors, personality traits, lifestyle, and physical condition (e.g. Riihimäki, 1991).

Disorders of the neck and upper limbs are more common among women than men (Ohlsson, 1995). Afflicted women often work in light industry or clerical work where the tasks have a repetitive and monotonous character. These disorders also seem to be increasing as evidenced in the Swedish national statistics on occurrence of occupational diseases (Malker *et al.*, 1990). This increase is difficult to explain since there has been an increased level of consciousness about the importance of a good work environment among employers, employees, the unions, and the occupational health services. Winkel (1989) suggests that one reason for the increase may be that even though the higher degree of automation has reduced workloads such as heavy lifting, there are strong demands for increased productivity with a resulting increase in work pace and maybe work stress. There seems to be ample evidence that these problems can only be understood by an interactive model which takes into account the individual susceptibility, the physical work environment, and the psychosocial work environment (Ohlsson, 1995). To this one might add that within these categories there are many variables. Thus, for instance, individual susceptibility may include both physical condition, lifestyle habits, personality, attitudes, and so forth, which correlate to these disorders.

Depression

Mrs F (55 years of age) is married with grown children. At the time when she experienced the 'empty nest', she also lost her job owing to factory closure. She has lived all her life for others, especially the children and her dominant husband, seeking love, recognition, and admiration. When she lost her work she became deeply depressed. She found no reason to get out of bed in the morning, felt great apathy and sense of meaninglessness. Her husband's cheerful order to pull herself together had no effect. She could not rid herself of the feelings of worthlessness and self-blame.

Depression is a condition which affects many women at different stages in life. The reasons for depression may be psychological and social as well as biological. Depression may occur in response to strong psychological stress or may be due to some important life event such as a relative's death, divorce, or job loss, which brings about a dramatic change in the person's life situation.

The depressed person feels apathetic, down, a failure, and finds it difficult to show interest in the things in which he/she would normally be involved; the experience of life has ceased to be meaningful. The depressed person may also experience self-disgust, helplessness, anxiety, or psychosomatic problems.

One way of understanding depression is through the theory of 'learned helplessness' (Seligman, 1975). Helplessness is defined as a condition which results from repeated failures by the individual to gain control and to be able to affect one's own life. The person has had repeated experiences of not being able to influence his situation, experiences where other factors and other people have been in control, rather than the person himself. After such repeated experiences the person comes to adopt an attitude of fatalism characterized by sentiments such as: 'It does not matter what I do. Things just happen. I can't do anything to control or influence these things, but since other people seem to succeed where I fail I must have some of the blame'.

Interviews with people who are depressed indicate that feelings of apathy and helplessness are common. Seligman's (1975) theory of learned helplessness postulates that experiences of helplessness leads to depression. A vicious circle develops, where the person's tendency to react with helplessness in a situation of crisis or conflict leads to feelings of depression, which reinforce the feeling of helplessness and in turn deepens the depression.

It is well documented that women suffer from depression more frequently than men. Eliasson and Carlsson (1989) provide an analysis of depression as a typical 'women's disease'. They suggest that sex role identity is a crucial factor. Through traditional sex role socialization processes, women run a greater risk of being socialized into helplessness. This traditional female sex role is associated with passivity and dependency, subordination, and feelings of guilt. Thus the tendency to react with help-

lessness in difficult situations is incorporated in many women through the socialization process.

Eliasson and Carlsson (1989) also discuss the social situations of women, in which they run greater risks of finding themselves in real situations of helplessness. Many women are victims of unwanted pregnancies or unwanted childlessness which may lead to feelings of helplessness. They refer to a Norwegian study which indicated that housewives experienced psychological problems to a greater extent (43%) compared to career women (19%) (Westman-Berg, 1979). In particular, women who were caring for young children at home without social support were at risk of depression.

Another explanation for women's greater tendency toward depression can be found in the cultural environment. It is more acceptable for a woman to show weakness, to be in need of help, to be depressed. Depression is tolerated more in women than in men. The reactions of guilt and passivity can be understood more easily in the context of the female sex role identity discussed above. When women show weakness they will be understood, and they expect others to take over the responsibility for handling the problem. Eliasson and Carlsson (1989) point out that it is important that the woman actually solves her problem by her own initiative and power. Naturally, she can have support from people around her, but they must not take over. If other people actually solve the problem, the woman's sense of helplessness will be reinforced. The real help to a depressed woman must aim at breaking the vicious circle of depression and learned helplessness.

Activating Psychological Resources in Patients

Illness will affect most of us sooner or later. To be ill has been labeled a 'risky opportunity' by Brudal (1995). Most illnesses in adult life are associated with dangers and challenges, but also with the opportunity to get to know oneself better, to find out new sides of one's personality. Brudal (1995) claims that this human knowledge is not valued in society, and suggests that health care personnel must become more aware and knowledgeable about the ways in which they can support the patients' understanding of themselves. When patients come in contact with their psychological resources, they may realize that they can actively contribute to improving their condition.

Brudal (1995) suggests that the traditional curative medical model is not sufficient to handle many of the lifestyle-induced conditions afflicting people. She advocates a 'promotive' model of health care, which emphasizes autonomy for the patient, close interpersonal relationships, a holistic approach, and an awareness among health professionals of the many paradoxes of human nature. She expands the notion of the 'paradoxical person' who is not 'either – or' but 'both'. For example, one is not either logical or intuitive but both logical and intuitive. The message is that we must stop thinking in a dualistic, categorizing way and become more flexible and creative in the way we think about people. Our thinking about patients must incorporate both health and illness, and help the patient find him/herself and new strength.

What are the psychological resources which may be latent and unused in the patient, which can be activated? Brudal (1995) examines some of the research which has a bearing on this question. She notes the research on vulnerable but resilient children as one example. These children developed exceptionally well despite poverty, illness, divorce, drug dependence, and other challenges in their home environment. Werner's (1989) study of high-risk children indicated that a third of them showed good adjustment where the contrary might have been expected. By comparing those who developed well with those who had failed to develop well by becoming criminal or mentally ill, Werner found two distinguishing characteristics: behavior in infancy and development of a close relationship with a care-giver. The well-adjusted children had been active and lovable, easy to take care of as infants and had had the opportunity to develop a close bond with the care-giver, who had given them love and positive attention. The significance of this research is that it challenges our ideas of what brings strength and quality of life. Regardless of difficult external circumstances, some individuals have the inner resources to overcome the physical and material barriers in their lives. The research points to the very important factor that close human relationship is essential for the child, not only to cope with difficult life situations, but positively thrive in them.

Other examples of an individual's capacity to bring forward unknown strength in order to survive are war, accidents, and catastrophies. Malt (1982) claims there are four conditions which make adjustment possible for the victims: (a) controlling one's feelings so that an assessment of the situation can be made; (b) protecting one's sense of integrity; (c) maintaining ability to make one's own decisions through retaining independence and avoiding passivity; (d) maintaining social relationships. Malt (1982) emphasizes that if the sense of independence is stimulated through opportunities requiring choice, the person will be able to make his own decisions, which in turn strengthens his/her sense of self. The ability to mobilize effective coping strategies seems to be the key to controlling ones emotions. By activating resources to control the emotions of anxiety, aggression, and helplessness, which might overwhelm us in a crisis situation, we regulate the emotions so that they are kept within the boundaries of tolerance. We have seen how adverse situations bring out unexpected resources in the individual. Strong positive experiences may also bring out the individual's latent abilities. Experiences of this kind, so called 'peak experiences', have been described by Maslow (1964). Maslow suggests that the releasing stimulus for a 'peak experience' may be nature, childbirth, art, creative activity, or death. However, the 'peak experiences' have certain common elements. Characteristic of these experiences is a feeling of harmony (absence of conflict) and transcendence which creates optimism and courage.

The opportunities inherent in fantasy are also being explored as ways to activate inner resources. Popular psychology advocates the power of positive thinking, mental training and visualization. Some of the techniques involved have been described by Siegel (1986). These techniques, which have been employed successfully in sports psychology and childbirth, utilize fantasy and ability to create symbols in one's mind. For example, mental preparation before an important sports event involves visualizing and concentrating on doing all the right things in order to achieve that optimal result, including actually achieving the new record or whatever the goal is. Similarly in preparation for childbirth the mother-to-be imagines a good birth process and a successful outcome, concentrating on what she will do at any one point in the birth process, such as breathing, pushing, and so forth. In the treatment of cancer Siegel (1986) describes the work of the Simonton husband and wife team. One often-cited case study involves a young boy with a brain tumor. Simonton suggested to the boy that they should try to use fantasy and together they decided that the boy should imagine he had a kind of video game in his head and that he could direct missiles against the tumor. After several months the boy one day said to his father that he could not find the tumor any longer which turned out to be true. The research on visualization techniques in sports and medicine shows that they can have positive effects on achievement and health (Brudal, 1995).

Brudal (1995) recommends that more effort must go into providing the positive counterforces to the negative forces released by illness and disability. She suggests more training on the part of health professionals in use of the techniques which could help patients cope by activating their own positive resources. She claims that it is not enough to nurse or to make the patient comfortable, but the opportunity must be used to strengthen the patient's sense of self, to afford opportunities for self-knowledge. The idea of activating the patient's resources is consistent with the rehabilitation approach. Physical and occupational therapists are trained to focus on the abilities of the patient – not just disabilities – and in discussion with the patient set goals to work toward. In this process many opportunities for increased self-knowledge must also afford themselves.

Summary

This chapter emphasizes that psychological development takes place not only during the first 20 years of life, but all throughout the age span. The adult person continually faces new developmental tasks; new challenges to his/her psychological growth to cope with.

The seventh stage of Eriksson's (1982) theory of psychosocial development is referred to with its critical contrast of generativity versus stagnation. Generativity includes procreativity, productivity, and creativity, while stagnation is the failure to be involved in generative activities. To care for other people is the characteristic virtue of adulthood, the essential generative task. Other authors such as Levinson (1978), Vaillant (1977), and Gilligan (1982) are also cited on adult development.

Havighurst (1973) lists major developmental tasks associated with adulthood as: selecting a mate, starting a family, rearing children, holding a job, establishing and maintaining a home, and participating in civic affairs. In this chapter, parenthood and work are selected for more in-depth discussion as the two major universal developmental tasks of adulthood.

Life-patterns of men and women during the adult years are illustrated with the categories described by Sheehy (1976). The concept of mid-life crisis which occurs for many around the age of 40 is explained and exemplified.

A brief summary of some of the health problems in adulthood is provided. The thesis is that many of these are associated with lifestyle and by implication the individual himself has the possibility to assert some influence over the course of events. The concepts of internal locus of control and self-efficacy, are cited in this connection.

Since many of the lifestyle influenced illnesses of adulthood are believed to be caused by stress, this chapter also gives a brief overview of this concept and its relationship to type A personality and heart disease.

A final section of this chapter discusses the possibility of activating psychological resources in patients. This idea is consistent with the rehabilitation approach where the emphasis is to bring out the patient's abilities and resources. Those resources may be psychological as well as social. The importance of family and friends to provide the network of support cannot be overemphasized, neither can the importance of increased self-knowledge.

References

Arnetz, B (1995) Stressreaktioner i informations-samhället: Fysiologiska och psykosociala aspekter. In: Sivik, T, Theorell, T (eds) *Psykosomatisk Medicin*. Lund: Studentlitteratur.

Bailey, R, Clarke, M (1989) Stress and coping in nursing. London: Chapman and H.

Bammer, G (1990) Review of current knowledge – musculoskeletal problems. In: Berlinguet, L, Berthelette, D (eds) *Work With Display Units 89*. North-Holland: Elsevier Science publishers BV.

Bandura, A (1986a) Self-efficacy mechanism in physiological activation and health promoting behavior. In: Madden, IO, Mathysse, S, Barchas, J (eds) *Adaptation, Learning and Effect*. New York: Raven Press.

Bandura, A (1986b) *Social Foundations of Thought and Action: A Social Cognitive Theory*. Englewood Cliffs, NJ: Prentice-Hall.

Banus, BS (1979) Development and occupation. In: Banus, BS, Kent CA, Norton YS, Sukiennicki DR, Becker ML (eds). *The Developmental Therapist*, 2nd edn. Thorofare NJ: Charles B. Slack.

Barefoot, JC, Dahlström, WG, Williams, RB, Jr (1983) Hostility, CHD incidence, and total mortality: a 25-year follow-up study of 225 physicians. *Psychosomatic Medicine* 45: 59–64.

Berg, M, Arnetz, BB, Lidén, S, Eneroth, P, Kellner, A (1992) A psychophysiological study of employees with VDU-associated skin complaints. Journal of Occupational Medicine 34: 698–701.

Blomdahl Frej, G (1988) *Toward a Holistic View – An Existential Relationistic Approach.* Doctoral Dissertation, University of Göteborg, Department of Social Work.

Brudal, LF (1995) *Hälsopsykologi. Aktivering av Psykiska Resurser vid Sjukdom.* Lund: Studentlitteratur.

Collins, A, Landgren, B-M (1994) Reproductive health, use of estrogen and experience of symptoms in perimenopausal women: a population-based study. *Maturitas* 17:

Eliasson, M, Carlsson, M (1989) *Kvinnopsykologi.* Stockholm: Natur och Kultur.

Erikson, EH (1982) *The Life Cycle Completed.* New York: WW Norton.

Friedman, M, Rosenman, RH (1974) *Type A Behavior and Your Heart.* New York: Knopf.

Gilligan, C (1982) *In a Different Voice.* Cambridge, MA: Harvard University Press.

Gurin, G, Veroff, J, Feld, S (1960) *Americans View Their Mental Health.* New York: Basic Books.

Hansson-Scherman, M (1994) *Refusing to be Ill: A Longitudinal Study of Patients' Relationship with Their Asthma/Allergy.* Doctoral Dissertation, University of Göteborg, Göteborg Studies in Educational Sciences 95.

Havighurst, RJ (1973) *Developmental Tasks and Education,* 3rd edn. New York: David McKay.

Holmström, E (1992) *Musculoskeletal Disorders in Construction Workers. Related to Physical, Psychosocial and Individual Factors.* Doctoral Dissertation, Lund University, Dept of Physiotherapy.

Jacque, E (1965) Death and the midlife crisis. *International Journal of Psychoanalysis* 46: 203–214.

Jenkins, CD, Zyzanski, SJ, Rosenman, RH (1971) Progress toward validation of a computer-scored test for the Type A coronary-prone behavior pattern in employed men. *Journal of Chronic Diseases* 20: 371–379.

Koster, A, Garde, K (1994) *Övergång–inte Undergång. Om Kvinnans Klimakterium – och Mannens.* Stockholm: Natur och Kultur.

Kvarnström, S (1983) Occurrence of musculoskeletal disorders in a manufacturing industry, with special attention to occupational shoulder disorders. *Scandinavian Journal Rehabilitation Medicine Suppl* 8: 1–112.

Levinson, D (1978) *The Seasons of a Man's Life.* New York: Knopf.

Lomi, C, Burckhardt, C, Nordholm, L, Bjelle, A, Ekdahl, C (1995) Evaluation of a Swedish version of the arthritis self-efficacy scale in people with fibromyalgia. *Scandinavian Journal of Rheumatology* 24: 282–287.

Lundberg, U (1994) Beteende, stress och hälsa. In Törestad, IB, Nystedt, L (eds) *Människa–omvärld i Samspel.* Stockholm: Natur och Kultur.

Malker, HSR, Hedlin, M, Malker, BK, Weiner, JA (1990) Occupational musculoskeletal disorders. Identification of risk by ISA statistics. *Arbete och Hälsa* 29: 1–122.

Malt, U (1982) *Og Livet går Vidare ... Festskrift till Leo Eitinger.* Oslo: Universitetsforlaget.

Malten, A (1992) *Grupputveckling.* Lund: Studentlitteratur.

Maslow, A (1964) *Religions, Values, and Peak Experiences.* Columbus: Ohio State University Press.

Melin, B (1992) *Stress, Health Related Behaviors, and Biological Risk Factors: Psychobiological Studies of Healthy Men and Women.* Doctoral Dissertation, University of Stockholm, Department of Psychology.

Nachemsson, AL (1991) Spinal disorders. Overall impact on society and the need for orthopedic resources. *Acta Orthopaedica Scandinavica* 62(Suppl 241): 17–22.

Neugarten, BL (1973) Adult personality: a developmental view. In Charles, DC, Looft, WR (eds) *Readings in Psychological Development through Life.* New York: Holt, Rinehart, & Winston.

Ohlsson, K (1995) *Neck and Upper Limb Disorders in Female Workers Performing Repetitive Industrial Tasks.* Doctoral Dissertation, Lund University, Sweden, Dept of Occupational and Environmental Medicine.

Plesner, R (1981) *Övergångsåldern – Myt och Verklighet.* Stockholm: Bokförlaget Trevi.

Richter, A (1994) *Kvinnor Mitt i Livet.* Stockholm: Bonniers.

Riihimäki, H (1991) Low-back pain, its origin and risk indicators. *Scandinavian Journal of Environmental Health* 17: 81–90.

Rosenman, RH, Brand, RJ, Sholtz, RI, Friedman, M (1976) Multivariate prediction of coronary heart disease during 8.5 year follow-up in the Western collaborative group study. *American Journal of Cardiology* 37: 903–910.

Rotter, JB (1966) Generalized expectancies for internal versus external control of reinforcement. *Psychological Monograph* 80: No. 609.

Seligman, MEP (1975) *Helplessness: On Depression, Development and Death.* San Fransisco: WH Freeman.

Selye, H (1936) A syndrome produced by diverse nocuous agents. *Nature* 138: 32.

Sheehy, G (1976) *Passages – Predictable Crises of Adult Life.* New York: EP Dutton & Co.

Siegel, BS (1986) *Love, Medicine and Miracles.* New York: Harper & Row.

Sievers, K, Klaukka, T (1991) Back pain and arthrosis in Finland. How many patients by the year 2000? *Acta Orthopaedica Scandinavica* 62 (Suppl 241): 3–5.

Vaillant, GE (1977) *Adaptation to Life.* Boston: Little Brown.

Vaillant, GE, McArthur, CC (1972) Natural history of the adult male psychologic health. I. The adult life cycle from 18–50. *Seminars in Psychiatry* 4: 415–427.

Wallston, KA, Wallston, BS, De Vellis, R (1978) Development of the multidimensional health locus of control (MHLC) scales. *Health Education Monograph* 6: 160–171.

Wallston, KA, Smith, RA, King, JE, Forsberg, PR, Wallston, BS, Nagy, VT (1983) Expectancies about control over health: relationship to desire for control of health care. *Journal of Personality and Social Psychology* 9: 377–385.

Werner, EE (1989) High-risk children in young adulthood: a longitudinal study from birth to 33-years. *American Journal of Orthopsychiatry* 59: 72–81.

Westman-Berg, K (1979) (Red.) *Gråt Inte–forska! Kvinnovetenskapliga Studier.* Stockholm: Prisma.

Winkel, J (1989) Why is there an increase in the occupational disorders? *Nordisk Medicin* 104: 324–327 (in Swedish).

7

Normal Aging

Shulamit Werner

Introduction
•
Biological Theories of Aging
•
Psychosocial Theories
•
Normal Aging Versus Successful Aging Versus Pathological Aging
•
Gerontological Research, Dimensions, and Problems
•
Psychological Aspects of Aging
•
Social Aspects of Aging
•
Health, Health Assessment and Health Promotion
•
Impairment, Disability, and Handicap in Old Age

Introduction

'Remember your Creator in the days of your youth,
Before the days of trouble come and the years approach
When you will say, "I find no pleasure in them" –
Before the sun and the light and the moon and the stars grow dark,

When the keepers of the house tremble, and the strong men stoop,

When the grinders cease because they are few, and those looking through the window grow dim;

When the doors to the street are closed and the sound of grinding fades
When men rise up at the sound of birds, but all their songs grow faint;
When men are afraid of heights and of dangers in the streets;
When the almond tree blossoms and the grasshopper drags himself along and desire no longer is stirred,
Then man goes to his eternal home and mourners go about the streets.'

Ecclesiastes 12:1–5.

Ecclesiastes portrays old age as an unavoidable stage of life, something all men will experience. He considers old age to be a time for reflecting on the past, for settling one's affairs and for preparing for the day of reckoning. His very vivid picture of man's physical decline, with the dimming of sight, the deterioration of hearing, the trembling of the limbs, the stooped posture and the loss of teeth, is accompanied by feelings of sadness, fear, and despair. These are the years in which man finds no pleasure. There is no mention of the joys and blessings of old age.

This negative picture of old age has been presented throughout the ages; sometimes as an isolated image, such as in Ecclesiastes and King Lear, or as part of the life cycle as in Sophocles' *Oedipus* and Shakespeare's '*As You Like It*'. In modern times, with its strong regard for youth and youthfulness, a conscious effort is being made by gerontologists all over the world to soften this baleful impression of old age. Not only the professionals and scientists involved in the study of aging, but many old people themselves have moved away from the notion that negative physical and behavioral changes are necessarily a part of growing old. Today it is considered that the ravages of the aging process can be prevented in the course of life, and sometimes remedied, even in old age. We talk of 'successful aging' as opposed to 'normal aging', of 'healthy aging' as opposed to 'pathological aging'. The study of aging in all its aspects has become one of the most highly regarded fields of research in the biological and social sciences. How have the actual lives of old people all over the world improved as a result of the extensive research and funding which have been invested in the subject during the last three decades? Do old

people perceive themselves differently? Has society changed its attitude toward them? Has the general health and overall function of elderly people improved? Have all the helping professions found more and better solutions to the physical, mental, and psychological problems of the aged? To what extent do legislation and government policies in most countries of the world meet the needs of the elderly? All these questions will have to be asked, even if satisfactory answers cannot as yet be found.

Why should health professionals learn about old people and the aging process? First, because we, and those close to us, will all grow old. This last stage of life is inevitable, if we are fortunate enough not to die young. If we know more about how others grow old, perhaps we will have a better chance of coping with our own old age in a way that will bring us, and those around us, a sense of fulfillment, satisfaction, and acceptance.

Second, most of our target population, the clients of health services, are old people and their numbers will increase in the future. By the year 2000 the proportion of people over 65 in the world population will be about 10%. In the developed countries this proportion will be even higher. As the numbers of very old people age 85 and above increases, there will be more frail and handicapped among them. The older people get, the more they will accumulate impairments which will limit their functional ability. For example, it has been estimated that the number of visually impaired people over the age of 85 in the USA will be over 1 200 000 in the year 2000. In a study by Crews in 1984, it was found that almost 53% of the visually impaired over the age of 85 had difficulty in walking, compared ·

with 39% of those with no visual impairment. Of this visually impaired group, over 24% had difficulty getting in and out of bed, compared to 19% of the group with no visual impairment (Crews, 1994).

All these people will need special facilities and services which the various health professionals will have to supply. We have to prepare ourselves to be able to meet these numerous new needs, both professionally and administratively.

Finally, we need to know more about the aging process in order to be aware of, and able to rid ourselves of all the negative stereotypes concerning aging and old people which are so prevalent in developed cultures. In our society today we worship all that is new, fresh, and youthful. Childhood and adolescence are considered more worthy of our consideration and study than the later stages of life. Many focus on the negative aspects that are common in old age, such as illness, dependency, and mental deterioration, assuming that they are all interrelated, and the inevitable result of the aging process. This grim attitude is often adopted by society at large, emphasized by the media, and reflected in the paucity of public funding for health and social services for the elderly. Learning more about aging will enable us, as responsible members of the society in which we live, to consider aging as a part of the developmental sequence, and give due attention to this most significant period of the human lifespan. We will be able to challenge the current myths about old people and be better prepared to address their special needs.

What are the causes of human aging? Why do people and domestic animals grow old while animals in the wild are either killed by predators or die of hunger, and trees and bacteria can live for ever provided they have the right environmental conditions? What are the basic physical, emotional, and social changes that occur during the aging process? Do these changes follow a common, universal pattern or are they influenced by the society and culture within which the individual lives? Aging as a total phenomenon comprises biological, psychological, and social aspects, each having different theoretical concepts. A theory, in its broad sense, is a model of how the world functions. Over the years, scientists from many academic fields have striven to arrive at a comprehensive theory that will cover the various aspects of aging and explain the process. Several biological and psychosocial theories have been proposed, each explaining one feature but not others. The challenge is to arrive at a theoretical concept which will enable us to understand the various aspects of the aging process, how they are interrelated and how this should influence our professional approach.

Biological Theories of Aging

Biological theories can be classified into several different categories according to an organizing premise such as the developmental – genetic theories. These are based on genetic predetermined changes within the cell nucleus itself. Another category of stochastic, or non-genetic theories attribute the aging process to both extrinsic and intrinsic causes. The Hayflick limit theory (Hayflick, 1987) is an example of the former, which suggests that there is a limit to the number of cell replications. Also the free radical theory (Harman,

1987) states that free radicals cause accumulating damage in important cell structures; the Walford's caloric restriction theory (Walford, 1981) states that a high nutrient – low calorie diet will positively influence disease susceptibility and aging rate.

The stochastic theories of aging all refer to insults to the cells caused by extrinsic or intrinsic factors. Among these are:

1. *The error theory* This attributes the aging process to the accumulation of errors in the synthesis of proteins as a result of environmental factors such as radiation.

2. *The cross–linkage theory* This states that large molecules will be linked together by some free radical or by their own side chains.

3. *The transcription theory* This is concerned with the faulty replication of DNA.

The latest theory of aging is the opoptosis theory which states that the cell is equipped with a pre-programmed suicide mechanism which will cause the aged cell to die at a pre-programmed stage.

All these biological theories will support some of the phenomena of aging, but fail to explain them all. An integrated theory is needed that combines the two fundamental hypotheses, and that would support the pre-programmed human life span theories on the one hand, and explain the individual differences on the other.

Psychosocial Theories

During the last 30 years, several different theories have been proposed which attempt to explain the behavior of older people. All are based on extensive research performed mainly in Western cultures. Like the biological theories, they are far from comprehensive. These include the disengagement theory, the activity theory, the exchange theory, and the lifespan development theory.

The disengagement theory

This classic theory was first described by Cumming and Henry (1961). Although circumstances and ideas have changed in the last three decades, many still think that disengagement is the norm, and 'good' both for the old person himself, and for society. The theory proposes that old people, when they feel that their life is drawing toward its end, choose to disengage from life, to turn inward to their inner selves. They are no longer interested in the outside world, not even in their close families. They choose to disengage from society just as society disengages from them at the same time, in an attempt perhaps, to prepare for the final disengagement of death. The theory emphasizes the mutuality of the process between the old person and society, and highlights the equilibrium achieved between the deterioration in functional capacities of the old person and the decrease in his social roles. As the older person grows weaker, both physically and socially, it is 'right' that less should be expected of him, in all respects.

Case 1: Mary

Mary lives in an old age home on the outskirts of a big city. The large building resembles an old family mansion, with its spacious rooms and wide corridors. Large glass doors lead out onto the spacious grounds with its rolling lawns and manicured flower beds. Old people in wheelchairs are sitting in small groups, some playing parlor games, some watching TV and some engaged in the activities organized by the recreational therapist. A few are sitting by themselves, reading, listening to music, engaged in needlework or just enjoying the beautiful balmy day. Mary is sitting on the porch, her head dropping onto her chest. Her eyes are closed but she is not asleep. The nurses report that she sits like this for hours, not talking to anyone, not doing anything. She never complains or requests anything, does not get excited or angry or happy. Even the prospect of seeing her grandchildren does not seem to elicit any reaction from Mary. She seems to be quite content to be left alone. Mary, a widow of 20 years with two married children, was a primary school teacher, a job she had held for 30 years. In the past, she was very much involved in community affairs, and busy with various hobbies such as reading, singing in the local choir and tending her beautiful garden. Soon after she retired 15 years ago, her health deteriorated suddenly. She suffered a severe heart attack after which she never returned to her former level of functioning, limiting her activity to the house and its immediate surroundings. Her children helped as much as they could, visiting her several times a week and seeing to the heavy cleaning and the shopping. Soon she began to lose interest in all the things that had previously given her pleasure, never opening a book, not listening to music or even watching TV. The few friends she had stopped coming or phoning. Gradually she ceased to see to her daily needs, forgetting to eat or to wash, hardly ever getting out of bed. Finally there was no choice but to make some alternative arrangement, such as finding somebody to live with her or to move to an old age home. Mary did not seem to care either way, so it was decided that she come to this place. Here at least she is cared for, cleaned and fed. As to her mental condition, the doctor cannot find anything specifically wrong with her. She is lucid, though not alert, devoid of affect, though not depressed, aware of time and place, though totally disinterested in her surroundings. Mary seems to be in the process of disengagement.

The disengagement theory was widely criticized because it claims to present a universal, inevitable process. This mutual disengagement does not occur in all old people in every state of health or physical function, and not in all societies. We see elderly statesmen continuing to function in very senior capacities almost to the day they die. In simple societies today, as in rural South Africa, the old people continue to serve as the advisors and leaders of their communities just as in the past. However, if the disengagement theory is adopted by policy makers and planners of services for old people, it might serve as justification for the minimal services and sub-standard treatment often provided for old people (Lewis, 1984; Hazan, 1988).

The activity theory

The activity theory is the polar opposite of the disengagement theory. Whereas in the latter theory old people are supposed to slowly detach themselves from the life they led before, the activity theory postulates that people behave in a totally different manner. They and their care-givers strive to maintain and encourage activity for activity's sake. They believe that in order to be happy in old age, elderly people should remain active and continue to be involved socially. Sometimes this philosophy can be carried to extremes. People who seem to emulate this theory are those who participate in every possible course, engage in every occupation offered, just to 'keep busy'. Very often we see older people encouraged to take part in activities which are not necessarily meaningful for them and do not give them satisfaction or pleasure, just to 'be doing something'.

The activity theory originated in the USA as a contraposition to the disengagement theory probably because some old people and their care-givers were trying to treat the symptoms rather than attack the cause. We seem to have a conundrum. When one is forced to give up previous social roles in favour of those that are considered by society as appropriate for older people and when a gradual slowing down occurs which is normal when one grows older, a period of uncertainty results. A feeling of having to change together with a wish to continue along the same path exist simultaneously. These feelings may lead a person towards a driving force to 'keep going', to 'remain active'. For those who adopt this theory as a basis for planning services for old people a danger exists that they will arrange for a series of occupations and courses thought to be appropriate for old people, without asking the people whether they would like to participate. Thus we find long lists of activities offered in elder centers or old age homes, in which very few people participate.

The exchange theory

The exchange theory is based upon the relationship between old people and the society in which they live, suggesting that we expect to receive some reward for our investment in human relations, just as we expect to be rewarded for any other investment. The world is one big market place, where relationships are based on give and take, one has to pay a price for all that is received. The old person usually cannot, and is not expected to invest, so his position within his social environment is necessarily one of weakness and dependency according to this theory. The only thing the old person can give in exchange for what he receives is his acquiescence, his submission to the dictates of the society around him.

Case 2: Jim

Jim suffered a stroke six months ago. After a prolonged period of rehabilitation, he was moved to a nursing home as he has no immediate family. Jim is confined to a wheelchair and requires assistance in most activities of daily living. The nurses and orderlies like Jim for he never complains and is always very grateful for anything that is done for him. Several things in the nursing home aggravate him, like the blaring radio, the lack of privacy, and not being able to stay up after the official bedtime, but he never complains. Jim is always very considerate of the staff and does his utmost to please them. He is always polite to all staff members, even when they neglect him and disregard his wishes. Jim is a model patient! We often see elderly patients in nursing homes and hospitals where they are dependent on the good will of the staff, acting in a manner consistent with the exchange theory. It is impressive to see how old people adapt their behavior, to become acquiescent and submissive in order to survive in an environment in which their position is one of powerlessness.

The lifespan development theory

This is the most comprehensive of all the psychosocial theories mentioned previously. The concept of life as a continuum with many phases was the accepted way of thinking since the days of antiquity. In art and literature we find many examples of life as a series of steps or stages. In several old engravings such as *Ten Ages of Man* by Jorg Breu the Younger, or *The Life Cycle of Man and Woman* by Jan Houwens, one can follow man along the course of life from budding youth, through the power of manhood to the drooping of old age (Cole, 1993). Jaques in Shakespeare's *As You Like It* compares the world to a stage where the play-

ers each play seven parts, the seven stages of life, and the seventeenth-century English epigrammist, Thomas Bancroft, compares life to a staircase one ascends during childhood and youth and descends as one grows old.

We climbe the slippery stairs of Infancy,
Of childhood Youth, of middle age' and then
Decline, grow old, decripit, bed – rid lye,
Bending to infant – weakness once agen'
And to our Cophines (as to Cradles) goe,
That at the stair – foot stand, and stint our woe.

In all these examples, old age is the end of the journey of life which began at birth, the final stage, a time for reckoning and repentance for one's sins.

This philosophy, so familiar in the art and religion of mediaeval times, has been integrated into modern developmental theories, some of which are now described. Buehler's model, based on more than 400 interviews, depicts a sequence of five phases: from progressive growth in childhood and puberty, to regressive growth and decline in old age (see Box 1).

Box 1
The five phases of life according to Buehler

Phase	Age
Child at home; before self determination of goals	0–15
Preparatory expansion and experimental self-determination of goals	15–25
Culmination: definite and specific self-determination of goals	25–45
Self-assessment of the results of striving for these goals	45–65
Fulfillment of goals or experience of failure; previous activities continue but late in life there may be a re-emergence of short-term goals focusing on satisfying immediate needs.	65 and above

Buehler bases her theory on goal-related psychological expansion and regression which are in a parallel sequence with the biological development in childhood, and the physical deterioration in old age. She concludes from her studies that the feeling of not having achieved one's goals is perhaps more frustrating in old age than the confines of physical decline (Buehler, 1968).

Unlike Buehler, Carl Jung based his developmental theory on his experience as a clinical psychologist. The first stage of life is youth, according to Jung, for he does not believe that normal children have problems of their own even if they are a problem to their parents. In old age, Jung found some deep changes in the psyche. He believed that older people changed into their opposites: that men become more 'feminine' in their old age, and women more 'masculine'. Jung argued that there is always a purpose in life, even in old age. He suggested that the 'turning inward' in old age is an inner exploration of the self which might help people to find meaning in their lives and thus be able to accept their approaching death (Jung, 1971).

Erikson, who together with Jung, studied with Freud, presents life as a series of crucial turning points which divide the lifespan into eight stages. Each stage represents a conflict between two opposite tendencies. According to Erikson the two opposite qualities resolve into one of the basic human strengths, such as hope, purpose, fidelity, or wisdom (see Box 2).

Life's last stage according to Erikson, is the time of reckoning, of summing up. In old age, the concept of integrity gives to the struggle between the two opposites the sense that life was worthwhile and meaningful; despair, on the other hand, gives the feeling that life was wasted and should have been different from what it actually was. From these opposing attitudes arises wisdom, the understanding of oneself and life itself. (Erikson, 1976)

Box 2
The eight stages of life according to Erikson

	Opposites	Period	Basic strength
1.	Trust versus mistrust	Infancy	Hope
2.	Autonomy versus shame	Early childhood	Will
3.	Initiative versus guilt	Play age	Purpose
4.	Industry versus inferiority	School age	Competence
5.	Identity versus identity confusion	Adolescence	Fidelity
6.	Intimacy versus isolation	Young adulthood	Love
7.	Generativity versus stagnation	Maturity	Care
8.	Integrity versus despair	Old age	Wisdom

The essence of Erikson's lifespan development theory is that at each of life's crises, when passing from one stage to the next, there are appropriate rites of passage and those elements that have to be left behind. But as one advances into the new stage, one acquires new experiences and new insights. When approaching old age, just as at any other stage of life, one has to relinquish some social roles, such as that of the stressed executive, and accept new ones, such as that of the pensioner with time on his hands. One might miss the excitement of the busy workplace, but one can look forward to the peaceful stroll in the woods.

Case 3: Morris

Morris, aged 76, lives alone in a sheltered housing project on the outskirts of the city. Morris is a self-made man. He came to Israel by himself at the age of 18, leaving his whole family behind in Germany, the country of his birth. Four years later they were all wiped out, his parents, two brothers, his sister, her husband, and their little daughter. Morris was left alone in the world. He met Hannah, his future wife, on his first job in a textile factory. After they were married, they moved to a small town in the north, where they opened a small dress shop. Gradually the little town grew, and with it their business. Their three sons were born and Morris became quite affluent. The small shop grew into a large department store and Morris and his wife enjoyed several happy years, watching their children grow up, serving in the army, and furthering their education. Twenty years ago the blow fell. Morris will never forget that evening when the army jeep stopped at their gate and two officers descended from it. His youngest son, Gideon, had been killed in action. For Morris and his wife the world had come to an end. The two older children tried to comfort them but to no avail. Both Morris and Hannah felt as though a limb had been amputated and the wound was continually bleeding. Hannah could not stop crying and Morris could not concentrate on anything. It took them about two years to regain some kind of emotional equilibrium. Morris claims that Hannah's health began to deteriorate after Gideon's death. At the age of 60, Hannah died suddenly of a massive coronary. Morris tried to stay in the old house but the emptiness and loneliness drove him crazy. His two sons, their wives and children did their best to cheer him up and see to his needs but Morris came to a decision. He turned the business over to his sons who had been working with him all along, sold the house and bought a small flat in the sheltered housing project. Looking back at his long eventful life, with its joys and its sorrows, he decided that a new stage was ahead of him, a period when he would be alone and have to see to his own needs without being dependent upon his children, financially or emotionally. For him the sheltered housing seemed the ideal arrangement. He was not entirely alone but still had his privacy. Morris participated in many of the activities, such as a music appreciation class and a Bible class, and seemed very content. Every now and then he visited the department store, but felt rather out of place there, even though everybody was very glad to see him. Morris said that his working days were over and now he had the leisure and opportunity to pursue his hobbies, something he had had no time for in all the years in which he brought up his family and built his business. When summing up, Morris came to the conclusion that life, in spite of all the difficulties and sorrows was worthwhile. He weighed the gains – a loving family, a sense of achievement at having taken part in the establishing of a new state, against the losses – the loss of his family in the Holocaust, the loss of his son and of his beloved wife. He made up his mind to make the most of the time left to him.

Normal Aging versus Successful Aging versus Pathological Aging

Over the past few decades research in gerontology has attempted to define what is normal to the aging process and what is pathological. This differentiation is important in order to combat the stereotype of aging as a collection of diseases. Several basic understandings have been reached.

1. Though universal and common to all people in the different parts of the world, aging is a highly individual process, influenced by many different variables, both intrinsic and extrinsic. Among the intrinsic factors are the genetic, physical, and intrapsychic components. The extrinsic factors comprise the cultural, sociologic, and lifestyle components.

2. Not all age-associated changes are necessarily age-determined. It is true that with the increase in age there is a rise in the rate of morbidity, but that does not necessarily mean that disease is an integral part of old age.

3. Psychosocial factors and physiological processes are always interrelated, in old age even more so than in other age groups. Several studies have demonstrated that bereavement influences immunological functions such as lymphocyte and T-cell responses (Bartrop, 1977; Schleifer, 1979). On the other hand, enhanced control over one's life may produce gains in health status as well as increased activity and life satisfaction. (Schulz, 1977; Avorn, 1982).

4. In general, aging involves a reduction in the efficiency of the organism to respond to stress of all kinds, both physiological and psychological. In old age the state of equilibrium is more precarious, and it takes the self-regulating mechanisms longer to return to pre-stress homeostasis. Examples of this reduced response to physiological stress is the slow increase in pulse rate during exercise, and its slow return to normal, or the reduced reaction to extreme temperature changes often resulting in hypothermia. Stressful life events such as bereavement or relocation can cause severe reactions resulting in disease and even death.

During the last three decades numerous longitudinal and cross-sectional studies have demonstrated the effects of age on physiological variables such as systolic blood pressure and immune function. More recently the effects of aging have been associated with psychological variables such as cognitive and behavioral function. In populations which had been carefully screened for disease, certain changes occur which are 'normal' to the aging process. These physiological and psychological changes may be precursors of disease, and may influence the disease process, the possible outcome of treatment, and the likelihood of complications. Two examples are the need to monitor carefully the dosage of narcotic drugs because of the reduced renal function in old age; and the necessity to prevent pressure sores which develop easily in elderly patients because of their decreased blood supply and the trophic changes in the skin. Serious complications may occur.

The non-diseased elderly population, both within and across cultures, has great heterogenity. When we look more closely, we can see the immense differences in people's health status and quality of life in old age, in their physical, psychological, and social function. Old people who do not experience those physiological declines considered 'normal' in their age group, are viewed to have aged 'successfully'. That which is considered usual and normal in elderly people living in prosperous urban areas may be virtually non-existent among those living in poorer rural areas. To state one example, risk factors for cardiac disease such as elevated cholesterol levels and increased body weight are common in some urban societies, and are rare in simple rural communities.

'Normal' aging is not without risk. Each society must develop and implement measures to prevent possible disease processes and promote the general health of elderly people. Early diagnosis and early intervention are vital. This is true not only of definite disease processes but also of non-specific functional decline owing to general weakness, that results in a decrease in speed and distance of walking, and in the performance of various instrumental and advanced activities of daily living.

Research indicates that the 'normal' process of aging can be modified by paying attention to extrinsic factors such as diet and exercise. One example is that osteoporosis, a painful, crippling, and expensive condition, often considered to be 'normal' in the process of aging, can be prevented to a certain degree by eliminating risk factors such as smoking and alcohol, and by instituting programs of moderate exercise (Rowe and Kahn, 1987). There is a strong association between the health of elderly people and extrinsic, interrelated factors such as the level of education, the quality of the living arrangements, and the general economic status (Kitagawa et al., 1973).

Psychosocial factors such as family and social support are known to contribute to the health and general well-being of older people. Enhancing older people's sense of autonomy and control of their lives on the one hand, and increasing their social networks and feeling of connectedness on the other, has been shown to be important to the achievement of successful aging. Modern medicine has already achieved a dramatic increase in the lifespan; the next goal is an accompanying increase in health status and functional ability.

Gerontological Research, Dimensions, and Problems

The scientific disciplines comprising the study of old people are numerous and diverse. Multifaceted as the aging process itself, gerontology incorporates knowledge from the humanities, the biological and the behavioral sciences. All the social sciences are represented; gero-psychology is the study of inter and intra psychic processes, gero-sociology deals with the social aspects of the aging process and the changing roles of people as they grow older, gero-anthropology studies old people and their way of life in different cultures, and economics deals with the impact of the aging population on the society in which they live and, conversely, how they are affected by the economic situation of that society. Even seemingly unrelated subjects such as architecture, art, history, and literature have a place in gerontology.

In addition, the various health and welfare professions which care for elderly people and provide services for them, have developed into scientific disciplines with bodies of knowledge and empirical research of their own. Geriatrics, a fairly new branch in medicine, has developed only during the last five decades. Geriatricians, like pediatricians, have adopted a holistic approach to the elderly patient unlike the organ specialists of other medical branches. Other health professions such as nursing, physical and occupational therapy have also developed specialities in geriatrics. All these professionals and scientists study human aging from different perspectives using different scientific nomenclature and concepts. In order to arrive at comprehensive conclusions it is imperative that a common scientific language be developed. This lack of communication between the various disciplines might be one of the main reasons why interdisciplinary studies concerning the subject of aging are so few.

Most gerontological research was performed in the developed countries. It is virtually impossible to transfer information from these studies to the developing world. The social status, economic conditions, lifestyle, and result-ing health status in these societies are totally different. Only during the last few years have studies dealing specifically with the aged in developing countries been published.

Research designs involving elderly populations encounter several problems.

1. Cross-sectional studies investigating the effect of variables on the process of aging by comparing different age groups, need to consider the effect that time and historical events have on people living in different places at different times. For example, when comparing 20 year olds and 70 year olds in any country in Europe today in terms of physical factors such as height, one has to remember that the older subjects were young children during the second World War, and that their height would certainly be affected by their poor nutrition during their growing period. The same would be true for psychosocial variables, such as a sense of security, for the traumatic experience of the war in their childhood would certainly have an effect many years later.

2. Cohort studies present other difficulties. One has to remember that a cohort of elderly people may not necessarily represent the whole of the study population, for many would have died, and the remaining sample might represent only the survivors.

3. Longitudinal studies, where the same group of people is followed for many years, are suitable for measuring changes occurring over time: for example the study of how personality traits like assertiveness, or attitudes such as life satisfaction, are affected by the aging process. However, one must bear in mind

that, though abiding by the demands of validity, longitudinal studies are very expensive and not easy to perform. It might be difficult to contact and follow all the subjects over a protracted period of time, subjects might drop out of the study and if there is a selective drop-out, the results might be totally distorted. For example: in a longitudinal study on the effect of aging on health practices in rural Africa, those subjects who are better educated and more affluent may have dropped out from the study because they moved away and could not be located. Another problem encountered in longitudinal studies is that some measures which might have been relevant at the beginning of the study, are not relevant 30 years later. For example a variable such as job satisfaction, which is very important in young adulthood, will not be relevant in old age. The same problem occurs with the use of research instruments. For example, the Barthel Index which was the instrument of choice for functional assessment 20 years ago has been proved to be of low reliability, and is rarely used today. (Lewis and Bottomley, 1994). In summary, gerontological research is beset with many pitfalls and requires careful planning and considerations if these are to be avoided.

The ages of man

In a study of old people one must remember that chronological age is only one dimension of the aging process. A person's *biological* age indicates his state of health and physical condition; his *social* age reflects his passage through life's social roles, and his *psychological* age indicates his intellectual and emotional functioning.

There is usually very little correlation among the different aspects of aging: one 70-year-old man might be in excellent physical health and have the constitution of an average 40 year old, but judging by his social function he might be 90 years old as he has abolished all his social roles and does not interact with any of his family members or former friends. On the other hand we might encounter a 95-year-old man, who is totally 'with it': involved in family affairs and professional matters, keeping up to date with what is going on in the world through the media and computer networks, but is unable to see to his most basic physical needs.

Physical aspects of aging

The distinction between aging and disease has intrigued scientists and philosophers since ancient times. Aristotle who lived between 384 and 322 BC noted that 'aging is not a disease, because it is not contrary to nature' (Guillerme, 1963). Nevertheless, because of the high incidence of disease in old age and the difficulty of separating it from the effects of physiological, psychological, and social factors, it is tempting to equate aging with disease. As people grow older they are more prone to chronic conditions such as arthritis and osteoporosis. In addition, they experience sensory deficits such as decreased hearing and sight, and social losses such as the death of a spouse and friends. Some suffer slight to severe cognitive deterioration. All these factors tend to interact and become the underlying causes of distinctly pathological conditions, such as fractures and depression. Many studies of healthy elderly people have succeeded in isolating factors that are typical of normal aging, such as muscle weakness, synaptic delay, and a decline in peristalsis, vital capacity, and cardiac output. These changes are usually slight and do not compromise the older person in everyday life, but as soon as the organism is put under physiological or psychological stress, problems in function may occur. These changes do not necessarily appear in all physiological systems or in all individuals. Many of them can be prevented or postponed by adopting appropriate lifestyles which will promote and improve general health. Nonetheless, it is important for health professionals to be aware of the common physical changes which occur, as they complicate disease processes and have an important effect on the implementation and results of the treatment.

Case 4: Elsa

Elsa, an 80-year-old widow, was referred to the geriatric rehabilitation center. She has suffered from Parkinson's disease for the past ten years. She had been coping fairly well, but lately a sharp decline in her physical and mental condition has been noted. At the staff meeting after the first week, the physical therapist reported that Elsa was not concentrating and was not responding satisfactorily to treatment. The occupational therapist also reported that she was uncooperative and seemed to be disoriented. But when the social worker reported that Elsa's husband, to whom she had been happily married for 55 years, had died suddenly only two months ago, it was understood

that she was still in the process of mourning. In addition, the speech therapist reported a slight hearing deficit, which might explain some of Elsa's distracted behavior. The physical and occupational therapy departments were large open spaces with a lot of background noises, such as music on the radio, conversations between the other patients and the staff, and the lawn mower in the garden. It was decided that Elsa should be treated in a separate quiet room. More opportunities would be provided to help her to work through her grief by talking about her deceased husband to the therapists, who would lend a sympathetic ear during the process of their specific treatments. At the staff meeting two weeks later, a distinct improvement in her physical and social function was reported.

Psychological Aspects of Aging

Psychological aging can be defined as

'the process of adaptation to a changing internal and external environment' (Shanan, 1991).

This includes the different intellectual functions and emotional reactions to disease or disability, which have an important impact on the way older people cope in everyday life.

Cognitive functions

Information processing Information processing can be defined as the understanding, reaction, and response to a single stimulus, such as a flashing light. It may also be defined in terms of the perception, analysis, storage, and retrieval of information. Both sets of capabilities are affected by aging, though usually not to an extensive degree. Several studies have shown that there is a distinct slowing in reaction time, regardless of the type of sensory input or the motor response. In ordinary circumstances this general 'slowing down' is not of great importance and often can be compensated for. But in some complex situations, as in driving a car, or when crossing the street, it might be crucial. This increase in reaction time, is more pronounced in the more complex functions. It is believed to be caused by synaptic delay, but is also attributed to the 'speed – accuracy trade-off'. Here it is presumed that older people subconsciously prefer to ensure an accurate response at the expense of speed. It is interesting that this slowing down does not occur in all functions. In those areas where the individual has achieved expertise, the organism will find ways to compensate. Salthouse (1984, 1987) found no difference in the typing rate of older typists despite slower responses in other activities, Arthur Rubinstein was the same magician of the piano in his later years as earlier in his career.

Health professionals such as physical and occupational therapists must take this delayed response into account when planning treatment programs in which elderly people participate. As the pace common for younger people needs to be slowed down, especially in the more complex exercises, it should be carefully considered whether to combine older patients in the same group with patients who are much younger.

Intelligence and memory Many longitudinal studies of intelligence and memory have shown that there is a slight decline after the age of 60 in measures such as the speed of adding columns of numbers or visualization of objects in a two-dimensional plane (Schaie, 1983). How important are these slight changes? How do they affect the function of elderly people in everyday life? Research indicates that older people who are experts in their field have the ability to use their cumulative experience to compensate for the decline in fluid intelligence, which is dependent upon reaction time. They seem to 'encapsulate' processes such as attention, memory, and reasoning, with the products of these processes, such as knowledge in a specific domain. This form of intelligence, called crystallized intelligence, not only does not decline in old age, but might even increase (Rybash *et al.*, 1986). Much of the recent research in the psychology of aging has focused on memory, usually adopting the information processing model, which includes encoding, storage, transformation, and retrieval of information. A decline in all these processes occurs in elderly people when tested in a psychological laboratory. Different types of memory have been described: sensory memory concerned with visual or auditory information, primary short-term memory concerning information that is retrieved after a very short time, secondary memory concerning newly learned information, and tertiary memory concerning remote memories of past events. It seems that secondary memory is most affected in old age (Kimmel, 1990).

Decline in memory functions does not affect all older people, and a great variability in memory performance exists. Many old people perform very well in memory tests, such as the immediate recall of pictures, and react to memory enhancing cues just as younger adults do.

The perceived decline in everyday memory which causes many older people much anxiety, is controversial. It seems that exercises to improve memory such as playing bridge or memory games, can have as great an effect on old people as on younger people. On the other hand, many old people complain of forgetfulness, of not remembering people's names, of going to fetch something and forgetting what it was. Several strategies can be learnt to compensate for these lapses in memory, such as making shopping lists, having a specific place for objects such as car keys and reading glasses, or developing a set routine of actions before leaving the house: first checking the stove, then closing the windows, locking the kitchen door, etc. Older people who are forgetful are encouraged to concentrate on the task and focus on performing it, to 'switch off the automatic pilot' while performing everyday activities.

Learning Learning is closely associated with memory. It is defined as a change in behavior as a result of the acquisition of new information or a new skill; this change will often be measured by improvement in task performance or by retrieval of stored information. Thus, learning will be useless without memory. It is believed that there is a gradual decline in learning ability, involving the encoding of new information, after the age of 60, but we have seen that elderly people are very serious students in university programs and compensate for their slower pace by their higher motivation (Kimmel, 1990).

The learning ability of older people is highly affected by external conditions, such as distractions in the environment, sensory deprivation, and unsuitable teaching strategies. As rehabilitation following illness or injury is mainly a learning process, therapists must do their utmost to enhance the learning abilities of their patients by applying the following principles:

1. Demonstrate that the information or skill to be learnt is relevant to the needs of the patient.
2. Allow enough time for the information to be absorbed.
3. Present the information in a structured form to facilitate its encoding and storage.
4. Make the new knowledge consistent with the existing knowledge.
5. Use all possible senses in the learning process.
6. Provide immediate and encouraging feedback.
7. Reinforce the verbal learning process with written instructions and reminders.

Wisdom Perhaps the most important aspect of cognitive function in old age is wisdom. This is defined as

'the ability which enables the individual to grasp human nature, which operates on the principles of contradiction, paradox and change' (Clayton, 1982).

In contrast to intelligence, which enables the individual to think logically and to conceptualize – both of which are non-social and impersonal abilities – wisdom is an essentially social, interpersonal skill, involving insight, knowledge of oneself and understanding of other people. It seems that this ability is not affected by the aging process, but is often enhanced by the person's life experience. Wisdom comprises the ability to grasp the relative importance of life situations, to make good judgments in conditions of uncertainty, and to solve problems of a social and interpersonal nature. These qualities earned older people the respect and honor of the community in traditional societies; for example we learn from the Old Testament that the leaders and judges of the People of Israel were the elders of the tribe.

Intrapersonal perspective

Personality changes in old age The definition of personality focuses on three main aspects:

1. Uniqueness, those special qualities which make a person different from other people.

2. Stability, those traits which are relatively stable over time.

3. The way the person interacts with the physical and social environment in which he lives.

All three dimensions pertain to the subject of personality in old people. The elderly have diverse personalities; the longer they live and the more they interact with their environment, the more unique they become. Therefore it is more difficult to categorize old people into distinct personality types than any other age group. Aging is a developmental process. Does a person's personality change as he passes through life, or will it remain fairly stable? Which are the personality traits that are more stable? What are the aspects which change over time?

Personality has two distinct facets: change and stability, and both may exist simultaneously, incorporated in the concept of continuity. This suggests that

'many personality traits change slowly and by imperceptible degrees, so that at any time the individual is recognizably the same' (English and English, 1958).

From our observations of everyday life we see the veracity of this definition. Older people resemble themselves as they were when they were younger, more than they resemble each other. The likeable little old lady was probably a pleasant, outgoing person when she was young, and the cantankerous old man probably was unsociable and complaining in his earlier days as well.

Several longitudinal studies have focused on personality types and how they change over time. Shanan and his colleagues followed 224 subjects for over 20 years, attempting to answer the question 'Who ages how?'. Two important measures of ego functioning were chosen in order to arrive at a typology of personality: styles of coping behavior and internal consistency. Four distinct personality types were identified:

1. The active integrated copers, who constituted 42% of the subjects. These were well adjusted, hard working, socially integrated individuals. This group preserved their type identity with only minor changes throughout the study period.

2. The dependent passive copers, who constituted 38% of the subjects. These seemed insecure, easily dominated by others, lacking in initiative and imagination. This group, like the active copers, retained their identity over time.

3. The failing over-copers, who constituted 8% of the sample. These were people over-involved in work, compulsively orderly, dis-

satisfied with themselves and their achievements, and far from happy. They derived little satisfaction from family life and social interaction, being totally involved in their careers.

4. The self-negating under-copers. These constituted 12% of the sample. These were rather moody, unhappy loners, lacking in self-confidence and personal ambition.

The last two types did not remain consistent over time; new and different personality types emerged in their place. On follow up, the over-copers changed into 'the tired heroes', who though still rather unhappy, compensated for their loneliness by trying to attract attention as 'heroes', demonstrating pride in the way they dealt with their life and their aging. On the other hand, the self-negating under-copers appeared tense, extremely unhappy and depressed. The fact that they appeared to be complacent and accepting of their fate, earned them the name of 'disenchanted moralists' in this study.

One of the conclusions of this study is that about 80% of the people do not change very much in their personality traits as they grow older. Most people cope with life events in a fairly satisfactory way. Those who demonstrate extreme unhappiness and dissatisfaction with life in their old age were probably not very happy individuals in their younger years.

Case 5: David

David suffered a massive stroke which left him totally paralyzed on the right side of his body.

The first few weeks were complete agony for him. He had been self-sufficient and independent all his life. Now, when he needed help in the simplest activities, he felt that he would have been better off dead. He hated being washed and fed like a baby and was extremely impatient with himself, his family, and the hospital staff. After a while, he was transferred to a geriatric rehabilitation center where he received intensive therapy. Slowly he recovered his spirits and began to participate actively in his rehabilitation program. He made sure to be on time for his appointments and worked extremely hard, not only with the physical and occupational therapists but also by himself after they had left. His sons and daughters-in-law visited regularly, offering support and encouragement. Very gradually David improved. Soon he was able to dress himself and walk short distances with the aid of a tripod cane. He started making plans to return to his little apartment in the sheltered housing project. His son wanted him to move in with him, but was met with blunt refusal: David was going to live by himself, and resume his former life pattern as far as possible. David's recovery was better than anyone expected.

Based on the research literature and our own observations, it seems the coping mechanisms developed throughout the lifespan are those that will follow individuals into their old age. Morris had to deal with several difficulties in his life, including tragic losses. He had started out alone in a strange country, without the support of family or friends, with no financial backing, and had succeeded in establishing himself as a successful business man, well respected in his community. He established a loving family and enjoyed the blessings of life.

He also had his share of life's tribulations and tragedies: the loss of his whole family in Europe, the untimely death of his son, and lately, the death of his beloved wife. Morris always managed to come through, and coped well. The best predictor of a person's ability to deal with a difficult situation is the way he coped with previous critical life events.

Sexuality and aging Sexuality is a complex term which means many things to many people. Here we refer to sexuality as the actual biological function of sexual intercourse and the accompanying desires, fantasies, and emotional responses. Many myths and misconceptions have to be dispersed when discussing the sexuality of older persons. Some of the mythology suggests that sexual desire and activity is limited to young adulthood and that older people lack the interest and the ability to be sexually active. In fact, the opposite is true. In spite of some physiological, age-related changes in the urogenital system, most healthy elderly people retain their sexuality and their capacity for enjoying sexual relationships, provided they have a suitable partner. Small adaptations to facilitate the sexual act, such as increased manual stimulation for men, or vaginal lubrication for women, might be necessary. With increasing age, intercourse may becomes less frequent and may be viewed as less important, with the emphasis usually shifting towards the non-coital aspects of a loving interpersonal relationship. Touching, caressing, and bodily nearness are extremely important, as they make one feel loved and cared for by one's partner.

Expression of one's sexuality among older people is strongly influenced by social mores and environmental factors. Women usually marry men older than themselves and live longer than their spouses, so many are left without partners in their old age. Expressions of sexuality in the form of intimate behavior in public with the opposite sex is often frowned upon by society. Older persons who show an interest in sex are considered 'dirty old men and women'. This poses a problem for some elderly people, especially for those living in institutions where the lack of privacy to pursue and develop intimate relationships and the frequently encountered negative attitudes of staff members might effectively limit or prevent them from satisfying one of life's most basic needs.

How can empathetic therapists who work with older patients in institutions enable human contact? It is important to acknowledge and respond to the need all humans have to touch and be touched, to give and receive affection and create an environment where this will be possible.

The impact of life events: retirement, bereavement and relocation Retirement marks the social transition point between the middle and later years of life. When Bismarck, the German Chancellor, created the Old Age and Survivors Act in 1889, it was considered one of the most advanced social laws of his time. He was advised to set the retirement age at 65 because, at the time, few people survived to that age. Today, with the increased life span, many who reach age 65, still have many years before them. The transition to retirement marks a major event in their lives. The reactions of people to retirement are closely linked to the values and beliefs of the society and culture within which they live. For many middle class, urban working people in the Western world, retirement at the obligatory age of 65 marks a time for more leisure with relative financial security. If they have a pension scheme and social security benefits they can begin to enjoy life and do some of the wonderful things they have always wanted to do, such as pursue favorite hobbies, travel abroad, or even start a new career. Others, for whom work provided the core meaning for their life, and who developed few if any outside interests, retirement marks a difficult transition. We find them trying to hold onto their jobs even though they might not derive much satisfaction from them. For others, such as kibbutz members in Israel, work is a cherished value; they continue working for as long as they possibly can, very often well into their eighties, moving on to less physically demanding jobs as they grow older and more frail.

An individual's personality is also an important factor in the transition process into retirement. Mature, well-adjusted individuals, who have accepted the reality of their advancing age, will make the best adjustment to their retirement and enjoy it. Others, for whom their profession or job was the primary support of their self-efficacy, will view their retirement as the end of meaningful existence. Some of these over-copers suffer their first coronary immediately after retirement.

One of the more painful experiences in old age is bereavement and grief over the death of a spouse and close friends. The reaction to losing one's loved ones is deeply intense sometimes. Symptoms of incessant crying, loss of appetite, impaired concentration, and inability to sleep are common. Often a distinct decline

in general health will occur, resulting in an increase in physical complaints and visits from the physician (Parkes, 1987). Frequently rituals help to 'work through' the grief, such as the seven day mourning period in the Jewish religion, when it is customary to visit the bereaved and talk about the deceased. For others, this mourning period, during which the person's physical and social function is somewhat impaired, may last up to a year or two. When treating patients who are in mourning, it is important that health professionals be aware of the fact and take this into consideration when planning and supervising the treatment program.

Relocation is another event which might be traumatic for elderly people in Western cultures. After living in the same place for decades, elderly people may need to move to a more supportive environment, such as a retirement village, sheltered housing, or an old age home for a variety of reasons. When their health and functional ability deteriorates, some are obliged to move to a nursing home. Even when the move was by choice, the change is often a difficult experience. It takes time before one adjusts to the new environment. During this period of adjustment some people become depressed or even disoriented, others have difficulty in dealing with the separation from familiar places and old friends. In African and Eastern cultures it is customary that even very disabled old people remain within the extended family circle; they are not removed from the community in which they have lived for most of their lives. Sadly, this is rapidly changing with increasing urbanization and Westernization of these societies.

Social Aspects of Aging

Status and social roles

In primitive societies, the communal knowledge and experience necessary for survival was stored in the memory of the old people. Margaret Mead (1972) attributes man's comparative longevity to the need of the society to have long-living members who could remember important information, such as the location of water holes in periods of drought. It was the role of the younger members of the society to gather new knowledge and skills, and the role of the old members to conserve the existing knowledge. It is not surprising that in these cultures older people were honored and respected by all members of the community.

The development of symbolic language and writing changed the way knowledge and skills were stored and transmitted to the next generation. With the passage of time, the respected status of the old people declined. In modern developed societies the elderly are no longer perceived as the wise leaders of the community. Their 'social death' may precede their biological death by many years. This is in contrast to some African cultures where, until recently, the spirits of the deceased served an important social function long after death. As one ages in modern Western societies, people lose their previous social roles, such as head of the household and breadwinner. They are manuevered into new roles which society has designed for them, such as the role of the retiree (Hazan, 1988).

Today, older people in Western societies are a diverse group of individuals. The percentage of older people in the general population is steadily increasing; they enjoy better health and education and are more active politically and socially, but they usually do not occupy positions of power and many are victims of long existing-negative stereotypes. Many old people are below the average income level and experience a decline in lifestyle after retirement except for those who are financially well off and socially powerful.

In non-Western societies, the status of the elderly varies, and is closely related to other cultural norms and traditions. In some cultures old people enjoy great respect and honor, especially if they possess power, money or some special magic valued by that society; in others they are allowed to die if they are no longer productive (Beauvoir, 1972). People bring their attitudes, cultural norms, and practices regarding the aged when they move from one part of the world to another. Diversity in ethnic mores and practices poses a challenge to health professionals who seek to accommodate the treatment program to the specific social and cultural background of each patient.

Integration versus segregation, humanization versus dehumanization

Hazan (1988) proposed a social model that allows one to analyze the position of the elderly within a society along two perpendicular axes. The first axis, segregation versus integration, is a socially administrative concept. At one end we find the elderly completely separated from the general society; at the other extreme they are totally integrated and continue to fulfill their roles within the society. The humanization versus dehumanization axis is a socially symbolic concept. At one end we find old people who are complete human beings with distinct and unique identities; at the other extreme we will find the old people who have lost their identity and whose social roles are non-existent. Four distinct combinations will be found at the extremes, and in between innumerable possibilities can exist (see Figure 7.1).

The first combination is integration with humanization, in which older people are an integral part of the society, contribute to it, and are honored by it. They therefore regard themselves and are considered by others in their society as complete human beings. This combination is usually found in simple, rural, non-writing societies. People retain their power because of their knowledge and wealth and continue to function as the leaders and teachers of their society. In Western societies a parallel can be found in aging statesmen who are very powerful because of their social and political position.

An example of the second combination, integration with dehumanization, is found in newly retired professionals in developed countries. They continue to retain some of their social roles, but lose one of the main symbols of the 'complete person' based on Western standards. They are no longer involved in a profession. Upon retirement many of these people experience a severe identity crisis. They consider themselves, and are regarded by others as lesser persons than when they were part of the working community.

The third combination is segregation with humanization, which exists in some retirement villages. There elderly people have set up independent communities, separated from their families and the rest of society. The members of these communities are usually well off financially, and can maintain themselves without assistance from others. They retain their identity and have distinct social roles within the community. This segregation is voluntary, so these people are usually comfortable and content with their circumstances.

The last combination is segregation with dehumanization, a condition which is often found in nursing homes for the elderly. These places are actually 'total institutions' (Goffman, 1961) in which one group of people, the professional and administrative staff, are in control of every aspect of the lives of the other group, the patients. Many different institutions exist for the elderly, some very grand and expensive, others not fit for human beings; they all have in common staff members who set the rules, often for reasons of good management and efficiency, and patients who have to abide by them. Those patients who do not abide by the rules are termed 'non-functioning', or 'non-adapting'. These patients have to relinquish personal preferences and lifelong habits in order to conform to the regulations of the institution, thereby losing their individuality

Figure 7.1 Hazan's model of integration and humanization.

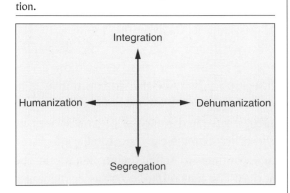

and uniqueness as human beings. Those working with institutionalized elderly people can often alleviate some of these dehumanizing factors by enabling some freedom of choice, and some bending of the rigid rules, thus enhancing the quality of life.

The model proposed by Hazan provides the dimensions to analyze the position of elderly people in a society within a social perspective.

Health, Health Assessment, and Health Promotion

Health as defined by Ivan Illitch is the

'adjustment to growth and development, to recovery after injury and illness, the coping with suffering and the calm expectation of death'.

This definition may be appropriately applied in the circumstances of the elderly, who are usually healthy, but may not be in a state of

'complete physical, mental, and social well-being'

as was defined by the World Health Organization in 1970. Both definitions have in common the concept that health is not only a physical state but also includes emotional and social aspects. The manner in which the elderly perceive their health is often more important than the objective evidence provided by physical examinations and medical tests. Indeed the number and severity of the medical diagnoses is not indicative of an elderly person's subjective state of health. We often encounter very frail and disabled old people who will profess to be 'quite healthy' while others, who have only a few objective pathological findings, will feel very ill.

The results of many studies identify the adverse effect of emotional factors on physical health. Loneliness, grief, and feelings of hopelessness frequently are translated into physical complaints that lead to unnecessary visits to doctors and therapists (Wack, 1982). Rodin identified that there is probably a link between a sense of control and the ability of the immune system to respond effectively in old people. (Rodin, 1986). Essential components of the treatment planning for health professionals therefore include attention to the emotional needs of the older patient with efforts to reduce the feelings of stress, and strategies to enhance control over one's life.

Impairment, Disability, and Handicap in Old Age

There is a distinct difference between the impairment caused by an injury or disease, the resulting disability, and the possible handicap this disability might entail.

Impairment is defined by the World Health Organisation (1980) as

'any loss or abnormality of psychological, physiological, or anatomical structure or function'.

This implies that impairment is the direct consequence of an injury or disease, a deviation from the norm, and the exterior manifestation of the loss or disease.

Disability, on the other hand, is defined by the World Health Organization as 'any restriction or lack (resulting from the impairment) of ability to perform an activity in the manner or within the range considered normal for a human being'.

Disability deals therefore, with functional problems rather than the pathological condition causing them. Often the main aim of our professional intervention with older people is to maintain their function and minimize the disability caused by the aging process itself, even without the presence of a specific injury.

The concept of the term 'handicap' is different. It is defined as

'a disadvantage for a given individual, resulting from an impairment or a disability, that limits or prevents the fulfilment of a role that is normal (depending on age, sex, and social and cultural factors) for that individual' (WHO, 1980).

A handicap is a very individual, culture-bound experience; that which is considered a handicap for one person is not necessarily a handicap for another.

When assessing the health status of an elderly person it is important to determine the physical impairments, correctly diagnose the various diseases, and to assess the physical, mental, emotional, and social function. Because of the existing discrepancies between the impairment, the disability, and the handicap, the comprehensive functional assessment is often the better indicator of an elderly person's general health. This assessment may have very little relationship to the older person's perception of quality of life.

Elderly people are prone to deconditioning, debilitating diseases, and injuries which have severe effects on their physical, mental, and social function. After a specific event such as a cerebrovascular accident or hip fracture, a process of rehabilitation may be instigated and continued until some degree of function has been restored. However, sometimes the general function of an elderly person may decline for no apparent reason. Family members or attending physicians may be aware of a slow, gradual downward spiral, which they attribute to 'just aging' and dismiss it. Dysfunction in the elderly, sometimes referred to as 'hypokinetic disease' is described as a distinct process of morbidity. A vicious circle, involving all systems, occurs. The older person frequently adjusts to the overall deconditioning and deterioration, limiting general activity accordingly. This may lead to severely restricted mobility and severe depression. Too often older people are referred for intensive, costly diagnosis and rehabilitation, when it is too late to reverse this process. Periodic, comprehensive functional assessment of the elderly would detect the early changes in function in a timely manner, making it possible to introduce suitable intervention. Thus the ravages of old age could perhaps be diminished and postponed, making Longfellow's optimistic outlook on old age possible:

'Whatever poet, orator, or sage
May say of it, old age is still old age.
It is the waning, not the crescent moon;
The dusk of evening, not the blaze of noon;
What then? Shall we sit idly down and say
The night hath come; it is no longer day?
Even the oldest tree some fruit may bear;
For age is opportunity no less
Than youth itself, though in another dress,
And as the evening twilight fades away
The sky is filled with stars, invisible by day.
Something remains for us to do or dare;'

Moritori Salutamus by Henry Wadsworth Longfellow.

References

Avorn, J, Langer, E (1982) Induced disability in nursing home patients: a controlled trial. *Journal of the American Geriatric Society* 30: 397–400.

Bartrop, RW, Lazarus, L, Luckhurst, E, Kiloh, LG, Penny, R (1977) Depressed lymphocyte function after bereavement. *The Lancet* i: 834–836

Beauvoir, S de (1972) *The Coming of Age.* New York: Putnam (translated by Obrian, P).

Bonder, BR, Wagner, MB (1994) *Functional Performance in Older Adults.* Philadelphia: FA Davis.

Buehler, C (1968) The developmental structure of goal-setting in group and individual studies. In: Buehler, Massarik (eds) *The Course of human Life,* pp. 27–54. New York: Springer.

Clayton, V (1982) Wisdom and intelligence: the nature and function of knowledge in the later years. *International Journal of Aging and Human Development* 15: 315–321.

Cole, TR (1993) *The Journey of Life.* Cambridge: University Press.

Crews, JE (1994) The demographic, social, and conceptual contexts of aging and vision loss. *Journal of the American Optometric Association* 65: 63–86.

Cumming, E, Henry, WE (1961) *Growing old: The Process of Disengagement.* New York: Basic Books.

English, HB, English, AC (1958) *A Comprehensive Dictionary of Psychological and Psycho–analytical Term* New York: David Mckay.

Erikson, EH (1976) Reflections on Dr. Borg's Life Cycle. *Daedalus* 105: 1–28.

Goffman, E (1961) *Asylums.* Chicago: Aldine.

Harmon, D (1986) Free radical theory of aging: role of free radical in the origination and evaluation of life, aging and disease processes. In: Johnson, JE, Walford, RL, Harmon, D, Miguel, J (Eds) *Free Radicals, Aging and Degenerative Diseases,* pp. 3–50. New York: Alan Liss

Hayflick, L (1987) Origins of longevity. In: Warner, HR, Butler, RN, Sprott, RL, Schneider (Eds), *Modern Biological Theories of Aging,* pp. 21–34. New York: Raven Press.

Hazan, H (1988) *Aging as a Social Phenomenon,* 2nd edn. Israel: University on the Air Publications.

Illich I (1976) *Medical Nemesis.* New York: Pantheon Books

Isaacs, B (1992) *The Challenge of Geriatric Medicine.* Oxford University Press.

Jung, CG (1971) The stages of life. In: Campbell, J (ed) *The Portable Jung,* pp. 3–22. New York: Viking.

Kane, RA, Kane, RL (1988) *Assessing the Elderly,* 12th edn. Toronto: Lexington Books.

Kimmel, DC (1990) *Adulthood and Aging,* 3rd edn. New York: Wiley & Sons.

Kitagawa, EM, Hauser, PM (1973) *Differential Mortality in the United States: A Study in Socioeconomic Epidemiology.* Cambridge, MA: Harvard University Press.

Lewis, C (1985) Psychological aspects of aging. In: Lewis, C (Ed) *Aging and the Health Care Challenge.* Philadelphia: Davis

Lewis, CB, Bottomley, JM (1994) *Geriatric Physical Therapy.* Connecticut: Appleton & Lange.

Mead, M (1972) Long living in cross-cultural perspective. *Paper presented at the meeting of the Gerontological Society of America, San Juan.*

Parkes, CM (1987) *Bereavement: Studies of Grief in Adult Life,* 2nd American edn. Madison CT: International University Press.

Rodin, J (1986) Aging and health: effects of the sense of control. *Science* 233: 1271–1276.

Rowe, JW, Kahn, RL (1987) Human aging: usual and successful. *Science* 237: 143–149.

Rybash, JM, Hoyer, WJ, Rodin, PA (1986) *Adult Cognition and Aging: Developmental Changes in Processing, Knowing and Thinking.* New York: Pergamon.

Salthouse, TA (1984) Effects of age and skill in typing. *Journal of Experimental Psychology: General* 113: 345–371.

Salthouse, TA (1987) Age, experience and compensation. In Schooler, C, Schaie, KW (eds) *Cognitive Functioning and Social Structure over the Life Course,* pp. 142–157. NJ: Ablex.

Schaie, KW (1983) The Seattle longitudinal study: a 21 year exploration of psychometric intelligence in adulthood. In: Schaie, KW (Ed) *Longitudinal Studies of Adult Psychological Development,* pp. 64–135. New York: Guilford Press

Schaie, KW, Willis, SL (1986) Can decline in adult intellectual functioning be reversed? *Developmental Psychology* 22: 223–232.

Schultz, R, Brenner, G (1977) Relocation of the aged. A review and theoretical analysis. *Journal of Gerontology* 32: 323–333

Shanan, J (1991) Who and how: Some unanswered questions in adult development. *Journal of Gerontology* 46: 306–316.

Starr, BD (1985) Sexuality and aging. *Annual review of Gerontology and Geriatrics* 5: 97–126.

Wack, JT (1982) Appraisals and patterning of effect in encounters with everyday stressors. *Dissertaion Abstracts International* 43:1601B (University Microfilms No. 82-22332).

Walford, RL (1981) Immunopathology of aging. In: Eisdorfer, C (Ed) *Annual Review of Gerontology and Geriatrics.* New York: Springer Publishing.

Wickler, W (1991) *The Biology of the Ten Commandments,* 7th edn. Munich: R Riper & Co.

WHO (1980) *International Classification of Impairments, Disabilities, and Handicaps.* Geneva: World Health Organization.

8

Aging With Illness

Cecelia Eales

Introduction
•
Population Aging in the Developed World
•
Population Aging in the Developing World
•
Disease in the Elderly Population
•
Treatment
•
Conclusion

Introduction

What does it mean to grow old 'gracefully' or 'successfully' in our society? The word 'old' is culturally defined, so each of us needs to look at the norms and definitions of our own country to find the meaning. One definition suggests that successful aging is a prolongation of minimal illness and disability coupled with a maximum participation in, and enjoyment of life (Baltes and Baltes, 1991). If we accept this definition we could go on to agree with Gonzalez-Aragon (1984) when he suggests that psychological factors are more decisive than chronological age, in the aging process, for quality of life during old age. Two

common life events cause stress in the elderly: the death of a spouse and the loss of physical health. Both may result in reduced feelings of self-worth and competence. The loss of health reduces the capacity to participate in daily activities, and this threatens the sense of control over environmental challenges leading to feelings of helplessness and despair.

We believe the aim of the health care system for elderly people should be to delay the onset of illness, reducing the final period of infirmity and illness to the shortest possible time. The most effective way to achieve this is health education and preventative medicine to maintain mobility and function. One should constantly bear in mind that changes in lifestyle even in late life may result in improved health, effectively decreasing the incidence of chronic diseases associated with advancing age (Rabbit, 1992).

In this chapter the elderly population in the developed and developing worlds is the focus of discussion. Some differences including social and economic factors will be highlighted. The implications of health care for patients with acute and chronic disease will be discussed using the models of cardiovascular disease and stroke because these diseases are the most prevalent in the developed as well as the developing worlds. Little information is available about disease incidence and treatment in the developing world. That which exists will be discussed and contrasted with what is known in developed countries. Disease prevention, health promotion, and the impact of physical disabilities that occur with aging are of great importance to every society. This chapter will include discussion related to problems of hospitalization and institutionalization for the elderly, dementia in aging, inactivity and exercise, psychological perspectives on providing health care, and some of the costs to caregivers of providing care to the elderly.

Population Aging in the Developed World

The population over the age of 65 is growing at a rate of 2.5 percent per year. This is faster than the rate for the total population. By the year 2020 the median age in Italy, Switzerland, and Germany will be 47 years. Unless the birth rate rises dramatically, these countries, and many other developed coun-

tries, face a future in which nearly half of the population will be 50 years old or more.

Within the population of the elderly, different age groups grow at different rates. The fastest growing segment in many developed countries is the 'old old', defined as people over the age of 80 years. Gains in life expectancy at age 65 now outpace increases in life expectancy at birth, in large part due to the reduction in heart disease and stroke in middle-aged and older adults. Men at age 65 can expect to live for another 15 years and women another 18 years (Suzman et al., 1992a). The quality of increased life expectancy is affected by two major factors – smoking and alcohol consumption. Life expectancy may be divided into three categories (Suzman et al., 1992b):

1. active life expectancy, free of disability.
2. disabled life expectancy.
3. institutionalized life expectancy.

Active life expectancy is characterized as life without a serious and chronic disability. There is a sharp decline in the active life expectancy between ages 65 and 85. Females live on average 5 years longer than males and have a corresponding longer period of disability and institutionalized care. In the developed world the elderly are a heterogeneous group. Two thirds of the population over 65 rate their health as good to excellent, 75 percent have no difficulties with activities of daily living. The majority of the people over the age of 60 live in urban communities (Barry and Eathorne, 1994). In the developing world the majority of older people live in rural areas, and die before reaching the age of 65 years.

In the developed world the ratio of older men to older women is generally higher in rural than in urban areas. Elderly women are more likely than elderly men to live in urban areas. This may be related to marital status, as elderly women are more likely to be widowed and prefer to live near their children and social services.

Education is an important component of health, economic achievement, and the ability to engage actively in all aspects of a modern society. Major differences in the educational status exist between the elderly and younger people. More than 90 percent of people between the ages of 15 and 34 years have completed primary school education; the comparable rates for people over the age of 65 is below 60 percent. In developed countries, the young old, who are 65 to 75 years old have a relatively higher level of education than do the old, who are 75 years and older. Education is strongly associated with health. Those with higher levels of education tend to live longer (Kitagawa and Hauser, 1973; Sagan, 1987). The reasons for this connection are many, including the fact that a well-informed and educated public is more receptive to public health campaigns and is better able to take more responsibility for maintaining personal health. Retirement is associated with loss of income and a resultant economic vulnerability. Income declines and so does the ability to replace assets. Social benefits thus become more important with advancing age.

More male than female babies are born each year and male mortality rates are higher at all ages. At the age of 30 there is usually a greater proportion of females. Because of the lasting effect of the Second World War, with high mortality rates for males age 15 to 25, the elderly male/female ratio is as high as 1:2. Thus the social, economic, and health prob-lems of this elderly population are largely those of women.

The marital status of the elderly is closely related to their living arrangements and eco-nomic, social, and psychological well-being. Marital status also directly influences how care is provided in coping with ill health and func-tional disability owing to chronic disease. Today we find a changing social structure in which more people are living together, they marry later or not at all, and there is a lower rate of childbearing. If these trends persist there will be more older people who are not married who have fewer children to support them. This has the potential to produce an increasing burden on the supportive services (Myers, 1990).

A number of factors affect the quality of liv-ing arrangements for older people, including marital, financial, health status, and the size of the family. Cultural values are also important. These circumstances that have an impact on the quality of living are set within a cultural context including the social and economic policies of a country. For example, at the social level there are broad policies that support the family, as well as specific policies that allow for social support, which will in turn provide spe-cial services to the elderly in the community to allow them to remain in the community although they can no longer manage inde-pendently. Over the past 30 years most devel-oped countries have witnessed an increase in the numbers of old people living alone. This phenomenon becomes a serious problem when the elderly become frail and can no longer manage alone. They then need super-vised care in a medical care facility or old age home. The 'warehousing' of the dependent elderly poses complex issues for many countries, regardless of social policies.

An increase in the absolute numbers of the aging population in both the developed and developing world is an accepted phenomenon. Patterns of disease and mortality become very important. The year before death is characteristically a time of decline in health status with an increase in problems associated with new diseases and chronic conditions. Morbidity and the health care associated with long-term illness is a serious concern in the last years of the twentieth century and will be a major economic issue in the twenty-first century (Brody, 1985).

The common causes of death are frequently divided into four broad categories: heart disease, stroke, cancer, and all other causes combined. As one ages, these disease processes become chronic and the incidence of coexisting chronic disease increases. One may argue that mortality is beneficial and necessary to society. But the same cannot be said about disability and impaired quality of life which pose serious social and economic costs to the individual and to society.

Population Aging in the Developing World

A decline in the crude birth and death rates is anticipated in all African countries and other developing countries so that by the year 2000 life expectancy at birth is projected to reach 55 to 65 years. At the same time it is expected that roughly two out of three of the world's 600 million elderly will be living in developing countries. Between 1980 and 2020,

the elderly population of the developing world will increase by 240 percent (Apt, 1996a). This increase has enormous economic and social implications for policy planning for the governments of those countries.

In most countries in the developing world aging has not presented problems up to the present time. Many of these countries do not consider poverty among the aged a special problem. It is certainly not a problem that is essentially different from the widespread economic deprivation found among the rest of the nation. The economic and social policy related to problems of the young usually take priority because populations of these countries are relatively young. Anthropologists have found that as societies develop and become more modern the status of the aged person declines (Tout, 1989). Old age is defined in terms of chronological age when a society becomes modern. Prior to modernization of a developing country, old age was associated with grandparenthood or succession to eldership. The elderly had a privileged position in the traditional family. Younger members of the family were made to stay and look after the elderly so that the elderly in turn could teach them basic household duties (Apt, 1996b). The bond between parent and child also does not weaken after the child marries and this continuity of relationships brings security in old age.

With the increased number of elderly in a population, a situation has evolved in which four or even five generations of a family are still alive. This places a heavy burden on the working adults who may be responsible not only for their children and grandchildren but also for their parents and grandparents. Modernization has made the skills of the elderly obsolete, and they lack modern education that would enable them to take on something new. Education has become the yardstick for power and prestige; the status of the elderly is seriously jeopardized because they lack a contemporary education (Apt, 1996b). Bondevik (1994) suggests that

'the role of the aged is no longer thought applicable in any society'.

Young people move in large numbers from rural areas to the cities, producing a decline in the rural communities. As societies in the developing world are becoming more modern and urbanized the traditional social welfare system of the extended family is being eroded. This is happening at the same time as the numbers of the aged are growing, with the result that they are losing their customary support (Grieco, 1996).

Few grandparents accompany these young migrants to the cities; they remain behind in the rural areas. Many elderly residents that relocated find themselves in impoverished community slum dwellings to become a burden to their families because of their lack of education and their lack of skills to cope with modern conveniences such as electricity. There is little they can do or are allowed to do so they spend their days unoccupied and in isolation. Younger family members living in these slum dwellings are severely stressed and the older person now becomes an unwelcome and unproductive burden (Tout, 1989).

In many developing countries the elder traditionally has absolute authority and in some cases an almost supernatural prestige. Elders are held in such high regard in part because it is believed they are living closer to the spirits than younger people. If the elder should die unhappy about the behavior of a younger member of the family, now being in a spirit world he could directly exercise an influence over past bad behavior. The isolation of elders because of modernization and mobilization is far removed from the traditional revered respect for the elder (Tout, 1989).

The opportunity to become involved in meaningful work is frequently an important value for older people in developing countries as well as in developed nations, irrespective of financial rewards. A contrary position is suggested by Partridge et al. (1996), that when the elderly work in the developed world it is regarded as a sign of financial need. Many elderly regard the ability to work as the important criterion. Remuneration does not seem to influence their productivity; they can achieve work of a high quality and become engrossed in the task. The incentive appears to be the fact that they are working.

Elderly women in rural areas have very little support. It is often more important for women to be economically independent when they are elderly than it was for them during their childbearing age. They are frequently the survivors and often have their children's families to support. As the younger members of families move to the cities in search of their fortune the healthy elderly that remain behind will look after the sick and disabled elderly.

The impact of AIDS has been described as the greatest crisis in the recorded history of Africa. AIDS will have a strong impact on grandmothers because they will become responsible for the AIDS orphans. The grandmothers will care for their terminally ill children, in the absence of adequate medical and hospice services. They will care for the critically ill with limited knowledge of the disease, trying to relieve the suffering. Finally they will arrange for their burials, and at the same time look after the grandchildren who remain in the family.

Disease in the Elderly Population

At the turn of the century mortality patterns were dominated by diseases such as smallpox, diphtheria, tetanus, and poliomyelitis. The decline of these acute diseases can be attributed to a number of socio-economic factors as well as increased knowledge and technology in health care.

Chronic diseases have replaced acute illness as major health threats.

'The practical focus on health improvement over the next decades must be on chronic instead of acute disease, on morbidity not mortality, on quality of life rather than its duration and on postponement rather than on cure' (Fries, 1980).

Fries goes on to say that the complex nature of the major diseases calls our attention to multifactorial influences on outcome, in particular social and psychological factors. Health outcome is related to choices of life style and treatment interventions, personal responsibility for those decisions, and obtaining the education necessary for making decisions about personal health. Ultimately the individual must have the ability to engage in self-care. These objectives are essential to changing health behaviors. The health professionals cannot make lifestyle changes for the individual, nor can they dictate treatment. The patient may experience discomfort, even anguish and resentment when encouraged to assume these

responsibilities. Therefore education becomes an essential part of patient care. Health education is even more important for children throughout their years in school and throughout life.

Few developing countries have information on the health and social conditions of the elderly. Nineteen African countries responded to a United Nations' questionnaire on aging and aspects of disease in 1985. The following chronic diseases were identified as important (Macfadyen, 1992).

1. Cardiovascular disease.
2. Hypertension and stroke.
3. Diabetes.
4. Diseases of the digestive system.
5. Cancer.
6. Rheumatic disease.
7. Opthamological disease.

The disease profiles in the developed and developing worlds differ. Little epidemiology research exists in developing countries but there seems to be less control of acute disease and a lower incidence of osteoporosis than in the developed world.

In the developed world the most common causes of death are heart disease, stroke and cancer. In both the developing and the developed nations, the two most prevalent causes of disease and death are cardiovascular disorders and stroke. These two diseases will serve to illustrate the impact of disease on the physical and psychosocial functioning of elderly patients.

Cardiovascular disorders

Cardiovascular performance deteriorates with advancing age. The decline in function may be a consequence of aging as well as a function of lifestyle and disease. Obscure disease may be overlooked but can cause severe functional impairments. Atherosclerosis is a good example of such a disease because it may be present in an occult form in as large a number of elderly patients as those who present a straightforward form of the disease.

Decreased physical activity affects not only the function of the heart but also the size of the heart (Lakatta and Gerstenblith, 1992). The extent of the decline in the maximum work capacity and maximum cardiac output with advancing age varies according to the physical condition of the elderly person, the presence of disease, and the level of physical activity prior to onset.

When activity and training is sustained or even increased, it is possible to halt the downward slope in cardiorespiratory function for at least 10 to 20 years (Astrand, 1988). The mythology associated with retirement leads to an expectation of 'slowing down' and 'enjoying a well-earned rest'. Exercise programs imposed by health professionals frequently face low levels of enthusiasm from those elderly who see this as contrary to their deserved withdrawal from work.

Cerebrovascular accident

The cerebrovascular accident (CVA) or stroke, is the second most common cause of death and disability in the elderly. While cardiovascular disease is responsible for an increasing number of deaths and disability in the older age group and accounts for almost 50 percent of deaths in people over the age of 65, stroke is responsible for 20 percent of all deaths from cardiovascular disease.

In the developed world the majority of stroke patients are over the age of 65 and half of this group are over the age of 75. As the proportion of older people in the world rises, health professionals will treat and manage an increasing number of older stroke survivors in the future (Brunton and McCullough, 1995). The predisposing factors in CVA in the elderly include hypertension, heart disease and impaired cardiac function, raised blood lipids, diabetes, obesity, race, and a family history of stroke. Cigarette smoking, alcohol misuse, and physical inactivity are lifestyle factors that contribute to CVA.

About 50 percent of all CVA survivors have some residual physical disability. Many need care and support at home; some are not able to cope at home with assistance and must move into a supported environment. When institutionalized care is not possible, caregivers experience serious stress in the demanding role of providing care.

Many patients who have had a CVA with a mobility disability experience depression associated with it. The quality of life may be severely affected owing to problems related to movement around the home and neighbourhood, or getting from home to anywhere else. If public transport is available they may not have access to it, or may not be able to get on it. Pavements are frequently uneven or unsafe, producing a hazard for ambulation. In the absence of pavements the ground surface is uneven. In remote rural areas of underdeveloped countries, CVA patients are sometimes brought in a wheelbarrow to collect their pensions or to attend medical clinics. The indignity of this 'curiosity' is overwhelming.

Much of the care is left to the voluntary sector and charity. Ideally individuals who are disabled as a result of a CVA should be in contact with day centres and self-support groups. But in developing countries these people may not be seen again after discharge from hospital unless they experience a health crisis. The CVA patients that survive are those who have become functionally independent.

A marked social deterioration often occurs when the patient has had a stroke of a severe nature, such that the quality of life is also severely affected (Astrom et al., 1992). In the study by Astrom et al. elderly stroke patients in Sweden were followed up over a period of three years. Compared to a general population of the elderly, they had more psychiatric symptoms, lower functional ability and reduced life satisfaction. They had maintained contacts with their children but their contact with friends and neighbours decreased. Their activities of daily living and somatic/neurological symptoms showed little change after three months but psychiatric symptoms showed change over time. If good life-satisfaction was restored it was maintained, but if life satisfaction was poor at one year, it remained so for the duration of the three years in which the study was conducted. The researchers concluded that depression experienced soon after stroke, the functional disability, and an impaired social network all contributed to reducing the life satisfaction of elderly stroke survivors.

We may use South Africa as an example of the developing world where we find that more than 3 million black people are hypertensive (Steyn et al., 1992). This number is greater than in any other racial group in South Africa. We can expect that the incidence of stroke is also much greater. In South Africa the circumstances of the aged person with chronic disease in impoverished urban areas is decidedly inferior to that in rural areas, owing large part to dissolution of the extended family (Scotch, 1960). In a community-based epidemiological survey of the socio-economic circumstances and functional abilities of elderly black people, researchers found that the magnitude of disabilities among the aged was not as great as expected (Bester et al., 1991). The authors hypothesized that this was probably due to the fact that only those people who were independent in ambulation, survive. There is no available information on lifestyle satisfaction or depression in elderly stroke victims in most developing countries.

Physical disability in older adults

Although diseases are the major contributing factors associated with disability, they are not the only factors (Fried et al., 1994). A small proportion of people without any disease reported difficulty in completing certain tasks related to activities of daily living, mobility, upper extremity function, and tasks dependent on cognition. Such difficulty in the absence of disease increased with age. These reports suggest contributions from aging-related physiological changes, though these are believed to be small. Other factors such as demographic and psychosocial characteristics contribute to these physical disabilities.

It is important in the care, management, and education of the elderly person that the health care professional be cognisant of the following potential problems:

1. Loss of mobility and function.
2. The presence of chronic pain.
3. Depression, physical illness, and disability.

These problems have a profound effect on the quality of life of the elderly and will be discussed in some detail below.

Loss of mobility and function Deconditioning is described as the multiple changes occurring in organ systems, which are induced by inactivity and restored by activity (Siebens, 1990). Deconditioning results from physiological changes caused by decreased activity or inactivity and leads to functional losses in activities of daily living. The most significant organ changes that health care professionals encounter occur in the cardiopulmonary and musculoskeletal systems (Vorhies and Riley, 1993).

Mobility is a basic human function essential for an individual's independence, to maintain social and intellectual interaction and the basic activities of daily living. Loss of mobility and the occurrence of falls are two of the major causes of a limited quality of life and increased dependence (Baker and Harvey, 1985). Falls are the leading cause of fatal injury in the population over the age of 75 years. Deconditioning, characterized by muscle weakness, and impaired gait and balance may contribute in important ways to the experience of falling and puts special importance on the role of physical activity in the management of this problem. Falls frequently produce minor injuries but often can result in hip fractures, head injuries, and death.

Mobility is dependent upon several factors including sensorimotor functions, joint flexibility, and overall conditioning. Diminished acuity in hearing and vision, orthostatic hypotension, and cardiovascular disease producing syncope are often related to falls. These age-related changes lead to the loss of mobility and function and a reduced capacity for protective reactions. There is also clear evidence of slower postural reflexes with the aging process. These are not in themselves the cause of the fall. However, combined with other biological and pathological changes they put the elderly at increased risk.

A decrease in proprioception and touch sensitivity also occurs with aging. It is possible that the impaired sensory function may contribute to the poor postural response, though there is no evidence of widespread neuropathy underlying this functional impairment.

Falls in older people can lead to hospitalization, disability, and premature death (Arfken et al., 1994). Fifty-two percent of deaths owing to domiciliary accidents in people over the age of 65 result from falls. One in three people over the age of 65 years and approximately one out of every two people over the age of 80 years fall at least once a year. Falling may also result in psychological trauma with resultant fear of falling (Tinetti and Speechley, 1989). This fear may lead to social isolation, through avoidance of activities that put them at risk of falling. Because they restrict their activities, debilitation will occur. Arfken et al. (1994) observed an association of fear of falling with decreased mobility and quality of life. This would suggest the need for effective interventions to prevent falls and limit the consequences of falls in elderly people. In this regard there is a major role for health professionals in both education for prevention and treatment. Several factors may contribute to a fall: transient ischemic attacks characterized by altered consciousness, light-headedness or vertigo, seizures, or cardiovascular conditions, and environmental hazards. The latter seem to be responsible for more than half of the falls in older people (Overstall *et al.*, 1977).

Falls frequently lead to fractures of the hip and the femoral neck which are among the major causes of mortality, morbidity, and loss of function. Poor functional recovery after hip fractures is due to co-morbidity, dementia and dependence, and clinical instability in the acute and intermediate care patients (Bernardini *et al.*, 1995). Co-morbidity and clinical instability have a strong effect on both improvement and the final rehabilitation result, but do not constitute insurmountable obstacles to rehabilitation. Their negative effects on outcomes can be overcome by an adequate and comprehensive approach.

Advancing age is associated with a loss of muscle strength. According to some cross-sectional studies the deterioration begins at approximately age 45 and progresses by at least 1.5 percent per year. Men are consistently stronger than women at the same age; for example the quadriceps strength of elderly men is 50 percent greater than that of elderly women. The strength to body weight ratio of weight-bearing muscles is almost 10 to 20 percent greater in men than women. Elderly men thus have a greater capacity for weight-bearing functional activities than women of the same age (Young, 1992).

Together with the decrease in strength, muscle power is also decreased. Power is defined as the rate of performing work. The slowing of muscle contraction as the person becomes older results in a decrease in maximal power. This decrease is greater than the decrease in maximal strength so that by the age of 80 there is a 45 percent decrease in power and only a 27 percent decrease in strength (Shock and Norris, 1970).

Decreased strength and power affect the elderly person's everyday life. A healthy 20-year-old female requires 50 to 70 percent of her maximal quadriceps contraction to rise from a low, armless chair. The healthy 80-year-old female has to use a maximal quadriceps contraction for the same movement. Healthy elderly women reach the 'threshold' for this activity at approximately the age of 80 years. Once a threshold has been reached only a very small decrease in strength or power results in insufficient strength to perform an activity. The functional implications are apparent when considering a low armless toilet, for example. The absence of a grab rail or other means of supplementing the failing quadriceps muscle results in the patient experiencing serious difficulty with this essential activity of daily living (Young, 1992).

The strength of muscles in the elderly can be increased by appropriate training. In elderly people it is not enough to strengthen the relevant muscles for certain functional activities: it is necessary to train the specific movements involved. The restoration of strength only may not be sufficient to restore a functional ability when the person has dropped below the 'threshold' for the activity (Young, 1992).

Pain in the elderly   Pain is a common symptom of disease experienced by the elderly. A number of medical conditions produce pain and may severely alter the person's quality of life and affect physical functioning.

The most common disorders producing pain in the elderly (Herman and Scudds, 1995) are:

1. Disorders of the musculoskeletal system. More than 50 percent of people over the age of 65 experience pain from arthritis.

2. Rheumatoid disorders such as fibromyalgia and myofascial pain syndromes.

3. Osteoporosis associated with the degenerative processes producing neck and back pain.

4. Malnutrition.

5. Lack of adequate physical conditioning and limited movement.

6. Neurogenic pain involving disorders of the peripheral or central nervous system.

7. Disorders of vascular origin such as migraine.

The experience of pain results in physiologic events that have an impact on the pain and the psyche. Release of norepinephrine at the sympathetic nerve endings sensitizes nociceptors, enhances pain transmission, and perception of pain. When pain persists, one effect is a mood of depression that results in part from changes in the monoamine metabolism of the brain. In addition, catecholamine levels and serotonin metabolism may change during the aging process, which may result in altered sleep patterns and depression. Both these factors have an effect on the patient's experience of pain. Emotional arousal such as fear, anxiety, and efforts to escape the source of pain occupy increasing amounts of time and energy, and contribute to the depressed mood as well. Pain frequently subsides with explanation, treatment, and reassurance. Health professionals are in a good position to ameliorate the effects of pain.

Alteration in sensory receptor function and a general slowing of transduction processes seem to underlie the functional deterioration of the sense organs (Harkins et al., 1990). A gradual decrease in pain perception and a higher pain threshold may be expected theoretically with old age. There are some indications that this may be the case when one considers incidence of silent myocardial infarcts, which seems to increase with advancing age (Bayer et al, 1986). 'Conditioned' pain behavior differs from 'respondent' pain that can be managed medically by identifying the cause of the pain and treating it with the appropriate means. Patients who complain a great deal, demand more medication, spend much of their awake time resting, and who talk about their symptoms, may be expressing 'conditioned' pain behaviour. When patients receive sympathy and attention in response to expressed pain behavior this behavior is reinforced. This illness behavior may result in more pain, increased dependency, and loss of self-esteem. Helme and Katz (1993) stress that behavioral strategies should be part of the pain management for patients with chronic disease to discourage inappropriate behaviors and encourage coping strategies.

Herman and Scudds (1995) point out that pain is a perceptual event. The experience and the intensity of pain is affected by what the individual thinks, feels and does. Older people differ considerably in the way they respond to pain. Symptoms of chronic pain may resemble the symptoms of depression to such an extent that it is not possible to distinguish between the two. Depression can interfere severely with the outcome of rehabilitation. Depression is present in 10 percent of adults over the age of 65 who are free of illness. The incidence is increased to 30 to 40 percent and can be as high as 83 percent in elderly patients suffering from disease or chronic pain. It appears that for older people symptoms of pain are looked on as more acceptable, and may be more treatable than the symptoms of their emotional distress. Uncertainty about the cause, duration, and outcome of the pain also causes fear and anxiety and has an affect on the outcome of treatment. The health care worker needs to provide frequent explanation and reassurance to reduce fear, and to enhance treatment outcome. The verbal interchange in itself has great therapeutic value, providing encouragement, enhancing problem solving, and increasing self-confidence. In the same way that thoughts can influence feelings and behavior, so behavior can influence thoughts and feelings. The manner in which people interpret their pain therefore influences the intensity of their pain as well as the outcome of interventions to treat the pain (Herman and Scudds, 1995).

The literature also suggests that the personality of an individual influences the response to pain and coping strategies employed. Therapists' interpersonal skills are critical and may be taxed while working with patients whose poor coping behavior has elicited attention and is thereby reinforced. The social support system available to patients influences the prognosis and rehabilitation outcome of elderly patients who are experiencing severe pain. (Herman and Scudds, 1995) The pain behaviour may be a way of drawing attention to one's predicament, especially in the absence of a strong support system. Group therapy may provide the much needed human contact and support, and may be a successful approach to some of the problems of elderly patients associated with loneliness.

The constant contact with people exhibiting pain behaviors in residents of old age homes frequently has a negative effect on their own pain behavior. The impact of modeling may be greater than the power of personality. The optimistic attitudes 'modeled' by the therapists may encounter overwhelming opposition from the negative input of the residents observed in the environment (Chapman and Turner, 1990).

Depression, physical illness, and disability
Depression has been defined as the loss of hope and faith (Carlsen, 1996a). The majority of old people believe that their lives have turned out better than expected and do not experience depression and are not unhappy or unfulfilled (Murphy *et al.*, 1988). It is important to recognize the signs and symptoms of depression as early as possible because it is treatable by various medical or social measures. Depressive symptoms are more common in older people, but depression does not become more common with advancing age. These depressive symptoms may be recognized by the appearance of a sad affect and a limited responsiveness to stimuli in the environment which presents as low energy most of the day (Reynolds, 1995).

A close association seems to exist between physical ill health and symptoms of depression in old age. Reactive depression may be a result of psychological reactions to physical illness and the process of adapting to the lifestyle changes that are required subsequent to disability and handicap. A depressed mood may lead to self-neglect, inadequate nutrition, and self-harm, which in turn leads to physical disease. Several physical illnesses have a particular association with depression that present as a mood disorder, such as a CVA. Many malignancies, cardiovascular disease, and metabolic and endocrine disorders are also linked to severe depression (Ouslander, 1982). The mortality rate of patients with depression is higher than that for the general population. This is perhaps due in part to poor physical health, though these health problems alone do not satisfactorily explain the higher death rate (Murphy *et al.*, 1988).

The relationship of chronic illness to depression was evaluated in a study on black Americans. This study is important because black Americans at age 65 experienced a disproportionate prevalence of chronic disease, illness, and disability. Depression was found to be greatest among patients with financial difficulties who experienced stressful life events and had less support from their friends (Bazargan and Hamm-Baugh, 1995).

In a descriptive, correlational study designed to examine the physical and mental health status of 80 year olds, depression emerged as a significant problem for 24 percent of the sample and was strongly related to physical health problems. However, the overall picture indicated that this group was optimistic, had high levels of life-satisfaction, happiness, and a sense of meaningful integration in the social structure (Heidrich and D'Amico, 1993).

The two common conditions of incontinence and sleep disorders are frequently neglected. Urinary incontinence is common, costly, and occurs frequently in older people and is a neglected problem. It leads to social isolation, depression, and a lack of self-esteem. It appears in 15 to 30 percent of all older people living in the community and can be as high as 50 percent in residents of old age homes (Diokno *et al.*, 1986). Incontinence is not an inevitable result of the aging process. Several interventions can be used to improve the condition substantially, if not cure it altogether. Urinary

incontinence is not a feature of normal aging and must be identified as a treatable, chronic disability in elderly people. Frequently medications prescribed for hypertension, such as diuretics, can magnify the problem of incontinence. Impaired mobility may also result in incontinence if the patient is unable to get to the toilet in time and if the patient lacks the manual dexterity necessary to remove clothing in order to use the toilet.

The accidental leakage of urine or faeces results in physical as well as psychosocial problems for the patient. The physical problems are those of perineal skin irritation, sores, and urinary tract infections. The elderly person who experiences incontinence is embarrassed by leakage. When the condition persists it may lead to the withdrawal from social interaction and the person may limit participation in physical activities such as walking and exercise classes, becoming progressively more isolated. Health care professionals should be aware of the available treatment for incontinence and acknowledge their role in educating the patient and the community about this problem (Tata, 1995).

The prevalence of sleep disorders increases with age and is one of the most frequently encountered problems in the geriatric population. According to Bliwise *et al.* (1992), insomnia can be divided into three categories: difficulty with falling asleep at the beginning of the night (initial insomnia), difficulty with returning to sleep after nocturnal awakenings, usually in the first two thirds of the night (middle insomnia), and awakening too early in the morning (early morning awakening). In practice many patients have a combination of these three categories. Current evidence suggests that physiological changes may predispose elderly patients to poor sleep, and may be associated with anxiety and depression. Physical illness also has a role in this complaint. Epidemiological evidence indicates that bronchitis and bronchial asthma are associated with middle insomnia, and musculoskeletal pain is associated primarily with initial insomnia (Gislason and Almqvist, 1987).

Hospitalization and institutionalization

Today the tendency is to enable elderly people to live in the community for as long as possible through support services in the community. Following an acute health care crisis requiring hospitalization the elderly individual may no longer be able to cope with independent living in the community in spite of support services. Placement may be sought in an institution that offers long-term care, if such a facility exists, and personal and public financial resources permit.

Hospitalization Increasing evidence suggests that greater attention needs to be given to the unique problems of the elderly, especially the frail elderly, when they experience hospitalization. Excess nosocomial infections, incontinence, confusion, activity limitations, skin breakdown and post-hospitalization mortality are identified as negative outcomes of hospitalization (Tappen and Beckerman, 1993). Older people have experienced an increase in surgical procedures in recent years because the negative bias is decreasing, though evidence of discrimination based on age continues, which influences treatment decisions in acute care. The average 70-year-old male and female can expect to reach the ages of 81 and

84 years, respectively. Age is considered a risk factor in most surgical procedures. Careful patient selection and monitoring make it feasible for even the very old to face surgical procedures with acceptable levels of morbidity and fatality.

Institutionalization A high probability exists that older people may spend some time in a nursing home before they die. In the USA, 43 percent of those who turned 65 in 1990 will spend time in a nursing home before they die, 55 percent of these will remain there for at least one year, and 21 percent will be there for five years of more (Kemper and Murtaugh, 1991). The increasing number of old people will result in health care, skilled nursing, and continuing care facilities being used increasingly. Owing to the severe economic constraints on social services in some developing countries, old age homes are no longer supported by government funding. The elderly find themselves unable to afford to stay in nursing care facilities because the costs far exceed their very small pensions. The plight of these elderly people is distressing and creates serious problems for those countries.

Long-term care is provided for frail elderly people primarily in nursing homes or old age homes. Frailty is defined by the older person's chronological age as well as by their dependence in one or more of the following areas: psychological, social, physical, cultural, or economic. It is evident that not all frail elderly are institutionalized (Bloom, 1993). Most nursing home residents require assistance with activities of daily living including transfers from bed to chair and ambulation. One of the major reasons for placing elderly people in long-term care is because they require medical attention. The elderly needing medical attention can be divided into two groups. One group who are younger and medically ill, and those who are older, experience chronic diseases, and are more confused. Lack of social support and lack of caregivers are other reasons for institutionalization. Social support from children is valuable as it helps the elderly parent cope with illness. Many of the residents in institutions have children who live too far away and cannot care for the elderly relative. Children are only one kind of social support that is important to older people. The support from family, friends, and neighbors is also very important following retirement, but when there are changes in social status or health and well-being the support of adult children is especially important (Silverstein and Bengston, 1994).

It is important to maintain as well as to optimize living for elderly people living in institutions. Baltes (1994) identified four areas that lead to optimization of life: health, personal control, independence, and social relationships. If these areas that include both the physical and psychological well-being of the elderly person are optimized, then the quantity and quality of their lives will be enhanced and this is the essence of successful aging according to Baltes. Personal control is identified as a basic need by Rodin and Langer (1977) but many institutions for the aged continue to foster an environment in which the resident is denied the right to make their own decisions and have virtually no control. When elderly residents engage in dependent behaviors such as demanding personal care, they are utilizing a strategy to exercise some control in their social environment that improves social contacts and avoids isolation. The staff and family who provide care for the elderly must be taught and encouraged to help the elderly maintain their independence and reinforce their strengths and competencies instead of emphasizing their weaknesses. The attitudes and actions of all care-givers should be to help the elderly person toward self-help.

Dementia

Dementia is defined by Friedland (1992) as an acquired impairment of intellectual and memory functioning caused by organic disease of the brain. It is not associated with disturbances in the levels of consciousness but is of such severity that it interferes with social or occupational functioning (Friedland, 1992). Dementia is not a normal occurrence. It is a clinical syndrome with various etiologies. Most people with dementia show progressive decline that is not reversible. The incidence of this illness increases with advancing age. The most common cause of dementia in the USA and Europe is Alzheimer's disease. In the USA, new cases of Alzheimer's disease between the ages of 75 and 85 is as common as myocardial infarction and more common than stroke (Katzman et al., 1989). As the world's population is aging rapidly and the incidence of myocardial infarction and stroke is brought under control, dementing illnesses will become a much greater problem in the future.

Alzheimer's disease is responsible for between 50 and 60 percent of cases of dementia in adults. In most instances it occurs sporadically, but in 10 to 15 percent there is a family history of the disease. The first symptom that people complain of is memory loss, which is difficult to detect during a clinical examination. Initially, memory for recent events is lost with relative preservation of long-term memory. Memory impairment may be the only dysfunction, but in the middle stages of the disease the cognitive deficits are apparent, such as intellectual decline and language disturbances. In the late stages of the disease the elderly person is incapable of self-care and speech, and loses the ability to attend to individuals and events in the immediate surroundings. In a survey that studied patients with irreversible dementia, 60 percent had Alzheimer's disease. The four most dominant characteristics identified were memory disturbance, catastrophic reactions, suspiciousness, and making accusations (Schunk, 1993). Alzheimer's disease is accompanied by a marked weight loss apparently not related to dietary intake or increased exercise. The disease is progressive.

Alzheimer's disease and Parkinson's disease have overlapping features. In 25 to 40 percent of patients with Parkinson's disease, they may also experience dementia. In 15 to 30 percent of patients with Parkinson's disease there may be concurrent symptoms of Alzheimer's disease. Many of the features of Parkinson's disease such as rigidity and bradykinesia appear in patients with Alzheimer's disease.

Psychosocial aspects of older people with dementia

According to Pomeroy (1995) there are a number of undesirable effects as a result of inadequate and inappropriate communication between people with dementia and others. These effects include: disempowerment, infantilization, intimidation, labeling, outpacing, and objectification. Each is described briefly here.

- *Disempowerment* is the process that results in not being allowed to complete tasks for oneself because care-givers find it easier and quicker to do it themselves.
- *Infantilization* results from talking to the individual in a manner similar to the way one would address a child.
- *Intimidation* results from not being told or given the opportunity to understand what another is doing that has an impact on oneself.
- *Labeling* an individual with words that are derogatory and discriminatory lead to a self-fulfilling prophecy – the individual becomes labeled.
- *Outpacing* occurs when the individual is not given adequate time to complete a task, and is left behind in thought, during the performance of the task.
- *Objectification* results when the individual is treated as an object and not as a person.

The treatment goals for people with dementia are the same as those for other elderly people – to maximize function. The main factor that complicates rehabilitation is impaired memory and the resultant difficulty in retaining the learning of new concepts. These patients have the same right to rehabilitation as any other, but have special needs which require that instructions be presented in a clear and uncomplicated manner. Instructions are most effective when delivered in a manner that is simple and consistent and accompanied by demonstrations, criticism is avoided, sensory cues are strongly emphasized, and patients are given adequate resting time (Mace *et al.*, 1989). Skills and activities engaged in on a regular basis before the onset of the dementia, such as eating, walking, and dressing, are relearned with a higher degree of success than new skills. The long-term care of the elderly person with dementia is frequently dependent upon family members and community support. The education and training of these care givers is also of great importance.

Treatment

Locomotion is a top priority in a therapeutic program for older people. The most important challenge to health care systems in all cultures is the declining functional capacity of the elderly. The single most cost-effective way of addressing the issue of maintaining function may be a well-designed exercise program of low to moderate intensity. Recent evidence suggests that many of the health benefits resulting from physical activity occur at moderate intensity levels. This is significant for the elderly, who are at an increased risk for injuries and sudden death, when engaged in vigorous exercise (Pescatello and DiPietro, 1993). For many elderly people a simple walking program is probably the safest and most effective form of exercise (Barry and Eathorne, 1994). The elderly population of the developing world has no access to transport in general; they have to rely on their ability to walk in order to deal with their tasks of daily living. For these people, exercise programs such as a walking program have little value, but education programs are vital. The elderly in the developed world are generally better educated, but their lives are increasingly sedentary. For these well elderly people, exercise programs are essential.

One benefit of exercise is an immediate elevation of mood which in turn has a favorable influence on one's perception of health status, enabling the older person to tolerate minor aches and pains more easily, with a resultant decrease in demand for medical services and an increase in the functional capacity and level of independence (Shephard, 1993). Physical activity has the potential to decrease the progression of a number of chronic diseases. Astrand (1992) maintains that,

'As a consequence of diminished exercise tolerance, a large and increasing number of elderly people will be living below, at, or just above "thresholds" of physical ability, needing only a minor illness to render them completely dependent.'

Maintaining or increasing one's level of physical activity can increase physical ability and improve physical functioning. As physical function improves, the quality and the quantity of life can be extended (Caspersen et al., 1994).

Older people's recommendations for treating symptoms

Limited evidence suggests that when the elderly engage in self-care decisions, the decisions are generally appropriate and the self-treatment is helpful. Self-care decisions seem to alleviate symptoms and reduce the duration of the illness (Stoller et al., 1994). It also appears that older people manage many symptoms on their own without consultation with health care professionals. Hickey and Stilwell (1991) report that older people have more symptoms than younger people but when they visit the doctor they report fewer of their symptoms. Lay decisions on treatment are rarely made in isolation. The decisions and care are embedded in the family value system and extended networks of friends. Older people frequently discover a pool of potential experts who, like themselves, experience symptoms of long term illness and chronic diseases. A strong internal health locus of control more frequently results in behavior that leads them to manage their own health and gather information to improve their health status than people with an external health locus of control. People with an external health locus of control are more likely to attribute responsibility for medical management to health care providers. The media provide an important source of medical information for the elderly. Older people were asked to respond to 15 commonly experienced symptoms and identify the required treatment (Stoller *et al.* 1994). The most frequently suggested advice was over-the-counter medication. Only in the case of diarrhea and chest pain did the respondents believe that one should seek medical help. Few respondents considered bedrest a form of treatment, and then only in the cases of fever, fatigue, and dizziness.

Prayer was mentioned most frequently for depression and sleep difficulties. Frequently their advice was to ignore the symptom especially in the case of depression, sleep difficulties, nausea, and cough. People with a broader repertoire of lay knowledge had higher levels of education and were more likely to emphasize personal responsibility and control over their own health. They were also more likely to experience a larger number of symptoms. In designing programs to enhance ability to self-manage illness it is important to recognize that the older person has a bank of information based on a lifetime of experience. New information will be added to the existing knowledge and will be modified to conform with existing beliefs. In order that these pro-grams should be presented in a successful manner it is essential to have insights into the belief system and the basic information held by the individual.

Myths about the elderly

Kastenbaum (1982) identified three assumptions about the aged that have a particularly lethal quality and reflect the mixed feelings on the part of members of society towards aging and the aged. These are:

1. Very little can be done to relieve the miseries of old age and it is the most helpless of circumstances.

2. The elderly themselves realize that they 'have had their day' and they only desire the opportunity to age gracefully and wait for the end to come.

3. Health care is already so expensive that it would be foolish to donate even more to geriatric care because it would simply absorb all the funds available and very little would be gained from it.

The concluding assumption is there is little that can or should be done to improve health care services for the elderly.

Kastenbaum believes that adults in Western societies behave as if they will never grow old and lack a clear and convincing image of how one develops through the stages of life to old age. Being old reminds one of death and brings a painful awareness and dread. There is an aversion to recognizing the continuity between the present and future selves which leads to distancing oneself from those who are the aged at the moment.

A tendency exists to project on to the older person fatalistic attitudes about life and death because of a lack of intimate contact and real knowledge. These sentiments, expressed by Kastenbaum, are not applicable in the developing world.

Cost to the caregivers

Caring for the elderly is accomplished primarily by families, particularly daughters and daughters-in-law. They provide the day-to-day care and health services of the disabled and frail elderly (Brody, 1985). Approximately 25 percent of people over 65 are functionally disabled to some degree and require assistance with the activities of daily living. Care is provided in the home for 80 percent of disabled people, 85 percent of which is provided by the family. Families find it increasingly more difficult to function in this capacity because of socio-economic factors and lifestyle. Most caregivers are spouses or children and female. Lifestyle changes in our society have resulted in many women who were traditionally the caregivers being employed outside the home. This added care of an elderly relative increases stress on family members with consequences for their own health and well-being.

Elderly spouse caregivers live with the chronic stress that is without respite and of long duration, making them more susceptible to cardiovascular disease (Vitaliano et al., 1994). As the life expectancy of the population increases, the older caregiver becomes even more important. In the developing world the healthy elderly take care of the ill and disabled elderly because of the migration of the younger adults to the cities in search of economic survival. These caregivers provide emotional and financial support and frequently share their household with the elderly person.

In any society caregivers may derive benefits from their responsibility because they have the opportunity to express their affection and give back something to the elderly person for what has been given them in the past. On the other hand, those who give care often feel guilty that they are not doing enough for the older person and feel angry at finding themselves in a situation where they need to do more than they feel capable of doing.

The health and well-being of caregivers is receiving attention in developed nations. These family members need education on how to maintain their own mental and physical health and how to cope with the physical stress. Providing adequate information about the disease or disability can decrease stress inherent in giving care.

Conclusion

Growing old is described by Willing (1981) in the following way:

'We know that we grow older; we don't know when we become old. I think it may be said that we become old when we declare ourselves old – and that is why I think it is so important to stop speaking prematurely of ourselves as old'.

The health professional must always bear in mind that many older people do not feel different just because they are advanced in years. Their identities are not negatively influenced by the fact that they are of such an age, and they do not feel old or different or disconnected from their younger selves. They have a well-developed sense of who they are. On the other hand, they are so markedly different from one another that we cannot generalize about them. The fact is that the longer we live the more different from each other we become because our life experiences are different. So two young children could be compared more easily to one another than two 80 year olds.

We can see the wisdom in a comment by Neugarten when she refers to the older person as a

'translator and interpreter of experience, a person who creates a future and recreates a past' (Neugarten, 1972).

Those who are successful and survive into old age are individuals made stronger by a wide variety of conditions that life has presented. We can admire them for their courage to grow old and in doing so acquiring the real wisdom that only age can teach.

References

Apt, NA (1996a) Aging in Africa. In: The South African National Council for the Aged Conference papers: *New Trends, Care for the Aged*, pp. 1–12.

Apt, NA (1996b) The Ghanaian tradition: kin, clan and informal caring systems. In: Apt NA (ed) *Coping with Old Age in a Changing Africa*, pp. 16–33. Aldershot: Avebury.

Arfken, CL, Lach, HW, Birge, SJ, et al. (1994) The prevalence and correlates of fear of falling in elderly persons living in the community. *American Journal of Public Health* 84(4): 565–570.

Astrand, PO (1988) Exercise physiology in the mature athlete. In: Sutton, J, Brock, RM (eds) *Sports Medicine for the Mature Athlete*. Indianapolis: Benchmark.

Astrand, PO (1992) Physical activity and fitness. *American Journal of Clinical Nutrition* 55: 1231S–1236S.

Astrom, M, Asplund, K, Astrom, T (1992) Psychosocial function and life satisfaction after stroke. *Stroke* 23(4): 527–531.

Baker, SP, Harvey, AH (1985) Fall injuries in the elderly. *Clinics in Geriatric Medicine* 1: 501–512.

Baltes, M (1994) Aging well and institutional living: a paradox. In: Abeles, R, Gift, HC, Ory, MG (eds) *Aging and Quality of Life*. New York: Springer Publishing Company.

Baltes, P, Baltes, MM (1991) *Successful Aging*, pp. 397. Cambridge: Cambridge University Press.

Barry, HC, Eathorne, SW (1994) Exercise and aging: issues for the practitioner. *Sports Medicine. Medical Clinics of North America* 78: 357–376.

Bayer, AJ, Chadja, JS, Farag, RR, et al. (1986) Changing presentation of myocardial infarction with increasing old age. *Journal of the American Geriatric Society* 34: 263–266.

Bazargan, M, Hamm-Baugh, VP (1995) The relationship between chronic illness and depression in a community of urban black elderly persons. *Journal of Gerontology: Social Sciences* 50B(2): S119–S127.

Bernardini, B, Meinecke, C, Pagani, M, et al. (1995) Comorbidity and adverse clinical events in the rehabilitation of older adults after hip fracture. *JAGS* 43: 894–898.

Bester, FCJ, Weich, DJV, Albertyn, EW (1991) Socio-economic circumstances and functional abilities of elderly black persons in the Orange Free State. *SAMJ* 82: 110–113.

Bliwise, DL, Pascualy, RA, Dement, WC (1992) Sleep disorders. In: Evans, JG, Williams, TF (eds) *Oxford Textbook of Geriatric Medicine*, p. 508. New York: Oxford University Press.

Bloom, SN (1993) The frail and institutionalised elderly. In: Guccione, AA (ed) *Geriatric Physical Therapy*, pp. 378–390. St Louis: Mosby.

Bondevik, M (1994) Historical, cross-cultural, biological and psychosocial perspectives of ageing and the aged person. *Scandinavian Journal of Caring Science* 8: 67–74.

Brody, J (1985) Prospect for an ageing population. *Nature* 315: 463–466.

Brunton, K, McCullough, C (1995) Stroke. In: Pickles, B, Compton, A, Cott, C, et al. (eds) *Physiotherapy with Older People*, pp. 230–254. London: WB Saunders.

Carlsen, MB (1996) *Creative aging: a meaning–making perspective*, pp. 11–28. New York: W.W. Norton & Company Ltd.

Caspersen, CJ, Kriska, AM, Dearwater, SR (1994) Physical activity epidemiology as applied to elderly populations. In: *Bailliere's Clinical Rheumatology* 8(1): 7–27.

Chapman, CR, Turner, JA (1990) Psychologic and psychosocial aspects of acute pain. In: Bonica, JJ (ed) *The Management of Pain*, 2nd edn, pp. 122–132. Philadelphia: Lea and Febriger.

Diokno, AC, Brock, BM, Brown, MB, et al. (1986) Prevalence of urinary incontinence and other urological symptoms in the noninstitutionalized elderly. *Journal of Urology* 131: 474–479.

Fried, LP, Ettinger, WH, Lind, B, et al. (1994) Physical disability in older adults: a physiological approach. *Journal of Clinical Epidemiology* 47: 747–760.

Friedland, RP (1992) Dementia. In: Evans, JG, Williams, TF (eds) *Textbook of Geriatric Medicine*, pp. 483–489. New York: Oxford University Press.

Fries, JF (1980) Aging, natural death, and the compression of morbidity. *The New England Journal of Medicine* 303: 130–135.

Gislason, T, Almqvist, M (1987) Somatic diseases and sleep complaints. *Acta Medica Scandinavica* 221: 475–481.

Gonzalez-Aragon, J (1984) In: Tout, K (ed.) (1989) *Ageing in Developing Countries*. New York: Oxford University Press.

Grieco, M (1996) In: Apt NA (ed) *Coping with Old Age in a Changing Africa*, foreword. Aldershot: Avebury.

Harkins, SW, Kwentus, J, Price, DD (1990) Pain and suffering in the elderly. In: Bonica, JJ (ed) *The Management of Pain*, 2nd edn, pp. 552–559. Philadelphia: Lea and Febriger.

Heidrich, SM, D'Amico, D (1993) Physical and mental health relationships in the very old. *Journal of Community Health Nursing* 10(1): 11–21.

Helme, RD, Katz, B (1993) Management of chronic pain. *The Medical Journal of Australia* 158: 478–481.

Herman, E, Scudds, R (1995) Pain. In: Pickles, B, Compton, A, Cott, C, *et al.* (eds) *Physiotherapy with Older People*, pp. 289–304. London: WB Saunders.

Hickey, T, Stilwell, DL (1991) Health promotion for older people: all is not well. *The Gerontologist* 31(6): 822–829.

Kastenbaum, R (1982) Healthy, wealthy and wise? In: Sanders, GS, Suls, J (eds) *Social Psychology of Health and Illness*, pp. 307–323. London: Lawrence Erlbaum Associates.

Katzman, R, *et al.* (1989) Development of dementing illness in an 80 year old volunteer cohort. *Annals of Neurology.* 25: 189–198.

Kemper, P, Murtaugh, CM (1991) Lifetime use of nursing home care. *New England Journal of Medicine* 324: 595–600.

Kitagawa, EM, Hauser, PM (1973) *Differential Mortality in the United States.* Cambridge: Harvard Press.

Lakatta, EG, Gerstenblith, G (1992) In: Evans, JG, Williams, TF (eds) *Oxford Textbook of Geriatric Medicine. Cardiovascular Disorders*, pp. 271–284. New York: Oxford University Press.

Mace, NL, Hardy, SR, Rabins, PV (1989) Alzheimer's disease and the confused patient. In: Jackson, O (ed): *Physical Therapy for the Geriatric Patient.* New York: Churchill Livingstone.

Macfadyen, DM (1992) The developing world. In: Evans, GJ, Williams, TF (eds) *Oxford Textbook of Geriatric Medicine*, pp. 20–24. New York: Oxford University Press.

Murphy, E, Smith, R, Lindesay, J, *et al.* (1988) Increased mortality rates in late life depression. *British Journal of Psychiatry* 152: 347–353.

Myers, G (1990). Demography of aging. In: Binstock, RH, George, LK (eds) *Handbook of Aging and the Social Sciences*. New York: Academic Press.

Neugarten, B (1972) Personality and the ageing process. *The Gerontologist* 12(1): 9–15.

Ouslander, JG (1982) Physical illness and depression in the elderly. *Journal of the American Geriatrics Society* 30: 593–599.

Overstall, PW, Exton-Smith, AN, Imms, FJ, *et al.* (1977) Falls in the elderly related to postural imbalance. *British Medical Journal* i: 261–264.

Partridge, C, Johnston, M, Morris, L (1996) Disability and health: perceptions of a sample of elderly people. *Physiotherapy Research International* 1: 17–29.

Pescatello, LS, DiPietro, L (1993) Physical activity in older adults An overview of health benefits. *Sports Medicine* 15: 353–364.

Pomeroy, VM (1995) Dementia. In: Everett, T, Dennis, M, Ricketts, I (eds) *Physiotherapy in Mental Health: A Practical Approach.* Oxford: Butterworth–Heineman.

Rabbit, P (1992) Ageing gracefully *The Lancet* 339: 1157–1158.

Reynolds, CF 1995 Recognition and differentiation of elderly depression in the clinical setting. *Geriatrics* 50: S-6–S-15.

Rodin, J, Langer, E (1977) Long-term effects of a control-relevant intervention among the institutionalized aged. *Journal of Personality and Social Psychology* 35: 897–902.

Sagan, LA (1987) *The Health of Nations.* New York: Basic Books.

Schunk, C (1993) Cognitive impairment In: Guccione, AA (ed) *Geriatric Physical Therapy*, pp. 140–148. St Louis: Mosby (Year Book).

Scotch, NA (1960) A preliminary report on the relation of sociocultural factors to hypertension among the Zulu. *Annals of the New York Academy of Science* 84: 1000–1009.

Shephard, RJ (1993) Exercise and aging: extending independence in older adults. *Geriatrics* 48: 61–64.

Shock, NW, Norris, AH (1970) Neuromuscular coordination as a factor in age changes in muscular exercise. *Medicine and Sport* 4: 92–99.

Siebens, H (1990) Deconditioning. In: Kemp, B, Brummel-Smith, K (eds) *Geriatric Rehabilitation*, p. 177. Boston: Little Brown.

Silverstein, M, Bengtson, VL (1994) Does intergenerational social support influence the psychological well-being of older parents? The contingencies of declining health and widowhood. *Social Science and Medicine* 38: 943–957.

Steyn, K, Fourie, J, Bradshaw, D (1992) The impact of chronic diseases of life style and their major risk factors on mortality in South Africa. *SAMJ* 82: 227–231.

Stoller, EP, Pollow, R, Forster, LE (1994) Older people's recommendations for treating symptoms: repertoires of lay knowledge about disease. *Journal of Urology* 131: 1022–1025.

Suzman, R, Kinsella, KG, Myers, GC (1992a) Demography of older populations in developed countries. In: Evans, GJ, Williams, TF (eds) *Oxford Textbook of Geriatric Medicine*, pp. 3–14. New York: Oxford University Press.

Suzman, R, Harris, T, Hadley, E. *et al.* (1992b) The robust oldest old; optimistic perspectives for increasing healthy life expectancy. In: *The Old.* Oxford University Press, Oxford.

Tappen, RM, Beckerman, A (1993) A vulnerable population of multiproblem older adults in acute care. *Journal of Gerontological Nursing* November: 38–42.

Tata, GE (1995) Incontinence. In: Pickles, B, Compton, A, Cott, C, *et al.* (eds) *Physiotherapy with Older People.* London: WB Saunders.

Tinetti, ME, Speechley, M (1989) Prevention of falls among the elderly. *New England Journal of Medicine* 320: 1055–1059.

Tout, K, (1989) *Ageing in Developing Countries.* New York: Oxford University Press for Help Age International.

Vitaliano, PP, Dougherty, CM, Siegler, IC (1994) Biopsychosocial risks for cardiovascular disease in spouse caregivers of persons with Alzheimer's disease. In: Abeles, RP, Gift, HC, Ory, MG (eds) *Aging and Quality of Life*, pp. 145–155. New York: Springer Publishing Company.

Vorhies, D, Riley, BE (1993) Deconditioning. *Clinics in Geriatric Medicine* 9: 745–763.

Willing, JZ (1981) *The reality of retirement: the inner experience of becoming a retired person.* New York: William Morrow.

Young, A (1992) Strength and power. In: Evans, GJ, Williams, TF (eds) *Oxford Textbook of Geriatric Medicine*, pp. 597–601. New York: Oxford University Press.

9

Long-Term Care: Living with Chronic Illness

Cheryl Cott

Introduction
•
Functionalism and the Sick Role Theory
•
Interactionism and Chronic Illness
•
Comparison and Reconciliation: Functionalism and Interactionism

Introduction

Chronic disease is the irreversible presence, accumulation, or latency of disease states or impairments that involve the total human physical and social environment for supportive care, maintenance of function, and prevention of further disability (Strauss *et al.*, 1984). Epidemiological information indicates that chronic diseases are and will continue to be of major concern to the health care system, particularly in view of the aging of the Canadian population. The prevalence of disability is considerable according to recent data. The

Canadian Health and Disability Survey indicates that 12.8 percent or 2,448,000 individuals reported some level of disability, defined as some limitation to one's major activity. Despite evidence of the extent of chronic illness within the population, few health professionals demonstrate either an interest in working in this area or an understanding of the social psychological processes involved in the experience of chronic illness.

By definition, chronic illness is a long-term event in a person's life (Bury, 1991) and involves ongoing, long-term care. However, most health professionals are educated using an acute care model and subsequently have difficulty when they encounter people who have chronic illnesses that do not fit into their traditional treatment models. The purpose of this chapter is to provide the student with a better understanding of the experience of chronic illness by reviewing the concept of role theory from two theoretical perspectives – functionalism (or structural functionalism) and interactionism (or symbolic interactionist).

This chapter will proceed under the premise that while functionalism and interactionism may operate at different levels of analysis, they supplement rather than contradict each other (Heiss, 1981). First, the functionalist approach to role theory will be discussed with particular reference to sick role theory and the limitations of its application to chronic illness. It will be argued that it is the inappropriate application of the sick role to the chronically ill by health care professionals, in particular, that strongly influences the experience of being chronically ill. Limitations and gaps will be identified in functionalist theory that restrict its usefulness in the understanding of the experience of chronic illness.

Second, the interactionist perspective on chronic illness will be discussed. It will be argued that because of the characteristics of chronic illness, the interactionist approach is more suited to understanding the chronic illness experience. However, this theory also leaves gaps in our understanding of the chronic illness experience, particularly in that it does not account for the broader structural influences of culture, politics, and economics. Finally, the integration of these two theories will be discussed in terms of how they complement each other and, in combination, increase our understanding of the chronic illness experience.

Functionalism and the Sick Role Theory

The roots of role theory can be traced to four different theoretical perspectives which can be broadly classified as interactionist or functionalist (Turner, 1985). According to the functionalist perspective, society is a stable and orderly entity within which there is a consensus on goals and behaviors and within which there are persistent patterns of behavior in the form of roles, formal organizations, or institutions. A role is a metaphor coined from the theatre that denotes conduct or behavior of a certain 'part' rather than to the players that are in them. Very simply, functionalism sees roles as institutionally defined and serving the purpose of regulating and constraining the behavior of whatever specific people are incumbent in the role. Norms and values that underlie the roles are internalized through socialization and the role incumbent therefore self-regulates his or her behavior.

Sick role theory (Parsons, 1951) was defined and described by Talcott Parsons in the 1950s and reflects the predominantly functionalist view of the times. The sick role concept is commonly used by medical sociologists and health professionals (although not always appropriately by the latter). Sick role theory as applied to acute illness is still of some relevance today, but its inappropriate application to the chronically ill is of most concern to this discussion.

Parsons initially viewed illness as a form of deviance. Health is important to the functional needs of the individual and, therefore, of society, because illness interferes with the performance of social roles. When a person violates societal norms by becoming sick, equilibrium of the system must be restored. According to Parsons, the classic doctor–patient relationship functions in this manner.

Obligations and exemptions

Parsons describes four aspects of the institutionalized expectation system as related to the sick role. They consist of two exemptions and two obligations. The *first exemption* is from normal social role responsibilities and requires legitimation by a direct legitimizing agent such as a physician. The *second exemption* is that the sick person is exempted from responsibility for being ill. The *first obligation* of the sick role is that the person must define the state of being ill as undesirable and want to get well. The role is conditionally legitimate on the person doing what he or she can to restore his or her health. The *second obligation* is that the person is obliged to seek technically competent help and cooperate with that help in the process of trying to get well.

Parsons' sick role is not only commonly used by medical sociologists and health care professionals, it represents the underlying view of sick people that is shared by members of society. It is based on the assumption that illness is temporary and therefore has limited application to the individual with chronic illness. Applying a framework of care designed for those with acute illness to the chronically ill can lead to fragmented care, incomplete information, overburdened caregivers, and isolated individuals (Charmaz, 1983). This becomes more apparent as each of the exemptions and obligations are examined from the perspective of chronic illness.

First exemption The first exemption is from normal social role responsibilities and requires legitimation by a direct legitimizing agent such as a physician. This exemption includes the usual work, family, civic, and other obligations (Gallagher, 1976). This exemption is not always appropriate in the case of chronic illness in that individuals may not be able to resume their social responsibilities in exactly the same manner that they were able to perform them prior to developing their illness.

This exemption may continue to be applied to the chronically ill long after it is appropriate. Mechanic's (1961) analytic distinction between disease, illness, and sickness is useful for this discussion. *Disease* refers to a disturbance in physiological equilibrium, whether or not this is recognized by the individual. *Illness* refers to recognition by individuals of the disturbance and their definition that they are 'not well', whether or not anyone else agrees with or recognizes their definition. *Sickness* refers to the social attribution of an illness state or a definition by others that an individual is 'not well'. In chronic illness there can be a number of situations when these definitions may not match. In some chronic conditions such as cardiac or renal illness, the illness may not be obvious so individuals may not be perceived to be sick and may not be accorded exemptions appropriately. In other chronic conditions such as spinal cord injury, individuals may be perceived by others to be sick when in fact, once they are past the acute phase, they are not ill but medically stable. These individuals may be inappropriately granted exemption from normal social roles such as employment.

Second exemption The second exemption is that the sick person is exempted from their responsibility for being ill. The person cannot help being ill and needs help to get better. This exemption of responsibility for the condition does not always apply in chronic illness as society does not always exempt chronically ill people from responsibility for their condition or from the consequences of their illness. Many people who have a chronic condition and are disabled are stigmatized. Goffman (1963) defines *stigma* as something that disqualifies individuals from full social acceptance, whether or not responsibility for their condition is imputed to them. Certain chronic conditions such as epilepsy (Scambler and Hopkins, 1986) and more recently AIDS (Carricaburu and Pierret, 1995) carry with them a stigma unrelated to the severity or degree of responsibility of the individual with the condition.

The notion of legitimation relates to the degree to which a condition is stigmatized. Freidson (1970) describes a typology of types of deviance or 'illness' for which the individual is not held responsible. The typology looks at how the imputed seriousness of the deviance (minor or serious deviation) relates to the consideration of the deviance as conditionally legitimate, unconditionally legitimate, or illegitimate and stigmatized. In the example of AIDS, responsibility for the condition is differentially stigmatized depending on whether the sufferer developed it through homosexual contact or through blood transfusion (Carricaburu and Pierret, 1995).

Parsons' sick role would only apply in situations where the deviance is considered serious and legitimation is conditional on the person seeking treatment and getting well. Of interest to this discussion is that chronic illnesses or disabilities tend to fall into either the classification of stigmatized or unconditionally legitimate (as long as they are identified as incurable), and do not correlate with Friedson's classification that corresponds to Parsons' sick role.

First obligation The third element and first obligation of the sick role is that the person must define the state of being ill as undesirable and want to get well. The role is conditionally legitimate on individuals doing what they can to restore their health (Gallagher, 1976). This obligation is unrealistic in chronic conditions in that individuals are not able to get well in the sense of returning to the state they were in prior to developing chronic illness. No matter how much individuals may want to get 'better', they will always have the condition.

The issue of legitimation also applies to the obligation to get well. In the case of chronic illness, legitimacy is not conditional on trying to get well, but on trying to improve oneself within the confines of the degree of 'incurability' of the condition (Freidson, 1965). The role of the physician is then to reinforce the patient's motivation to minimize his or her disability within the confines of the pathological condition (Coe, 1981). In rehabilitation, patients are expected to comply with the physicians' and therapists' goals and work toward 'functional independence' through a prescribed and monitored therapeutic regimen (Kaufman, 1988).

A further condition of legitimacy in chronic illness is limiting demands for privileges to what others consider appropriate. There are a number of examples in the literature of instances where legitimation is tempered if individuals (patients) are perceived by others (usually health care professionals) to be making unrealistic demands.

For example, Mizrahi (1982) describes how interns learn to label and categorize patients according a widely shared perspective which he refers to as GROP (Get Rid Of Patients). Many of the patients to whom this perspective is applied are chronically or terminally ill and for whom there are no cures. Under this perspective, the ideal patient is the one who can be 'gotten rid of'. Patients are actively disparaged by the interns and residents who feel that many of these patients are undeserving of the care that they are receiving.

Similarly, Rosenthal *et al.* (1980) describe how nurses in four acute-care hospital wards label 'problem' patients who do not fit with their perspective of the ideal patient. In general, these 'problem' patients tend to have behaviors or actions that are viewed as non-legitimate in some way, particularly if the behavior is linked to some demand of the nurse's job. Many of the labels such as controlling, non-compliant, career patient and inappropriate, manipulative, or demanding refer to behaviors not associated with the ideal behaviors of being grateful, cooperative, and not causing trouble.

Second obligation The fourth element and second obligation is the person's obligation to seek technically competent help and cooperate with that help in the process of trying to get well. In chronic illness, this philosophy of placing oneself in the hands of the doctor is of limited value in that it ignores the fact that it is more often the individual and their family who are actually providing the day-to-day care. Further, in the long term it could actu-

ally foster dependency because it fails to allow for the sense in which the person autonomously relates to the professional (Gallagher, 1976). There is a vast authority differential between the doctor and patient that is the single most important aspect of the traditional patient/practitioner relationship (Marshall, 1981). In chronic illness, it may be more appropriate for the physician to yield authority to the individuals with the chronic illness as the day-to-day management of chronic illness is by necessity and practice their responsibility.

An alternative model to the sick role model has emerged which is based on consumerism and authority challenges rather than authority acceptance (Haug and Lavin, 1981). This model focuses on the patient's rights and the physician's obligations rather than on the physician's right to direct and the patient's obligation to comply. This model implies a narrowing of the competence gap between the patient and physician. Haug and Lavin's (1981) research suggests that it is younger, better educated patients who tend to adopt a consumerist position but they also note that older people with long-standing chronic ailments may be sufficiently familiar with their own symptoms and treatments that they are also willing to adopt a consumerist stance. This consumerist model may also explain the tendency for some chronically ill individuals to 'shop around' for medical opinions, particularly if initial medical opinions are unacceptable in terms of prognosis and value of treatment.

The obligation to comply also fails to consider what 'cooperating with treatment' means for the chronically ill. Often cooperation with treatment involves following regimens prescribed by the physician or therapist that may be of questionable or limited benefit. Commonly, long-term medical regimens are not followed (Richardson, 1986) and when this occurs, individuals are labeled uncooperative (Strauss *et al.*, 1984) or non-compliant (Roberson, 1992).

Compliance   Compliance is commonly defined as

'the extent to which a person's behavior (in terms of taking medications, following diets, or executing life-style changes) coincides with medical or health advice' (Haynes *et al.*, 1979).

This concept is based on the assumption that, because of illness and lack of training, patients do not have the capacity to make decisions about appropriate medical or therapeutic care (Conrad, 1985) and therefore rational patients will always follow medical advice, which is always good for them (Roberson, 1992). It does not take into account that regimens sometimes present even more difficulties to the daily existence of the individual with chronic illness than the symptoms themselves would.

If regimens are not judged to be efficacious or legitimate they will not be automatically accepted (Strauss and Glaser, 1975). People will make decisions as to whether to follow medical or therapeutic regimens based on their personal priorities, the everyday demands of their lives, and their previous patterns of responding to crisis and disruption (Kaufman, 1988).

Parsons defined the sick role as being inherently universal in that there is generalized objective criteria to determine whether one is sick or not, how sick and with what kind of sickness. This assumption that types of illness conditions and the responses to them are undifferentiated has been identified as one of the major weaknesses of the sick role theory (Coe, 1981). The sick role is also affected by the nature of the illness and by social, cultural, and personal factors (Segall, 1976).

For example, in a study of workers in a pottery factory, Bellaby (1990) found that meanings of sickness are not universally applied; rather, age, gender, and class relations influence how and when sickness is acceptable. 'Genuine' sickness is negotiated between the sick individual and others in the work group, and sometimes with management and medical practitioners.

Summary

This review of the applicability of sick role theory to chronic illness illustrates the limitations of applying a model developed for acute illness to people with chronic, disabling conditions. To summarize, the limitations of Parsons' sick role theory stem from viewing illness as deviance (Gallagher, 1976). There are three main problems with the deviance conception: it fails to account for chronic somatic illness or disability; it fails to account for preventative health care as an element of normative lay conduct and of the professional responsibility of the physician; and it presents a relatively undifferentiated medico-centric picture of the social structure of health care.

There are a number of gaps in functionalist theory, then, that limit our understanding of the experience of chronic illness. In addition, because chronic illness represents an inherently ever-changing process of adaptation, the functionalist approach is limited in its application by its static approach to role theory that sees roles as social norms. It does not take into account other factors such as personal interaction and the ongoing process of socialization, both of which influence role and identity formation.

This brings us to a discussion of interactionism, an approach that stresses the importance of personal interaction in role performance and the influence of socialization as an ongoing, fluid process.

Interactionism and Chronic Illness

In contrast to the functionalist approach that views roles as laid down by society which provides a 'script' for the role performer, interactionists view role performers as active participants in the development of their role. People are agents, not simply

'the products of the contexts in which they live' (Bury, 1991: 452).

Interactionists view role as a much more fluid concept. Norms provide merely a set of broad imperatives within which the details of the role are negotiated according to attitudes, contextual demands, and the evolving definition of the situation as understood by the actors (Biddle, 1986). In performing a role, the individual conveys personal qualities that are role-appropriate and which provide the basis for the self-image of the role performer and the image that others will have of that individual (Goffman, 1961). Returning to the analogy of theatre, whereas functionalists see roles as scripted, interactionists see them as improvised.

According to the interactionist view of role, chronic illness poses a threat to the performance of role(s) that has implications for the person's self-identity and interaction with others. People with chronic illness have to negotiate to incorporate these changes in role performance into their everyday lives. The focus of interactionism with regard to chronic illness is therefore to understand the everyday lives of people with chronic illnesses (Strauss and Glaser, 1975). The interactionist perspective is concerned with the meaning of chronic illness both in terms of its consequences for the individual and its significance for how individuals regard themselves and for how others regard them (Bury, 1991). As such, it increases our understanding of the lived experience of chronic illness and the factors important to quality of life for people with chronic illness and disability.

The trajectory of chronic illness

One of the major differences between acute and chronic illnesses is the time-frame involved. Not only does the illness change over time, but, in addition, people will change as they move through the life course. For interactionists, having a chronic illness is seen as an 'unfolding' or 'emerging' process that occurs over time (Bury, 1988 a&b; Corbin and Strauss, 1988; Robinson, 1988).

Corbin and Strauss (1988) use the metaphor of a voyage of discovery to describe the unfolding of chronic illness. The concept of *illness trajectory* as opposed to course of illness is central to their analysis.

Course of illness is described as a common-sense, professional term, whereas *trajectory* refers 'not only to the physiological unfolding of a ... disease, but to the total organization of work done over that course, plus the impact on those involved with that work and its organization' (Corbin and Strauss, 1988:34).

Trajectory therefore focuses on the active role that people play in shaping the course of an illness. It involves not only the individual with the condition and clinical personnel, but also family and significant others. It implies a process of adaptation that is not only a physiological process but also a psychological, social, and economic process that involves interaction between individuals.

The concept of trajectory expands upon the notion of career proposed by Everett Hughes. Hughes (1971) distinguishes between 'objective career' and 'subjective career'. The former is a series of social statuses and clearly defined offices, while the latter is

'the moving perspective in which the person sees his (her) life as a whole and interprets the meaning of his (her) various attributes, actions, and the things which happen to him (her)'.

By referring to both the total organization of work done over the unfolding of the disease and the impact on those involved in that work and organization, the concept of trajectory incorporates both the objective and subjective aspects of career.

Different theorists have identified different stages of a chronic illness trajectory, beginning with the initial disruption of chronic illness and disability, followed by learning to manage the chronic illness, and finally adapting to living with chronic illness (Corbin and Strauss, 1988; Bury, 1991). Throughout these phases the person with chronic illness must deal with uncertainty, cope with stigmatization, manage

illness trajectories, do biographical work, and recompose a sense of identity (Carricaburu and Pierret, 1995).

The initial disruption of chronic illness or disability

Chronic illness is an unanticipated event, often with an insidious onset that has consequences for all aspects of the person's life. The concepts of biographical disruption (Bury 1982, 1991), biographical work (Corbin and Strauss, 1987, 1988), and identity reconstruction (Charmaz, 1987) have been used to conceptualize changes in everyday life, self-conceptions and personal relationships (Carricaburu and Pierret, 1995). The notion of biography is important because it

'suggests that meaning and context in chronic illness cannot easily be separated' (Bury, 1991:453).

Corbin and Strauss (1988) describe the initial phase of chronic illness after the onset of symptoms as the diagnostic quest, which they further subdivide into pre-diagnosis, the announcement, and the post-diagnostic or filling-in stages. This period can be quite traumatic, particularly if it concludes with the confirmation of disabling or life-threatening illness (Westbrook and Viney, 1982; Corbin and Strauss, 1988).

Uncertainty It is during this phase that the person with chronic illness first encounters one of the hallmarks of living with chronic illness: uncertainty. The trajectory of chronic illness is characterized by uncertainty, initially as symptoms manifest themselves, are recognized, and eventually diagnosed, and continuing as people try to cope with everyday life, not always knowing whether their symptoms will interfere with role performance, or what the long-term manifestations will be. Uncertainty is more pronounced in certain chronic illnesses characterized by exacerbations and remissions, such as multiple sclerosis (Robinson, 1988) and rheumatoid arthritis (Wiener, 1975). However, people with other chronic illnesses also describe uncertainty in terms of everyday planning of activities or tasks when they are not sure if their symptoms will allow them to follow through, and not knowing what the future will bring (Pinder, 1990).

Biographical work   After the onset and diagnosis of the chronic illness, individuals must come to terms with the failure of their bodies and resulting disrupted self-images. There is a separation of identity from past and present that occurs when a severe chronic illness comes into someone's life. Bury (1991) coined the phrase *biographic disruption* referring to changes not only to the physical self but also to the person's sense of identity.

'... who I was in the past and hoped to be in the future are rendered discontinuous with who I am in the present. New conceptions of who and what I am – past, present and future – must arise out of what remains' (Corbin and Strauss, 1988: 49).

Corbin and Strauss (1988) use the term *Biographical Body Conceptions* (BBC) to represent conceptions of self arising directly or indirectly from the body, as they evolve over time. The BBC chain represents the working together of these elements and can be disturbed or shattered by chronic illness.

George Herbert Mead's conception of self is central to an understanding of interactionism's approach to subjectivity (Wallace and Wolf, 1980; Petrunik and Shearing, 1988). He outlined two phases of self: the 'I' phase which consists of the unorganized response of the organism to the attitudes of others, and the 'Me' phase which consists of a set of organized attitudes of others that the individual assumes. The self-interaction which occurs between these two is the basis for role-taking.

Using a Meadian framework, Corbin and Strauss (1988) describe action as a process requiring both a body and a mind. Both are required for completion of the act or performance. However, performance requires a body in which mental and physical processes are working in harmony. The social actions of performance can therefore be affected by the physical limitations accompanying chronic disease, the appearance of the performance in the eyes of others and the physical appearance of the ill person. Perceived failure at performances that are important to one's sense of self can have strong effects on self-identity (see also Charmaz, 1983).

This conceptualization of the influence of the body on self-image is exciting because it attempts to conceptualize the totality of self-identity that incorporates the body. Until recently, the body has usually been ignored in social theory (Schilling, 1993). Although many roles may potentially be open to individuals, if they are unable to perform the role owing to characteristics of the body, they may be open to failure of performance with subsequent effects on self-image.

'Self is a cognitive construct that is constantly being reconstructed and which is expressed in the various narrative and autobiographical accounts which are offered by the individual in self presentation. Self is linked to body in so far as common-sensically self and body are experienced as one and the same thing. However, when bodily demands conflict with desired self-presentation the individual becomes acutely aware of the divergence between body and self' (Kelly and Field, 1996:245).

It is a basic assumption of role theory that each individual will perform more than one role (Goffman, 1961). Presumably the sum of these roles influences the person's self-identity. In chronic illness, the role of impaired or ill will tend to subsume all other roles and eventually lead to a loss or diminishment of self. This loss of self in chronically ill persons as their former self-images are destroyed, without the simultaneous development of equally valued new ones, has been described as a fundamental form of suffering for the chronically ill (Charmaz, 1983). These losses are most marked at the onset of chronic illness, but, over time, accumulated losses lead to diminished self-concept. How people with chronic illness reconcile their sense of self with their changes in body performance will be discussed further in the section on Living with Chronic Illness.

Managing the chronic illness

Once the diagnosis is made, decisions must be made by the physician, the individual, and their family members about the course of the condition and the best mode of management. This phase is made particularly difficult for individuals with chronic illness by the tendency for health professionals to withhold information about the projected course of the disease. For example, in *Timetables*, Roth (1963) describes how TB patients try to gain information about their progress and position in the recovery timetable from doctors and staff. Similarly, in *Passage through Crisis: Polio Victims*

and Their Families, Davis (1963) describes how doctors and health care professionals actually withhold information from families about the prognosis and outlook for their children with polio.

In a study of people who had suffered traumatic spinal cord injury, a participant describes the difficulty health care professionals had discussing his prognosis,

'I mean they (the doctors) are kind of reluctant to sit you down and say this is it for life. They feel that they are protecting you,' (Yoshida, 1994: 98).

Further, the participants in the study identified three important omissions in their rehabilitation process: they felt that they had not been adequately prepared for the outside or 'real' world, that insufficient attention had been paid to sexual concerns, and their individuality had not been considered (Yoshida, 1994).

The work of managing chronic illness In the book *Unending Work and Care: Managing Chronic Illness at Home*, Corbin and Strauss (1988) conceptualize the management of chronic illness trajectories in the home as consisting of three kinds of work: *illness–related work*, which includes regimen work, crisis prevention, and handling, symptom management and diagnostic related work; *biographical work*, which has been discussed earlier; and *everyday life work*, which encompasses the daily round of tasks that keep a household going. These types of work are linked and reciprocally interactive. Associated with each type of work are interactions with families, health care professionals, and others.

Managing treatment regimens The difficulties that people with chronic illness encounter following treatment regimens has been discussed earlier, but bears further emphasis. Although compliance with regimens may be of high priority for health professionals, people with chronic illness report that following treatment regimens can pose more difficulties for them than the actual health problem. Symptom control, social interactions, preventing medical crises, economic issues, and quality of life may take precedence for them (Strauss and Glaser, 1975; Gerber, 1986; Roberson, 1992). They may prefer treatment approaches that are manageable, livable with, and effective from their perspective (Roberson, 1992).

Over time, as they cope with the work of managing chronic illness, people with chronic illnesses may become more expert in the management of their own condition than the health care professionals with whom they come into contact. For example, people with conditions such as multiple sclerosis and arthritis may become experts on drug therapies in terms of medical effects and long-term usage and will make their own decisions about the relative costs and benefits (Robinson, 1988; Scambler, 1989, Bury, 1991). This can make it even more difficult for these individuals if they are recast into the sick role by an acute exacerbation and are expected to readopt a passive, compliant attitude in their interactions with health care professionals. A 'partnership' between patients and practitioners assumes even greater importance in these instances.

Living with chronic illness

Adapting to a life that includes chronic illness is the final stage of the chronic illness trajectory. Corbin and Strauss (1988) refer to this stage as that of 'putting life back together again'. It is at this stage that people with chronic illness reconstruct or recompose their identities to include the disabled self.

Recomposing a sense of identity Corbin and Strauss (1988) suggest that the BBC chain is put back together through four separate but overlapping biographical processes: *contextualizing* which involves incorporating the illness trajectory into one's biography; *coming to terms* which involves the person arriving at some degree of understanding and acceptance of the biographical consequences of actual or potential failed performances; *identity reconstitution* whereby the person integrates his or her identity into a new conceptualization of wholeness around the limitations of performance and *biographical recasting* which involves giving new directions to one's biography.

For example, Yoshida (1993) describes a pendular reconstruction of self and identity for adults following traumatic spinal cord injury in which they move back and forth between the disabled and non-disabled aspects of self until they eventually incorporate their disabled identity as an aspect of the total self. One of the participants describes this phenomenon:

'Initially, I sort of felt that I really wasn't a *whole person*. I also felt that I wasn't a *worthy person*. I must have done something *terribly wrong* to have this happen to me in my life. And I have sort of gotten over that and come to terms with that, if it happens, it happens. If you get run over by a bus, it happens. And I feel *good* about myself, I *like myself very much* and the fact that I am disabled, *is just another part of my life*, I don't like myself any *less* because of it. But I don't like myself *any more* because of it' (Yoshida, 1993:229).

Social isolation The self is developed and maintained through social relationships but, because of their chronic illnesses, individuals' self-identities suffer from leading restricted lives, experiencing social isolation, being discredited, and burdening others (Charmaz, 1983). Loss of social contact that may extend to social isolation is a very real problem for the chronically ill. It may be precipitated by the sick person him or herself, who may be unwilling or unable to maintain previous contacts or establish new relationships.

For example, in a study of individuals with Parkinson's disease, informants describe the shame that they feel as a result of the assumed rule-breaking character of the signs of the disease, such as shaking and drooling, particularly if the rules being broken are considered socially sensitive (Nijhof, 1995). One informant describes how he has gradually retreated and given up his participation in the public world:

'I used to like going out for dinner with the children, but I don't dare anymore. Then, I'm sitting there, fumbling, being all clumsy. You can do that at home, but not in a restaurant. No, I don't dare anymore. The children mind that I won't go anymore. But I already have towels which are used as a bib!' (Nijhof, 1995:201).

Dyck (1995) coins the phrase 'shrinking social and geographical worlds' to describe this phenomenon in her study of women with multiple sclerosis. She describes how they restructure their physical space and social relationships as they accommodate to their diminishing physical capacities.

Social isolation is also due to the tendency of others to withdraw from the sick person. Zola (1981) contends that the reasons for the distancing of the chronically ill and disabled in North American society is related to both the nature of society and the nature of people. He notes that the United States is built on the premise that there is no adversity (and therefore, no disease) that cannot be overcome. The chronically ill are visible reminders of the fallacy of this belief and the reality that we are all susceptible to the vagaries of disease, growing old, and death.

Coping, strategy and style Three concepts are important for understanding the process of learning to live with chronic illness: coping, strategy, and style (Bury, 1991). Although these terms are not always used consistently, Bury (1991) recommends the following definitions:

Coping refers to

'the cognitive processes whereby the individual learns how to tolerate or put up with the effects of illness' (Bury, 1991:460).

Strategy refers to

'the actions people take, or what people do in the face of illness' (Bury, 1991:461).

Style refers to

'the way people respond to, and present, important features of their illnesses or treatment regimens' (Bury, 1991:462).

Coping with stigmatization Unless individuals have been ill or disabled from birth or early childhood, they will probably share many of the negative attitudes of society toward the disabled (Davis, 1972). They will tend to value activities and pursuits now closed to them. Attempts to be accepted in these activities will be met with a sense of rejection by 'normals' that will be supported by the individuals themselves who share the 'normal' standards of personal evaluation.

Davis (1972) describes three alternative strategies that are open to the chronically ill or handicapped when they attempt to relate to 'normals': *passing, normalization,* and *disassociation.*

Passing When passing, individuals and those around them attempt to disguise the visible signs of the impairment. Because of the great rewards in being considered normal, almost all people who are able to pass will do so on some occasion intentionally using strategies such as concealment or disidentifiers, or presentation of the signs of the failing as representative of some other, less stigmatizing attribute (Goffman, 1963). However, even successful use of the stratagem of 'passing' results in high psychological costs despite the considerable benefits (Strauss *et al.,* 1984). Those who 'pass' have the anxiety that their secret will be found out, resulting in embarrassment, at the least, or loss of friendships or employment at worst.

Normalization In normalization, once again, the normal standard is used, but, instead of trying to pass for normal, those aspects of individuals that cause them to be different are rationalized or denied to be of any importance. Robinson (1993) describes how individuals and their family members construct the story of their lives as normal as a means of coping with chronic illness. They minimize the significance of the impact of the chronic illness and reconstruct the reference points by which the experience is judged. However, this normalization strategy can be very tenuous (Strauss *et al.,* 1984), requiring a balancing act

on the part of informants (Robinson, 1993). It requires considerable work on the part of the ill individual to maintain these tactics and very little to disrupt the performance.

Disassociation Unlike passing and normalization, disassociation involves relinquishment of the normal standard. In this situation, individuals and their families avoid situations that reinforce the fact that the person is 'different'. Disassociation may take other forms that include resentment and anger towards 'normals', passive acceptance of exclusion, retreat into a fantasy situation, and an attempt to recast and reformulate personal values, activities and associations in order to minimize the effect of the negative attitudes of normals (Davis, 1972).

Socialization to chronic illness To this point, the discussion has focused on the experiences of individuals who find themselves in the situation of being chronically ill, and the impact this has on their self-identity. However, there are other important influences that have profound implications on how the chronically ill eventually come to view themselves and be viewed by society. These influences relate to the process of *socialization to chronic illness.* The predominant social values in the society or culture in which a person lives influence socialization of the chronically ill.

A person's self-concept is acquired through the process of socialization in that one's image of oneself is based on one's perceptions of the evaluations of others of oneself, particularly if their opinions are valued. If individuals fall into a category of people perceived to be 'different' from the norm, a social identity related to those categories may be imputed to them.

Goffman (1963) refers to this characterization as a person's virtual social identity. The attributes that individuals in fact possess are their actual social identities. However, if individuals perceive the evaluations of their virtual social identity and internalize them as part of their self-concept, then this putative identity becomes a personal identity or their actual social identity. This process of role learning is termed *socialization.*

Scott (1969) describes the ways that blind people are socialized through personal interaction and in blindness agencies. Personal interaction with 'normals' has profound implications for the blind. The stereotypic beliefs of the sighted about the blind being dependent and helpless, reinforce these same behaviors in the blind. Like many chronic conditions, blindness stigmatizes and 'spoils' the person's social identity. Perhaps even more than many other chronic conditions, blindness itself affects the quality of personal interaction because the blind person is unable to maintain eye contact or get visual feedback during encounters. As a result, the conduct of these interactions is disturbed. In addition, relationships between the blind and the sighted are often ones of social dependency, in which the blind, by virtue of their dependency, are subordinate in the relationship.

Learned helplessness Learned helplessness (Seligman, 1975; Solomon, 1982) is another example of a situation in which stereotyping of a classification of individuals (in this case, the institutionalized elderly) by health care professionals in a setting in which there is unequal interpersonal exchange, leads to the adoption of behaviors on the part of the elderly that reinforce the stereotype. Older people in institutions are expected to be sick, confused, passive, and resigned to inactivity (Foy and Mitchell, 1991). Behaviors that fit with the stereotype are reinforced, while behaviors that do not are subtly, if not overtly, discouraged. Dependency behaviors are encouraged, albeit inadvertently, often under the guise of helping.

Summary

The interactionist approach adds to our understanding of chronic illness because it explains the effects of personal interaction and socialization on role formation. It provides a framework more suited to the experience of chronic illness in that it is fluid and changing, both characteristics that also apply to chronic illness. However, it too has gaps in that it also views illness as deviance and does not account for the broader social, political, and economic relationships that also influence the experience of living with chronic illness.

Comparison and Reconciliation: Functionalism and Interactionism

This chapter has examined the experience of chronic illness by reviewing the functionalist and interactionist approaches to role theory. Discussion of the functionalist approach led to the conclusion that, for a number of reasons, sick role theory has considerable limitations when applied to chronic illness. First, because it views illness as deviance and second, because it is static in that it views roles as prescribed and does not allow for the effects of personal interaction or the active participation of the role performer.

It was then suggested that the interactionist approach is more suited to the study of chronic illness experience because it does take personal interaction and socialization into account and through this analysis provides insight into the active and diverse ways that people respond to chronic illness and disability (Dyck, 1995). It is a more fluid approach that provides a framework that allows for a better understanding of chronic illness because it allows for flux and change – both characteristics of chronic illness. However, it too has limitations in that it does not take into account the broader structural contexts of culture, politics, and economics.

Is it possible to reconcile some of the limitations of the two approaches by integrating them? Do the strengths in one augment the gaps in the other?

Interactionism can augment the functionalist approach by analyzing how personal interaction and socialization affect role and identity formation. Although interactionism is thought to view roles to be in constant flux, it is not clear that the approach denies the existence and influence of roles brought to the interaction (Heiss, 1981). Interactionists concede that some identities have generally accepted norms attached to them and as such will form the starting point for interaction, although they can be modified by the individual. Functionalism can augment interactionism by providing the basis for defining what these preconceived norms and identities may be. This is particularly true in the case of chronic illness and disability where often the individual is imputed a social identity and role by virtue of their condition.

Using the theatre/drama metaphor, Goffman (1961) links the two approaches by describing the actor as playing out the 'prescribed' role but in a more varied way. In other words, role is neither totally spontaneous nor totally prescribed, and both interpretations are necessary for complete understanding of role performance.

The notion that within a culture or a society there are mutually shared sets of expectations as to the behavior of role incumbents provides a useful framework within which one can examine face-to-face interactions. At the same time, the idea that in each interaction we have the capacity to improvise or adapt our behavior according to our interpretation of the situation is critical. If we take the sick role to represent the social norms and expectations about illness and contrast that to the actual experience of people living with chronic illness, it helps explain the difficulties people with chronic illness experience as they interact with the health care system and try to reconstruct their everyday lives.

Understanding role from these two perspectives allows greater understanding of how society functions at both macro and micro levels. On the macro level, if we understand that there is consensus within society about certain roles, and that for these roles there are shared norms and values, then it begs the questions: how do we come to define these roles, and how do we come to share or internalize the underlying norms and values? On the micro level, how do these norms and values affect our face-to-face interactions, and why do some individuals adopt certain role behaviors while others do not?

The relationship between self and society is interactive in that it is possible to analyze not only how society affects the self-concept, but also how the self-concept affects society (Rosenberg, 1981). The self-concept is both a social product and a social force. For example, changes in women's self-concepts between the 1950s and the 1980s have had profound implications for the social system as a whole. The experience of people with chronic illness and disability is also an example in that, with changes in self-identity and self-concept, they are no longer willing to sit on the sidelines and be excluded from the mainstream. This has had implications for the broader social system in terms of ensuring accessibility, transportation, and employment opportunities, to name but a few.

Although it is possible for either of the two approaches to augment some of the limitations in the other, gaps remain. Functionalism and interactionism both reflect a disability as deviance perspective (Albrecht, 1992), and as such, neither approach adequately explains the interaction of chronic illness and disability with the broader structural influences in society related to politics and economics such as issues of gender, class, and access to and distribution of material and social resources (Dyck, 1995). However, despite these limitations, they do shed considerable light on the everyday experiences of individuals living with chronic illness.

References

Albrecht, GL (1992) *The Disability Business: Rehabilitation in America.* London: Sage.

Bellaby, P (1990) What is genuine sickness? The relation between work-discipline and the sick role in a pottery factory. *Sociology of Health and Illness* 12: 47–68.

Biddle, BJ (1986) Recent Developments in Role Theory. *Annual Review of Sociology* 12: 67–92.

Bury, M (1982) Chronic illness as a biographical disruption *Sociology of Health and Illness* 4: 167–182.

Bury, MR (1988a) Chronic illness as a biographical disruption *Sociology of Health and Illness* 4: 167–182.

Bury, MR (1988b) Meanings at risk: the experience of arthritis. In: Anderson, R, Bury, M (eds) *Living with Chronic Illness: The Experience of Patients and their Families.* London: Unwin Hyman,

Bury, MR (1991) The sociology of chronic illness: a review of research and prospects. *Sociology of Health and Illness* 13 (4): 451–468.

Carricaburu, D, Pierret, J (1995) From biographical disruption to biographical reinforcement: the case of HIV-positive men. *Sociology of Health and Illness* 17(1): 65–88.

Charmaz, K (1983) Loss of self: a fundamental form of suffering in the chronically ill. *Sociology of Health and Illness* 5(2): 168–195.

Charmaz, K (1987) Struggling for a self: identity levels of the chronically ill. *Research in the Sociology of Health Care* 6: 283–321.

Coe, RM (1981) The sick role revisited. In Haug, MR (ed) *Elderly Patients and their Doctors* pp. 22–33. New York: Springer.

Conrad, P (1985) The meaning of medications: another look at compliance. *Social Science and Medicine* 20: 29-37

Corbin, J, Strauss, A (1987) Accompaniments of chronic illness: changes in body, self, biography and biographical time. *Research in the Sociology of Health Care* 6:249-281

Corbin, JM. Strauss, A (1988) *Unending Work and Care: Managing Chronic Illness at Home.* San Francisco: Jossey-Bass Publishers.

Davis, F (1963) *Passage through Crisis: Polio Victims and Their Families.* Indianapolis: Babbs-Merrill.

Davis F (1972) *Illness, Interaction and the Self.* Belmont, Ca: Wadsworth Publishing Co.

Dyck, I (1995) Hidden geographies: the changing lifeworlds of women with multiple sclerosis. *Social Science and Medicine* 40(3): 307–320.

Foy, SS, Mitchell, MM (1991) Factors contributing to learned helplessness in the institutionalized aged: a literature review. *Physical & Occupational Therapy in Geriatrics* 9(2): 1–23.

Freidson, E (1965) Disability as social deviance. In: Sussman, MB (ed) *Sociology and Rehabilitation*, pp. 71–99. American Sociological Association

Freidson, E (1970) *Profession of Medicine.* New York: Dodd Mead.

Gallagher, EB (1976) Lines of reconstruction and extension in the Parsonian sociology of illness. *Social Science and Medicine* 10: 207–218.

Gerber, KE (1986) Compliance in the chronically ill. In: Gerber, KE, Nehemkis, AM (eds), pp. 12–24. *Compliance: The dilemma of the chronically ill.* New York: Springer.

Goffman, E. (1961) Role distance. In Goffman, E (ed) *Encounters*, pp. 85–152. Indiapolis: Bobbs-Merril,

Goffman, E (1963) *Stigma*. Englewood Cliffs, NJ: Prentice-Hall.

Haug, MR, Lavin, B (1981) Practitioner or patient – who's in charge? *Journal of Health and Social Behaviour* 22: 212–222.

Haynes, RB, Taylor, DW, Sackett, DL (eds) (1979) *Compliance in Health Care* p. 4. Baltimore: Johns Hopkins University Press.

Heiss, J (1981) Social Roles. In: Rosenberg, M and Turner, R (eds) *Social Psychology: Sociological Perspectives*, pp. 94–129 New York: Basic Books.

Hughes, EC (1971) Cycles, turning points and careers. In: Hughes, EC (ed) *The Sociological Eye*. pp. 1214–1231. Chicago: Aldine Atherton.

Kaufman, SR (1988) Stroke rehabilitation and the negotiation of identity, pp. 82–103. In: Reinharz, S, Rowles, GD (eds) *Qualitative Gerontology*. New York: Springer.

Kelly, MP, Field, D (1996) Medical sociology, chronic illness and the body. *Sociology of Health and Illness* 18: 241–257.

Marshall, VW (1981) Physician characteristics and relationships with older patients. In: Haug, MR (ed) *Elderly Patients and their Doctors*. pp. 94–118. Springer: New York.

Mechanic, D (1961) The concept of illness behaviour. *Journal of Chronic Disease* 15: 196–206.

Mizrahi, T (1982) Getting rid of patients: contradictions in the socialization of internists to the doctor–patient relationship. *Sociology of Health and Illness* 7: 214–235.

Nijhof, G (1995) Parkinson's disease as a problem of shame in public appearance. *Sociology of Health and Illness* 17(2): 193–205.

Parsons, T (1951) Social structure and dynamic process: the case of modern medical practice. In: Talcott Parsons, *The Social System* pp. 428–479. New York: The Free Press.

Petrunik, M, Shearing, CD (1988) The 'I', the 'Me' and the 'It': moving beyond the Meadian conception of self. *Canadian Journal of Sociology* 13(4): 435–440.

Pinder, R (1990) What to expect: information and the management of uncertainty in Parkinson's disease *Disability, Handicap & Society* 3 (1): 77–92.

Richardson, JL (1986) Perspective on compliance with drug regimens among the elderly. *Journal of Compliance in Health Care* 1(1): 33–45.

Robinson, CA (1993) Managing life with a chronic condition: the story of normalization. *Qualitative Health Research* 3 (1): 6–28.

Robinson, I (1988) *Multiple Sclerosis*. London: Tavistock/Routledge.

Roberson, MHB (1992) The meaning of compliance: patient perspectives. *Qualitative Health Research* 2 (1): 7–26.

Rosenberg, M (1981) The self-concept: social product and social force. pp. 593–624. In: Rosenberg and Turner (eds) *Social Psychology: Sociological Perspectives*. New York: Basic Books.

Rosenthal, C, Marshall, V, French, S, Macpherson, AS (1980) *Nurses, Patients and Families: Care and Control in the Hospital*. New York: Springer.

Roth, JA (1963) *Timetables*. New York: Bobbs Merrill Co.

Scambler, G, Hopkins, A (1986) Being epileptic: coming to terms with stigma. *Sociology of Health and Illness* 8: 26–43.

Scambler, G (1989) *Epilepsy*. London: Tavistock.

Schilling, C (1993) *The Body and Social Theory*. London: Sage.

Scott, RA (1969) *The Making of Blind Men*. New York: Sage.

Segall, A (1976) The sick role concept: understanding illness behaviour. *Journal of Health and Social Behaviour* 17(6): 163–170.

Seligman, M (1975) *Helplessness*. San Francisco: W.H. Freeman and Co.

Solomon, K (1982) Social antecedents of learned helplessness in the health care setting. *Gerontologist* 22(3): 282.

Strauss, AL, Glaser, B (1975) *Chronic Illness and the Quality of Life*. St. Louis: Mosby.

Strauss, AL, Corbin, J, Fagerhaugh, S, Glaser, BG, Maines, D, Suczek, B, Wiener, CL (1984) *Chronic Illness and the Quality of Life*. Toronto: CV Mosby Co.

Turner, R (1985) Unanswered questions in the convergence between structuralist and interactionist role theories. In: Helle, HJ, Eisenstadt, SN (eds) *Microsociological Theory: Perspectives on Sociological Theory*, Vol. 2, pp. 22–36. Beverley Hills, CA: Sage.

Wallace, RA, Wolf, A (1980) *Contemporary Sociological Theory: Continuing the Classical Tradition*, 2nd edn. Englewood Cliffs, NJ: Prentice-Hall.

Westbrook, MT, Viney, LL (1982) Psychological reactions to the onset of chronic illness. *Social Science and Medicine* 16: 899–905.

Wiener, CL (1975) The burden of rheumatoid arthritis: tolerating the uncertainty. *Social Science and Medicine* 9: 97–104.

Yoshida, KK (1993) The reshaping of self: a pendular reconstruction of the identity among individuals with traumatic spinal cord injury. *Sociology of Health and Illness* 15: 217.

Yoshida, KK (1994) Institutional impact on self concept among persons with spinal cord injury. *International Journal of Rehabilitation Research* 17: 95–107.

Zola, IK (1981) Communication barriers between the 'able bodied' and the 'handicapped'. *Archives of Physical Medicine and Rehabilitation* 62: 355–360.

10

Self-Efficacy

Monica Lehman & Beth A Roller

Introduction
•
Statement of Problem
•
Discussion
•
Case 1
•
Self-Efficacy Related to the Case
•
Implications for Treatment
•
Conclusion

Introduction

In this chapter, we will address the importance of assessing the level of a patient's self-efficacy in the physical therapy environment. We have arbitrarily chosen the topic of fear of falling in the geriatric population to give a context to this discussion of self-efficacy. Background information regarding falls in the elderly, as well as a general description of current treatment practices for these individuals, is included in the following sections. The objective is to discuss how treatment techniques may omit the vital component of assessment and treatment of low self-efficacy. Self-efficacy is defined and discussed within a theoretical framework, including several related concepts. A case study is presented to illustrate the importance of addressing low self-efficacy in geriatric patients. We conclude with several recommendations for incorporating a focus on self-efficacy within the treatment context of our physical therapy sessions.

Physical therapists, therapist assistants, and other health professionals understand that mobility is a vital factor in maintaining quality of life for the geriatric patient. Unfortunately for these patients, recurring falls or simply fear of falling, also known as *ptophobia*, can have significant consequences on quality of life. In this population, falling is widely recognized as a major health problem with life-threatening consequences. Tinetti and Powell (1994) estimated that over one third of all individuals over the age of 65 suffer falls each year, resulting in hospitalizations, nursing home admissions, and even death. Injuries resulting from falls in the geriatric population are predictable and preventable. Important physical and psychosocial factors associated with falls in the elderly can be addressed through prevention and intervention programs. These programs usually address the risk factors associated with falls, and how those risks can be minimized.

Researchers have identified many risk factors associated with falls in the geriatric population (Tinetti *et al.*, 1988; Brown Commodore, 1995). These risk factors have been categorized as either intrinsic or extrinsic factors. Intrinsic factors include changes in the individual's physical condition such as alterations in perception, memory, mood, decreased muscle tone, incontinence, mobility impairment, sensory changes, and/or decreased muscle mass. Extrinsic factors include aspects of the individual's environment such as poor lighting, inappropriate footwear, assistive devices, unsafe walking areas, and medication use (Bernstein-Lewis, 1990). Bernstein-Lewis suggests that approximately 55% of falls are caused by intrinsic factors and 40% by extrinsic factors. While the literature regarding intrinsic risk factors abounds with information related to the physical changes that may be present in the geriatric patient, little discussion focuses on the psychosocial factors that may be associated as a possible cause of falls.

Statement of Problem

A review of current literature pertaining to falls in the elderly reveals that most of the research addresses physiological changes in the individual and unsafe environmental factors which may increase the individual's risk of falling. Few studies approach falls from a psychosocial perspective. This is an interesting point when considering that studies have indicated fear of falling is quite common in the geriatric population, including those who have sustained falls and those who have not (Tinetti *et al.*, 1988; Tinetti *et al.*, 1994; Brown Commodore, 1995; Hill *et al.*, 1996). As a result of a fall or fear of falling, one may develop a decreased confidence in physical abilities leading that individual to withdraw from activities or on the wider scale, society. Tinetti *et al.*, (1988) found in one study that half of all individuals who sustained a fall reportedly avoided activities which they performed prior to the fall. Avoiding activities can have detrimental effects on the individuals in this age group. Aside from the obvious deconditioning that they will experience, this withdrawal can change the individual's perception of his/her capabilities. We will explore this aspect of self-efficacy, as it relates to withdrawal from activities in the geriatric patient.

A widely utilized physical therapy treatment for the individual who has a high risk for falls includes strengthening exercises, balance and coordination activities, gait training, and possibly education to prevent additional falls. Alternative methods of treatment such as t'ai chi, acupuncture and awareness through movement (ATM) are also used to prevent recurrence of falls in this population. Although there may be effective treatments that can address the physical components associated with falls, therapists rarely assess the patient's perception of their capability or self-efficacy. Therapists who do deal with low self-efficacy in treatment sessions tend to be using intuitive processes rather than cognitive strategies. We suggest taking a more deliberate approach in the clinic and including the assessment of self-efficacy in the evaluation of the patient.

Discussion

Corollary concepts

A brief presentation of corollary concepts will facilitate understanding of self-efficacy, and the discussion that follows. These related terms are: self-concept, self-esteem / self-confidence and motivation. Quite frequently these words are used incorrectly in everyday speech.

Self-concept, also referred to as 'ego', is an illusive term without a clear definition. Many theorists have promulgated different definitions leading one to conclude from the literature that these definitions are imprecise and contradictory. Byrne (1966) defines self-concept as an additive of two other concepts, self-as-object and self-as-process:

'Self-as-object is the total aggregate of attitudes, judgments and values which an individual holds with respect to his behavior, his ability, his body, his worth as a person, in short, how he perceives and evaluates himself. Self-as-process is defined in terms of activities such as thinking and perceiving and coping with the environment.'

Self-concept is a relatively stable set of perceptions that we hold of ourselves. Adler and

Towne (1996) propose that self-concept is almost totally a product of an individual's interaction with others, developed over time, and based upon the feedback about one's behavior as perceived by those others. Mead (1934) wrote of the social construction of self concept as a reflection of the opinions and attitudes that are communicated to us by our significant others.

Self-esteem, also referred to in the literature as self-confidence, is how favorably a person regards him or herself. Self-esteem is defined by Burns as

'The evaluation that the individual makes and customarily maintains with regard to himself: it expresses an attitude of approval or disapproval and indicates the extent to which the individual believes himself to be capable, significant, successful and worthy' (Burns, 1979).

It is the person's perception and evaluation, but not reality. Unlike self-efficacy, self-esteem is not task specific.

Motivation can be described from three different perspectives: biological, social, or cognitive. The latter construction of motivation is used in this paper. Cognitive motivation takes into account how our self-perceptions, interpretation of outside events, and degree of self-control have an effect on our level of initiative. Although a number of theories disagree about the origin and factors that affect motivation, they do generally agree that the end result is an arousal to action which involves physiologic mechanisms. There seems to be widespread misuse of the term 'motivation'. The concept identifies energy or a force in the individual, one which is internally driven. Therefore, a therapist can create an environment to facilitate a higher level of motivation in the patient, but it is not possible for the therapist to 'motivate' the patient to do something.

Self-efficacy

Many definitions of self-efficacy appear in the literature, dating from 1977 to the present. Among these, that of Albert Bandura's serves as the basis for this discussion because of his extensive work over many years on this concept. He defines self-efficacy as

'people's judgments of their capabilities to organize and execute courses of action required to attain designated types of performances' (Bandura, 1986).

Self-efficacy is an individual's subjective perception of this ability to perform the task in question. It is a specialized set of expectations that apply to the performance of a given behavior, not the outcome. Self-efficacy does not refer to the actual skills that an individual possesses, but rather to what that person believes about what can be accomplished with his/her skills. It is our perception of our own ability to cause or bring about a desired effect or event, a combination of our self-esteem, skills, and resources, and it is task specific.

Self-inefficacy, or a weak sense of self-efficacy, involves expectations of undesirable outcomes which leads to anxiety and avoidance of difficult or threatening situations. Bandura notes that a weak sense of self-efficacy results in

'low aspirations and weak commitment to the goals they choose to perform'.

Perceptions of self-inefficacy may explain why a person does not perform optimally even though he/she knows what to do (Bandura, 1982).

An individual's sense of self-efficacy in relation to one activity would carry over only to a similar activity because, as mentioned previously, self-efficacy is task specific. Individuals with a strong sense of self-efficacy tend to perform at higher levels, in part because they consider setbacks and difficult obstacles as challenges. Individuals with low self-efficacy, or feelings of self-inefficacy, view these situations as threats.

Work by Bandura (1985) indicates a physiological link to an individual's self-efficacy. He has demonstrated evidence of changes in catecholamine levels related to levels of self-efficacy. He found low levels of catecholamine release during activities that individuals felt highly efficacious. He also observed that catecholamine levels rose as individuals performed tasks about which they doubted their ability to be successful. After utilizing behavior techniques to help these individuals develop an increased sense of self-efficacy during these tasks, catecholamine levels were tested again. Bandura noted that the release of catecholamines was significantly less.

Bandura's self-efficacy model and the social cognitive theory

In his discussion of self-efficacy, Bandura speculates that behavior is influenced by two types of expectancy: outcome and efficacy (Scherer and Shimmel, 1996). Outcome expectancy is the belief that certain behaviors will result in certain outcomes. Efficacy expectancy is the belief that one can successfully execute the behavior necessary to produce the outcome. According to Bandura's (1977) earlier work, the strength of individuals' beliefs about their ability to produce a specific outcome determines whether or not they will attempt to deal with a difficult situation. Therefore, self-efficacy judgments play a major role in determining which activities or situations a person will perform or avoid. A person's level of expectations regarding self-efficacy is governed by four sources of information: performance accomplishment, vicarious accomplishment, verbal persuasion, and physiological status based on the social cognitive theory (Bandura, 1986).

Performance accomplishment refers to successful mastery of skills that results from personal experience. It includes a progression toward feelings of self-confidence as the individual performs and masters the task. Mastery of a task tends to increase perceived self-efficacy (Bandura, 1977). If a person has a high self-confidence in performance of a particular task, their self-efficacy as related to that task would also be high.

Self-efficacy may also be improved through *vicarious experience*. This occurs when an individual knows or sees someone similar to themselves achieve success at the task. Vicarious experiences may be fostered by exposing an individual to people of similar capabilities who have successfully performed a target behavior. Observations of others' successful performance enhance individual's expectation regarding their own mastery.

Verbal persuasion from an external source may affect self-efficacy by influencing a person's ability to complete a task through encouragement or discouragement. Used in a positive manner, it may convince individuals that they can perform an activity. The impact of verbal persuasion is determined by several factors related to both the persuader and the individual being persuaded. These factors are: the credibility of the messenger, the individual's prior experience, and the individual's other personal qualities. For example, verbal persuasion may be more effective for an individual who is outer-rather than inner-directed in terms of where they derive the energy to stimulate activity. Praise and encouragement are examples of verbal persuasion. We also call this positive reinforcement.

Physiologic status such as the experience of pain, fatigue, or illness will affect a person's perception of whether or not they can perform a task. Emotional states may lead to physiologic arousal and can also influence expectations about self-efficacy. Individuals rely on feedback from within themselves to judge their physical performance and capabilities. If an individual perceives pain, he/she may feel less able to complete a task.

Relationship of self-efficacy and corollary concepts

An individual's level of self-efficacy will determine whether or not he/she will attempt what they believe to be a challenging task. However, until that task is attempted and completed successfully, it is not possible to increase self esteem. If the person believes they are unable to complete a task successfully, that individual will not be able to generate the motivation necessary to perform it. Essentially, these components discussed above have a quasi-circular effect upon each other. When individuals experience task-specific successes, their self-efficacy grows. The more overall successes they experience, the higher their self-confidence and self-esteem (Fig. 10.1). On a wider scale, self-concept is altered as a result of how others may see the individual based on their successes and failures.

Figure 10.1

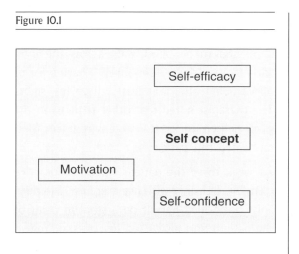

Case 1

Ms L.K. is a 76-year-old female referred to a subacute hospital by her physician because she is unable to ambulate. Three years ago this patient was diagnosed with adult onset diabetes mellitus. Her most recent hospitalization was due to anorexia. This diagnosis was questionable because the patient could eat and had an appetite; but she just had difficulty obtaining nutrition. Her older brother had found her dehydrated and unconscious in her apartment after he had been away on vacation for two weeks. For the previous eight months he had been getting her groceries and checking in on her occasionally to make sure she was preparing her own meals. She assured him that she would continue with meal preparation and would be fine while he was on vacation. She confided in her therapist that she had fallen on the second day of his absence but did not tell her brother about this so as not to ruin his time away. She reported that after the fall, her functional movement about the apartment decreased significantly, including her ability to prepare meals. Her visit to the hospital revealed peripheral neuropathy in both lower extremities and compromised vision. Ms L.K. reports a history of frequent falls and a fear of falling.

On initial evaluation this patient presented with mild obesity (120 lbs at 4'9"). She had normal range of motion in all extremities. Manual muscle testing revealed $4-/5$ to $4+/5$ throughout. Sensation to light touch as well as deep pressure was decreased in both lower extremities. The patient was independent in bed mobility and supine to sit transfers, but unable or unwilling to perform a sit to stand transfer. The therapist was unable to assess gait at the time of the evaluation. A diagnosis of ptophobia or fear of falling was added to the problem list. The psychiatry service was contacted to help plan and monitor the patient's treatment.

Week one of the patient's therapy consisted of strengthening and coordination exercises for the lower extremities. She also received instruction on activities that increased her awareness of the lower extremity positioning and movement. During these early stages she was given a lot of positive reinforcement in order to make her feel good about coming to and participating in therapy. By the end of the first week this patient was standing in the parallel bars with maximum assistance of two people for side support and blocking of the knees and a third person with wheelchair back-up. She did not necessarily need the assistance, but because of her fear of falling she would not even consider standing without it.

At week two this patient continued with these activities and was asked to begin pre-ambulation training. However, she continued to express a fear of falling whenever the word standing was mentioned. Halfway through week two, during a stand pivot sit transfer, both knees flexed and she was slowly lowered to the floor by her therapist. The therapist believed that the patient's knees did not 'buckle' from muscle weakness, because the results of the manual muscle tests and her performance of exercise indicated adequate strength. She also actually felt the patient pushing herself down. The therapist did believe, however, that the patient was truly afraid, based upon her widened eyes, increased respiration, and obvious perspiration. The incongruity prompted the therapist to confront the patient. The patient responded that she did not know why she fell, but she knew she was going to fall even before the transfer began.

The therapist reconsidered the approach she had been using with the patient. From the day of admission, Ms L.K. had been treated gently. The staff tried not to increase her fear by pushing her to do something she was not ready to do. Perhaps this approach served to encourage her to continue to avoid what she feared most – standing and walking. The therapist believed that forcing the patient to stand and walk would jeopardize the trust that was developing, so she decided to try a different approach. It started with a 'pep talk'. She told the patient that there was no physical reason why she could not stand and walk, she had good strength and coordination. Ms L.K. responded that she thought it might be because she could not feel her legs. The therapist agreed that the loss of feeling in her legs would make it scary to stand, but that did not mean that her legs would not work. This conversation took place in a quiet corner of the therapy gym, with the patient facing the center of the gym. As they spoke the therapist observed the patient watching a woman, who happened to be blind, walk across the gym with a cane. Ms L.K. exclaimed 'I have a lot of nerve being afraid, at least I have my sight.' The therapist noted that other patients in the gym helped to create an environment that motivated this patient.

At week three the patient agreed to practice transfers, but only with her therapist. The therapist positioned herself on a stool in front of the patient and instructed her on standing to a half squat position and sitting again, while maintaining a slow speed and control. This was the first time the patient actually pushed herself up from the chair with her arms. Initially, during transfer training she was actually pushing herself back into the chair. The therapist gave her a lot of positive reinforcement by saying things like, 'You are standing! You look great!'. By the end of week three, Ms L.K. could stand alone with the reassurance that the therapist would provide knee bracing and wheelchair back-up, if needed. Occasionally, her knees would buckle as she stood. At those times, the therapist gave clear, firm instruction to 'stand up straight'. During week three, the patient was introduced to the use of imagery. It was used for each activity progression the day before it was attempted. The patient reported that this worked well for her because as she sat in her room, alone at night, she visualized herself performing the suggested activity. She expressed a more positive attitude about her performance and even seemed eager to try new things as the days progressed.

When week four arrived, she was ready to perform the weight shifting and marching activities with a walker that she had been told about at the end of the previous session. To many of the staff members, this seemed to be a slow and drawn out process that would never end. The supervisor instructed the therapist to move on to gait training without further delay. Despite the therapist's calm demeanor and positive encouragement the patient regressed and promptly fell to her knees when a walk was suggested. This patient was going to progress at her own pace. The therapist opted for more time with the patient by explaining to the rehab director and the administrator how far they had come. They agreed to let the therapy continue when the therapist promised success.

In the two weeks that followed, the patient developed increased self-confidence in standing and walking activities. While standing she participated in flower arranging, laundry folding, cooking, washing dishes, and self-care. While walking she became quite comfortable maneuvering around obstacles, stopping short, turning, and stepping over articles of varying sizes. Her brother participated in the discharge plan for her to return home with his supervision.

Self-Efficacy Related to the Case

The patient in this case demonstrated an extreme case of ptophobia which caused her to avoid the activity she feared to such an extent that she endangered her health and required hospitalization. Tinetti and Powell (1993) described fear of falling as a lasting concern about falling that leads a person to avoid activities they are capable of performing. Self-efficacy is a concept that may shed some light on the etiology of and potential treatment for fear of falling. Self-efficacy, as discussed earlier, is an individual's perception of capabilities within a particular domain of activities.

It is difficult to determine if Ms L.K.'s decreased function led to a lower self-efficacy or a low self-efficacy led to decreased function, or both simultaneously. As her brother reported, her problem started with a slow but consistent decline in functional performance. It is quite possible that this was triggered by the onset of peripheral neuropathy in both lower extremities and the decreased sensation associated with it.

The therapist that worked with Ms L.K. did not follow any preconceived strategy about addressing the four aspects that impact upon a person's self-efficacy. As a matter of fact, she reported later, that she was not aware any such thing existed. The patient was going to be sent to a nursing home if she did not achieve independence in functional mobility. The therapist knew this, and also knew there was no physiological reason why the patient could not function in instrumental activities of daily living (IADLs). The therapist followed her intuition through the natural progression of treatment, which led to a successful recovery. We might speculate on where this intuition comes from, but that is beyond the scope of this discussion.

Upon admission to the subacute center, the patient's health was fairly stable. Her diabetes was under control following the episode of starvation and dehydration. She had a high anxiety level about functional performance, but that resolved as she progressed through therapy. Physiologically the patient was ready to work on performing tasks of IADLs.

Verbal persuasion started with the 'pep talk'. Until that interaction, the staff were very gentle with Ms L.K., by letting her set her own pace and activities. This strategy had a negative effect on her progression. She did not feel motivated to try activities she did not feel she could do successfully. Many factors may have an effect on the success of verbal persuasion. The *timing* of this 'pep talk' was fortuitous because the patient had already spent sufficient time with her therapist to develop some trust. The *message content* is important as well. The therapist explained the patient's condition to her and made it clear that there was no reason why she should not be able to perform functionally. This verbal persuasion was reinforced immediately by a *vicarious experience*.

The fact that Ms L.K.'s therapy took place in the physical therapy gym set the scene for vicarious experience to take place. The gym was an ideal environment because the patient was able to observe others, similar in age, participating in therapy. In addition the therapist taught the patient how to use imagery in learning a new task; this enhanced her ability to perform the activities successfully. Ms L.K. stated that this technique worked well for her.

The fourth aspect, as mentioned earlier, that has an impact on a person's self-efficacy is *performance accomplishments*. The patient's early successes with performing her exercise program and coordination activities helped to build her confidence and paved the way for her to exert a more consistent effort to continue in that vein. Perhaps if the therapist had been aware of the self-efficacy concept she could have assessed it and treated it more directly; this may have decreased the recovery time.

Implications for Treatment

Assessment tools

Self-efficacy and fear of falling seemed to have a strong relationship in this case study. We suggested that self-efficacy is an important component of evaluation and treatment of dysfunction in the elderly population. Measurement of self-efficacy is necessary in order to monitor the patient's condition objectively. Many self-efficacy measurement tools have been developed and are in use. Self-efficacy can only be measured on a task-specific level, therefore the measurement tools must be custom made to measure the problem at hand specifically. Some examples of self-efficacy measurement scales are the chronic obstructive pulmonary disease (COPD) self-efficacy scale (CSES), the multiple sclerosis (MS) self-efficacy scale (MSSE) and the Falls Related Efficacy Scale (FES). Because the case study illustrated physical therapy treatment and fear of falling, the falls related efficacy scale will be addressed in more detail here.

Tinetti and Powell (1993) found that 48% of people over the age of 75 years with a history of falling and 27% of people who did not fall admitted to a fear of falling. This discovery suggests that a fall is not necessary to develop fear of falling. A reduced self-efficacy in relation to falls and fear of falling, has been reported to be associated with a decline in activities of daily living (ADL), instrumental activities of daily living, and social functioning (Hill *et al.*, 1996). The Falls Related Efficacy Scale (FES) was developed by Tinetti and Powell in 1994, in order to measure fear of falling. The test is based on a ten point scale, varying from 'not at all confident' to 'completely confident'. The questions ask the respondent to identify how confident they feel about performing each of the activities without falling. Lower scores represent lower self-efficacy and higher scores reflect higher self-efficacy. The measurement scale is based on the operational definition of fear as 'low perceived self-confidence at avoiding falls during essential, relatively non-hazardous activities'.

The FES measures fear of falling during performance of activities that one may perform indoors. For that reason a modified falls efficacy scale (MFES) was developed to address outdoor activities for community dwelling individuals (Hill *et al.*, 1996). The FES and MFES are simple, quick, and easy to administer clinical evaluation tools that can be used to complete a comprehensive evaluation on older people who have any indication of balance or mobility dysfunction.

Ideal environment for treating self-efficacy

Both aging and declining health have been associated with alterations in self-efficacy levels (Johnson, 1995). Physical therapists and therapist assistants are in an ideal position to address easily and treat low self-efficacy, associated with functional mobility, in the elderly patient. Physical therapy intervention should target those functional skills necessary for safe transfers and ambulation and build from this baseline of ability. By improving upon those skills, the elderly individual will experience improvement in function, a decrease in fall risk, and improved confidence in performing those activities, which will result ultimately in increased activity participation (Tinetti and Powell, 1993).

In the course of treatment, the patient must feel they have some control over decisions being made and that they are responsible for setting and achieving goals. Johnson (1995) described *locus of control* as the degree to which individuals perceive events in their lives as being a consequence of their own actions and controllable (internal control), or as being unrelated to their own behavior and, therefore, beyond personal control (external control – fate). The feeling of control may result in an improved response with efficacy beliefs.

The learning environment that is inherent in rehabilitation treatment settings can be very threatening for patients because they must first admit that they are not fully competent at the task in question. This acknowledgment may be experienced as an assault on the learners' self-esteem, and in turn, their self-efficacy. The nature of the therapist – patient relationship may set the stage for a self-esteem building or self-esteem destroying experience, depending upon the environment that is created by the therapist. Self-esteem and self-efficacy can be enhanced through learning environments that are respectful of the learner and the learning experience. Under these conditions the environment is oriented toward success and relatively free of stigma against failure. The learner feels reassured and motivation can be focused to overcome problems with self-esteem.

In a clinical setting, a team approach is necessary for success to prevail. In order for self-efficacy to be treated comprehensively, all people who have contact with the patient must be aware of the issues and ways to address them. This includes family members and other healthcare providers. They must be able to provide the patient with verbal persuasion that encourages independence not dependence. Comments made out of concern such as 'don't do that anymore you might fall' and 'let me do that for you' may lead to self-doubt in the elderly person about their capability in specific tasks.

Performance accomplishment can be fostered by encouraging patients to set goals. Target behaviors are then divided into easily managed tasks that proceed in incremental steps to facilitate success. Success in turn will increase perceived self-efficacy.

Vicarious experience may be difficult for therapists to provide for their patients. Although successful demonstration of the task by the therapist may initially seem to be a vicarious experience, most patients will not see therapists as they see themselves. Examples of vicarious experiences include the use of videos, peer groups, tapes, books, and pamphlets.

The therapist can help to improve a patient's self-efficacy by educating the patient concerning their physiologic condition. Many people limit themselves out of fear of doing further damage to their already compromised health status. Having someone explain their medical condition may open the door for an increased and more accurate perception of their functional abilities.

Conclusion

Health care providers can aid their patients in achieving a greater self-efficacy. It is essential to address self-efficacy as we treat all populations, not just the geriatric patient who has a fear of falling. We must provide our patients with opportunities to make decisions about and take responsibility for their care. We can also help our patients understand how their health status, diagnosis or disability affect their functional performance. We must be careful not to set limits for our patients, but assure that they set realistic goals for themselves.

References

Adler, R, Towne, N (1996) *Looking Out Looking In: Interpersonal Communication*. Fort Worth: Harcourt-Brace College Publishers.

Bandura, A (1977) Self-efficacy: toward a unifying theory of behavioral change. *Psychological Review* 84: 191–215.

Bandura, A (1982) Self-efficacy mechanism in human agency. *American Psychologist* 37: 122–147.

Bandura, A (1985) Catecholamine secretion as a function of perceived coping self-efficacy. *Journal of Counseling and Clinical Psychology* 58(3): 406–414.

Bandura, A (1986) *Social Foundations of Thought and Action: A Social Cognitive Theory*. Englewood Cliffs, NJ: Prentice-Hall, Inc.

Bernstein-Lewis, C (1990) *Aging: The Healthcare Challenge*, 2nd edn, pp. 170–180, Philadelphia: FA Davis, Co.

Brown Commodore, B (1995) Falls in the elderly population: a look at incidence, risks, healthcare costs and preventative strategies. *Rehabilitation Nursing* 20: 84–88.

Burns, R (1979) *The Self–Concept*. London and New York: Longman.

Byrne, D (1966) *An Introduction to Personality: A Research Approach*. Englewood, NJ: Prentice-Hall, Inc.

Hill, K, Schwarz, J, Kalogeropoulas, A, Gibson, S (1996) Fear of falling revisited. *Archives of Physical Medicine and Rehabilitation* 77: 1025–1029.

Johnson, M (1995) Interactional aspects of self-efficacy and control in older people with leg ulcers. *Journal of Gerontological Nursing.* April: 20–27.

Mead, G (1934) *Mind, self and society*. Chicago: University of Chicago Press.

Scherer, Y, Shimmel, S (1996) Using self-efficacy theory to educate patients with chronic obstructive pulmonary disease. *Rehabilitation Nursing.* 21: 262–266.

Tinetti, M, Powell, L (1993) Fear of falling and low self-efficacy: A cause of dependence in elderly persons. *The Journal of Gerontology.* 48(13): 35–38.

Tinetti, M, Powell, L (1994) A multifactorial intervention to reduce the risk of falling among elderly people living in the community. *The New England Journal of* Medicine. 331: 821–827.

Tinetti, M, Speechley, M, Ginter, SF (1988) Risk factors for falls among elderly persons living in the community. *The New England Journal of* Medicine. 319: 1701–1707.

Tinetti, M, Mendes de Leon, C, Doucette, J, Baker, D (1994) Fear of falling and fall-related efficacy in relationship to functioning among community-living elders. *The Journal of Gerontology.* 49(3): 140–147.

11

The Relationship Between Health Practitioner and Patient

Judith Fadlon and Shulamit Werner

The Doctor–Patient Relationship as a Social Issue and the Parallel
Role of Other Health Professionals
•
Problems in the Doctor–Patient Relationship
•
Structural Elements in the Patient–Health Practitioner Relationship
•
Elements of Interaction in the Doctor–Patient Relationship
•
Communication

The Doctor–Patient Relationship as a Social Issue and the Parallel Role of Other Health Professionals

The doctor–patient relationship, in order to be fully understood, must be viewed in the context of both micro and macro sociology. Micro in the understanding of the mechanisms which construct situations such as symbolic interaction, verbal exchanges, and perceptions of status and role; macro in the sense that each situation is embedded in a social, cultural context which lays out the interpretative and behavioral repertoires to

which participants have recourse. The role of the health professional is no different from that of a doctor when interacting with a patient and is subject to the same criticisms and limitations.

What is in the relationship between health professionals and their patients that makes it the subject of such extensive discussion? On the most basic level, one may perceive this relationship as a professional interaction in which a qualified expert applies his expertise to help an individual who complains of physical discomfort.

Reality, however, is not so simple. If this were indeed the picture, we would not have to deal with the problem of non-compliance which is very common in health practitioner – patient interaction. For example, a patient might visit a doctor and receive a prescription or a referral for tests but will not bother to get the prescription filled nor the tests performed. The same holds true in the case of the relationship between other health professionals and their patients.

This situation is obviously detrimental to the patient's health, but also carries repercussions for the health system, as this type of patient is likely to engage in 'shopping' behavior, moving from one doctor to another, not complying with instructions and invariably causing unnecessary expense to the sick fund.

In the course of this chapter we shall be discussing views which originated mainly from examination of the doctor–patient relationship. Most of the literature on the subject of compliance focuses on the doctor as the caregiver and very little has been published on other health care professions such as nursing, physical therapy, and occupational therapy. This is interesting, since these professionals play an important part in rehabilitation, where the active cooperation of the patient is vital to the process and outcome of the professional intervention.

Problems in the Doctor–Patient Relationship

Understanding non-compliance can provide the key for understanding the problematic relationship between the health professional and the recipient of care. A common reason for non-compliance is the patient's feeling that his or her complaint has not really been understood by the caregiver who, therefore, cannot possibly know how to treat it. Stimson and Webb (1978) suggest that this feeling might stem from the patient's interpretation of the problem and the subsequent attempt to guide the doctor towards the 'right' diagnosis. A woman consulting her doctor because of headaches might ask: 'Could it be due to high blood pressure, Doctor?'. In this manner she is in fact negotiating with the doctor as to the cause of her symptoms and suggesting an explanation that could be supported or ruled out. If the doctor chooses to ignore this attempt, implicitly dismissing it and refraining from even taking her blood pressure, the patient will tend to feel dissatisfied and misunderstood and will probably seek a second opinion. Such situations can be attributed to the fact that the cues ventured by the patient have been categorized by the health practitioner as irrelevant.

Therefore, when a physical therapist interviews a patient who complains of pain radiating down her leg which she attributes to her shoes, it would not only be good professional procedure to examine her footwear (she might be right), but it would also indicate that the therapist has listened to the patient, placing her concerns, rather than those of the medical profession, foremost. This kind of behavior on the part of the therapist would be conducive to eliciting the cooperation and compliance of the patient.

The process of ignoring or phasing out 'irrelevant information' has been described remarkably well both by Waitzkin (1991) and Good (1994), respectively. Waitzkin shows how physicians serve as agents of social control by ignoring the personal or social cues that a patient might try to introduce into a medical interview. Good, on the other hand, illustrates the manner in which medical students learn to guide a patient's account of his or her illness in a manner that will be convenient to 'write up' in the patient's file, and thus be suitable for other physicians' perusal. Good's description admirably fits the situation often encountered by patients who are referred to physical therapy treatment and are not allowed to describe their condition in their own words because the 'intake' interview is structured to fit the closed precise questions appearing on the assessment form.

The dialogue between the parties involved is therefore bound to be problematic for several reasons:

1. The differing views as to what information is 'relevant' to the situation.

2. Embarrassment and intimidation felt by the patient in the interaction with the health professional.

3. Structural characteristics of the situation such as the time allotted to the consultation or the physical setting in which the consultation takes place.

In order to convert the patient into a partner and establish therapeutic collaboration, the caregiver must take into account the patient's socio-economic background and lifestyle; they must also consider how these factors might limit the patient's compliance, and how the therapist – patient alliance can be established under the given circumstances. When the patient is expected to perform a series of prescribed exercises at regular intervals or required to adjust his physical environment to enable optimal function with a disability, it is of utmost importance that the therapist be aware of the patient's physical environmental, and the social and psychological conditions.

These issues, then, are not only the patient's problem but the doctor's and the health practitioner's as well. The medical consultation often takes place in physical surroundings that do not make the patient feel comfortable or relaxed. The therapeutic situation is 'medical', as is the physical space which is strange to the patient, smells 'sterile' and often entails the use of instruments or equipment with which the patient is unfamiliar. Much of the interaction between patient and doctor or health practitioner, although privileged, is often not private, frequently taking place in the corridor, in a curtained cubicle or in an open space in the gym, with other staff members and patients coming and going or overhearing bits of information.

Non-compliance often results from the fact that the patient did not understand or could not remember the instructions, or that the instructions were in conflict with the patient's beliefs or values. For example, certain exercise positions such as kneeling down on all fours might be unacceptable in certain cultures. An elderly man of Iraqi origin, who is accustomed to receiving signs of respect from his children or acquaintances such as greeting with bowed head and hand kissing, might feel demeaned by the instruction to perform exercises in the kneeling position, especially when requested to do so in his own home. In such a case the therapist will have to find alternative positions in order to achieve the required movement.

Unrealized expectations will also shake the patient's confidence in the health professional and his/her instructions. This is especially relevant to rehabilitation when the results of compliant behavior are not immediate. Improvement in functional ability, increase in range of motion and reduction in musculoskeletal pain are gradual processes and the patient, discouraged by not seeing immediate results, might discontinue the prescribed regimen, thus terminating the therapeutic relationship prematurely.

Important, too, is the fact that in the patient–health professional interaction, the patient is ascribed a particular social role: that of 'patient'. This role overshadows any other role in which the patient might define himself outside of the therapeutic encounter. Health professionals often tend to talk down to patients without ascertaining what level of technicality may be adopted in the dialogue. The overall assumption seems to be that medical procedures are considered so technical and professional that they cannot be explained to the lay public, who are therefore not privileged with precise and detailed information concerning an ailment, its causes and treatment.

Zola (1980) illustrates this point very well in the following description of a dialogue between a patient and a doctor in a hospital:

'Looking down at the chart and not at the patient in the bed, the physician said jocularly: "Well Anne, how are you today?"

"Lousy, Robert, how are you?"

Taken aback he responded, "My name is Dr. Johnson, I only called you Anne to make you feel comfortable."

"Well," my friend responded, "My name is Dr. Greene, I only called you Robert to make *you* feel more comfortable."'

A similar case was recounted by an Israeli anthropologist of English origin who was admitted to the emergency ward of a large general hospital. In order to ensure that the patient did not understand what he was saying to the numerous medical students present, the attending physician discussed her symptoms in English which was far inferior to hers. Insulted, but not daunted, our self-assured anthropologist promptly corrected his English.

But not all patients are as assertive as these. In most cases they assume the role assigned to them by the doctor or health professional. The above examples provide evidence of the manner in which the temporary status of 'patient' can overrule any other aspect of an individual's identity (such as 'colleague' or 'anthropologist'), reducing him or her to a symptom or a disease ('the hip replacement in room number five'). Although the more educated or assertive individual might react on the spot and introduce other statuses into the situation, most patients will passively accept their depersonalization with a sense of humiliation, consoling themselves with the fact that it is only temporary. Health professionals often tend to use the transience of the medical encounter as an excuse for the affront caused to patients.

Such was the case in a discussion conducted with a group of student nurses following the complaint of a young woman who had been embarrassed by a young man peeking in through the screen while she was having an electrocardiogram examination. The nurses sympathized with the patient's feelings and conceded that the young man should have been waiting outside the examination room. However, one senior nurse remarked that although the woman's privacy had indeed been invaded, patients generally understood that in the long term the staff act in their best interests and that the medical imperative, as well as their health, take priority to 'minor discomforts' which should not be considered as a personal affront.

It would be well to remember that whilst many medical situations are indeed temporary, this does not give the staff license to disregard other aspects of an individual's personality. This holds true especially in long-term situations such as in rehabilitation after a stroke or a motor vehicle accident in which the patient's cooperation and his relationship with the health professionals who care for him is especially important.

In such cases, successful treatment calls for a therapeutic alliance between patient and caregiver which can only become possible when the patient as a person is brought into the encounter and not only the patient as a medical problem.

Structural Elements in the Patient–Health Practitioner Relationship

In order to promote a better understanding of the problems described so far, we would like to outline the sociological theory of social role and status, and illustrate the manner in which this theory can contribute to our understanding of the relationship between health practitioner and patient. Social status can be divided into ascribed and achieved status. Schaeffer and Lamm (1992) explain that

'an ascribed status is "assigned" to a person by society without regard for a person's unique talents or characteristics. Generally this assignment takes place at birth; thus, a person's racial background, gender and age are all considered ascribed statuses, since these statuses often confer privileges or reflect a membership in a subordinate group'.

It is important to emphasize, however, that an ascribed status does not have the same meaning in every society. For example, although gender is an ascribed status, women are not afforded the same position in society on a universal basis. To clarify this point, it is sufficient to compare equal employment opportunity legislation in the United States to societies in which women are denied all rights to participate in the public sphere.

On the other hand, Schaefer and Lamm point out that unlike ascribed statuses, an achieved status is obtained by a person largely through his or her own effort:

'Both "bank president" and "burglar" are achieved statuses, as are "lawyer", "pianist", "advertising executive" or "social worker". One must do something to acquire an achieved status: go to school, learn a skill, establish a friendship or invent a new product'.

An individual, therefore, is enmeshed in a web of statuses, some of which they were born with, such as gender or color, and others which were acquired along the way, such as university degrees or marital status.

While status denotes a given position in society, a social role denotes a set of behaviors and expectations from people occupying a given status. With each distinctive social status – whether ascribed or achieved – come particular role expectations. For example, the role expectations from a neurosurgeon might be, among others, manual dexterity, exercising good judgment, demonstrating empathy towards the patients, and the ability to teach students. An individual might, however, have difficulty fulfilling all roles associated with a specific social status with the same degree of success. For example, a surgeon might be gifted with superb manual dexterity, but not command the social skills necessary to communicate empathy towards patients. Whilst occupying the status of 'surgeon' and filling the accompanying roles, the doctor will most probably refrain from introducing any of his other social statuses into the situation such as 'father' or 'bridge player', for example.

On the other hand, however, an individual filling the rather subordinate role of 'patient' would probably be glad to project his other, more prestigious statuses such as that of 'lawyer' or 'millionaire' to bear on the situation, and thereby influence his interaction with the medical staff. Therefore, when a per-son fills a certain social role, they are in a state of mutual interaction with other people in different social statuses, each functioning in the role relevant to the particular situation (Figure 11.1). Thus, an individual can be viewed as enmeshed within a web of social roles and statuses, emphasizing or minimizing a particular role in accordance with the demands of the situation.

Role theory provides the theoretical basis for the Szasz and Hollender (1956) conceptualization of the doctor–patient relationship. Szasz and Hollender compare various types of interaction between doctors and their patients to stages in the relationship between parents and their offspring.

The first stage, that of activity–passivity, relates to a situation in which there is no real interaction between the two parties but rather one individual is doing something to another individual who is not able to actively con-

Figure 11.1 Elements of sociology (adapted and translated from Shapiro & Ben-Eliezer 1989).

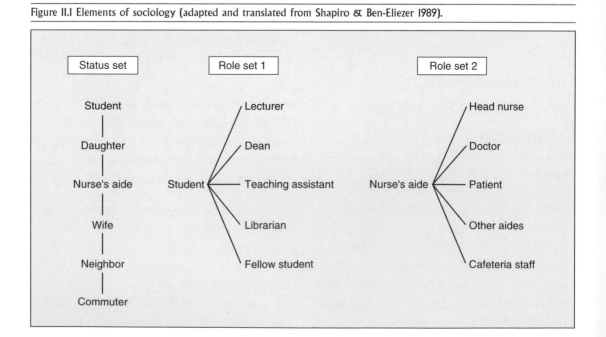

tribute to the situation. This is characteristic of treatment such as surgery, or intensive care, and comparable to a parent caring for an infant.

The second stage, that of guidance and cooperation, is employed in situations in which the patient is conscious and suffering from distressing symptoms which have led him to seek help and render him willing and able to cooperate. This stage is more 'active' than the preceding one since both parties actively contribute to the relationship, although the doctor, owing to his superior knowledge, is the more powerful of the two. The patient is expected to 'obey' his doctor and not argue with the treatment he receives. This model, according to Szasz and Hollender, has its prototype in the relationship between parent and adolescent child. Threats and other undisguised types of force are employed, presumably for the patient's or the child's 'own good'. This is indeed the model most suited to Parson's description of the 'sick role', which has been discussed in an earlier chapter of this book. This stage of interaction is also pertinent to the relationship established between health professionals such as physical and occupational therapists and their patients. Although a lack of symmetry exists, the patient's active participation is necessary for the alliance to produce therapeutic benefit. This stage exemplifies the existing concept of compliance – the health professional prescribes and the patient is expected to acquiesce.

The third and final stage in the Szasz and Hollender model is one of mutual participation in which equality between participants is assumed. A characteristic of this stage is the fact that participants have approximately equal power, are mutually interdependent and engage in activity that can be satisfying to both. This model is useful in the case of long-term treatment or chronic disease in which the patient becomes quite an expert on their condition and in which the patient's long-term cooperation and active participation are called for. In long-term rehabilitation, the patient's role as an equal participant in the process is dominant and should be recognized as such by the health practitioner.

The Szasz and Hollender model is valuable for its categorization of various types of relationship which may exist between health professionals and patients and the attempt to tie these relationships to various physical conditions. However, an interesting aspect of the model is what happens when the patient and the attending health professional have to progress from one stage of the relationship to the next. This can be illustrated by elaborating on the metaphor of the parent–child relationship. As some parents who obtain gratification from ministering to helpless infants find the transition to parenting adolescents difficult and fraught with conflict, other parents who find taking care of infants less rewarding, excel as parents of older children. When this metaphor is applied to the doctor–patient relationship the question arises whether the surgeon trained in open heart surgery can effectively deal with the day-to-day problems and fears encountered by the patient in the process of recuperation, when he is no longer a passive recipient of treatment but requires explanation and encouragement to ensure his cooperation. This difficulty in progressing from the first level of interaction is vividly illustrated in a novel by an Israeli author (Yehoshua, 1994). A surgical resident describes the moment in surgery in which the heart of the powerful chief administrator of the hospital is stopped and his blood circulation transferred to a heart–lung machine manned by a team of technicians. The surgeon performing his role, holds the chief administrator's heart, literally his life, in his hands while the surgical team looks on.

This situation of omnipotence leads one to ponder on the personality traits necessary to perform such a procedure, and then again, whether this same personality will be able to adapt to the type of relationship called for to steer the patient through the long and arduous process of convalescence and rehabilitation.

Although this dilemma is sometimes solved by the infinite specialization in modern medicine, enabling doctors to choose those fields of the profession more suitable to their personalities, other health professionals often guide their patients through all the stages of recovery. For example, in the case of spinal cord injuries, the nurses and therapists will start working with the patient when the latter is totally dependent upon them and cannot do anything for himself. At this stage the health professional will turn the patient every two hours, and feed and wash him as if he were a helpless infant, a condition which is very difficult for the patient but often gratifying to the staff members. This therapeutic relationship will continue until the patient achieves, with the aid and guidance of the various health professionals, a certain level of independence at which he can fill his own needs to a certain extent. Finally the stage arrives when the relationship between the patient and the health practitioners is terminated and the patient becomes independent. The manner in which

the therapeutic relationship progresses from one stage to the next and is finally severed is of utmost importance, especially when the patient is chronically ill or disabled and has become dependent upon the health practitioner for continued treatment, supervision, and even company. In some cases, the parties involved might have different expectations concerning recovery and functioning, thereby causing difficulties in the therapeutic relationship. One way to avoid this problem is to set up a workable therapeutic contract which is continually renewed as the patient moves from one level of independence to the next.

Elements of Interaction in the Doctor–Patient Relationship

Social status and social roles have thus far been used to illustrate problems inherent in the relationship between health professional and patient. We have shown that although an individual occupies many statuses, he is usually defined by means of the status pertinent to a specific situation. The question arises as to how these situations become constructed, how status is projected, and how a patient, for example, communicates to the doctor that he is educated and well off, or conversely, at a loss and destitute. The answer is to be found in the theoretical construct of symbolic interaction. Goffman (1959) defined encounters between people as a process of negotiation during which each individual attempts to control the situation by means of impressions created. Goffman divides impressions into two categories: impressions given and impressions given off. An impression *given* is the impression created by verbal means, what an individual says. An impression *given off* covers a broad spectrum of non-verbal behavior such as body language, the way a person dresses and the use of other status symbols in order to define a situation. A person filling the social role of 'patient' will do so using verbal and non-verbal behavior. If we expand the example that we cited earlier of the female patient consulting her doctor about headaches, we may observe that her behavior can be understood on the verbal as well as on the non-verbal level. On the verbal level she voices her complaint and also offers a tentative diagnosis: 'Could it be blood pressure?'. This is an attempt at negotiation in order to define the medical situation. On the non-verbal level, the way she dresses for the appointment, the amount of jewelry she is wearing and the manner in which she enters the room are all elements of non-verbal behavior which contribute to the negotiation conducted in the situation. If the doctor receives the impression that his patient is intelligent, assertive, well dressed, and upper-class, he might just go along with her tentative diagnosis, if only to placate her. If, however, the patient gives off a less assertive impression, the doctor might feel free to ignore the patient's attempts at negotiating the outcome of the situation and dictate his own interpretation. The doctor on his part, might also make use of certain status symbols such as the surgical mask or stethoscope dangling from his neck, or a paging device peeping out of his pocket, in order to give off an impression of being an important and busy doctor. Owing to the fact that much of the non-verbal interaction is conducted by means of symbols, it has been called 'symbolic interaction' (Goffman, 1959). It is, however, very important to remember that both giving off and interpreting symbols is context bound and culture specific. Symbolic currency varies from one culture to another and the process of giving off and interpreting symbolic cues depends on both parties understanding the symbolic code of a given culture. Misunderstanding can occur on the verbal as well as on the non-verbal level. Donna Lee Davis (1984) provides a poignant example of verbal misunderstanding in her description of a visit to a doctor by a poor, semi-literate inhabitant of a remote fishing village in Newfoundland. Intimidated by the doctor and his relative social status, the woman answers his query as to what is wrong with her with 'It's my nerves doctor, they're playing up something terrible'. The doctor responds by prescribing a tranquilizer. What he does not know is that among inhabitants of the village, the term 'nerves' serves to cover a wide span of physical as well as mental complaints and the patient was really suffering from sharp abdominal pain. If, however, the patient had engaged in specific non-verbal behavior such as clutching her abdomen and wincing in pain, perhaps the doctor would have interpreted these cues correctly and his response would have been more appropriate. Misunderstanding of cultural codes can create an impression entirely different from the one intended. For example, a patient, wishing to appear affluent and upper class, might resort to wearing a lot of gold jewelry in a culture where this is regarded as flashy and gaudy, thereby eliciting disdain rather than respect.

The issue of culture, therefore, is an additional element to be reckoned with in the medical situation and is also very important in achieving patient cooperation. Bloom and Summey (1978) have recognized the importance of this issue and have incorporated it in their models of the doctor–patient relationship.

The first, most basic stage in the Bloom and Summey conceptualization is that of the doctor and the patient engaging in a specific, goal oriented interaction which results in medical treatment which the doctor administers to the patient, regardless of his family status, cultural mores, or health beliefs (Figure 11.2).

The second stage acknowledges the fact that the patient, as well as the doctor, do not operate within personal 'vacuums'. The patient is usually part of a family whose members are concerned about his health and are also likely to suffer repercussions from his ill health or disability. The family, therefore, should be involved in any decision making and treatment strategy as they constitute an important element in the patient's cooperation. This is especially important in the process of rehabilitation, in coping with a chronic disease, and in coming to terms with long-term or permanent disability. On the other hand, the doctor and other members of the health team are not free agents but act as representatives of various health professions and are bound by sick fund or government regulations, such as sick leave policy, available options for treatment, and medical ethics. All these factors will influence the manner in which the medical treatment will be administered (Figure 11.3).

The third stage acknowledges the fact that the medical encounter takes place within a given social and cultural context. This context will dictate several aspects such as the relative status of the doctor within the society, and the degree of formality or informality with which the relationship between doctor and patient will be conducted. For example, a doctor who happens to be a member of a kibbutz in Israel, would be on a first name basis with the patients he treats within his community, but would be addressed by his official title when seeing patients at the university clinic. Both the patient and the attending health practitioner will change their behavior during the professional encounter depending on the social context in which the interaction takes place (Figure 11.4).

The fourth and final stage of their conceptualization acknowledges the fact that alongside the dominant cultural and social system within

Figure 11.2 The interaction model (from Bloom SW 1963 The doctor and his patient. Russell Sage Foundation, New York. Reproduced with permission).

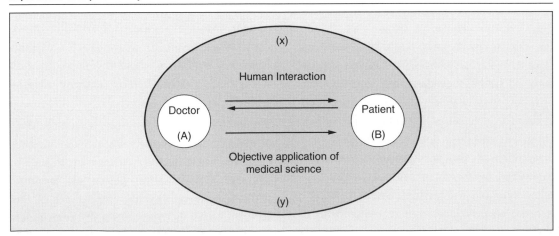

every society, a set of subcultures exits. These subcultures which might be constructed around ethnic origin, socio-economic level, or religious faith, all influence health beliefs and health behavior. Health professionals and patients, though members of the same society, often do not belong to the same subculture which can cause difficulties in communication, treatment, and cooperation, such as when a male patient from a traditional, conservative background might feel uncomfortable when examined and treated by a female health practitioner who happens to be young and attractive.

The final stage, therefore, describes the intricate social situation which encompasses the doctor–patient consultation. This is not merely an encounter between an individual sensing physical discomfort and another who will 'put it right', but an encounter of cultures, background, families, and aspirations. The final stage of the Bloom and Summey conceptualization also shows that the patient

Figure II.3 The doctor's view: a limited system (from Bloom SW 1963 The doctor and his patient. Russell Sage Foundation, New York. Reproduced with permission).

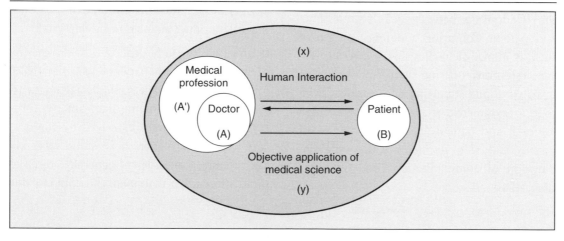

Figure II.4 The doctor–patient relationship as a social system (from Bloom SW 1963 The doctor and his patient. Russell Sage Foundation, New York. Reproduced with permission).

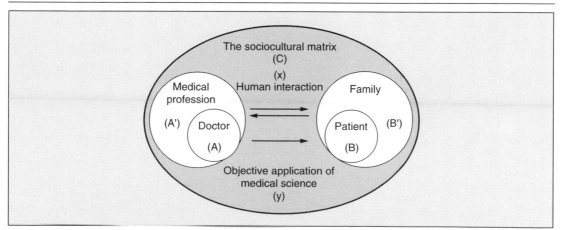

contributes actively to the instrumental encounter between himself and the doctor, who not only treats the patient, but also responds to his cues, suggestions, and reservations (Figure 11.5).

Communication

All the factors mentioned above influence not only the nature of the treatment, but also the manner in which the treatment is administered. Communication, a prominent factor in the relationship between health professional and patient, comprises a number of aspects such as intake of medical history, asking relevant questions, offering sympathy, explaining, instructing, and supplying information. Owing to the asymmetric relationship between professional and patient, it is usually the health professional who decides on the type and duration of communication conducted with the patient.

Providing information and the concept of informed consent

One of the decisions confronting the health professional concerns the nature and amount of information the patient should receive. This is not always in harmony with the amount and type of information the patient requires or expects. Although medico-legal practice requires patients to sign an official form of consent prior to any invasive procedure, it often happens that the patient lacks the necessary information to be able to make an educated decision. The patient's 'informed' consent actually depends on the information that the health practitioner finds suitable to be imparted.

In an extensive study dealing with the sharing of information with patients, Waitzkin (1985) found that well-educated, middle-aged patients received more information than others, probably because they were perceived by the doctors to be of a higher social status. Waitzkin also found that women generally received more information than men. This could be due

Figure 11.5 The total transactional system (from Bloom SW 1963 The doctor and his patient. Russell Sage Foundation, New York. Reproduced with permission).

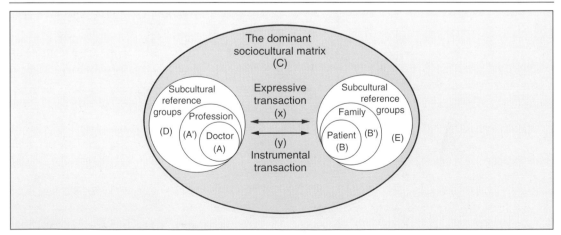

to the fact that women were more likely to engage in verbal communication and usually ask more questions. Waitzkin's results also indicated that physicians are relatively poor judges of the time they thought they were allotting to information. Whilst doctors thought that they had spent approximately 8 minutes imparting information, Waitzkin found that in a consultation averaging 16.5 minutes, only 1.3 minutes of the time was allotted to information. Although instructions and advice are not included in Waitzkin's definition of information, this would still appear to be a relatively short time.

In another study by Street (1991), based on the analysis of 41 videotaped medical consultations, it was discovered that information regarding diagnosis and health matters was primarily related to the patient's anxiety, level of education, and question asking. Street also found that it was the doctor's attitude that encouraged patients to ask questions and voice their concerns. 'Partnership building' utterances such as 'I can understand why you are worried' or 'I know it is difficult' encouraged patients to ask more questions and express their anxiety more freely. The study concludes that a physician's perceptions as well as the communicative styles of their patients will determine the nature and quantity of medical information imparted. We would like to remind the reader that the manner in which these perceptions are formed has been discussed in the section of this chapter relating to role theory and symbolic interaction.

The doctor as an agent of social control

As we have already shown, the consultation between doctor and patient cannot be regarded as a limited interaction which takes place between two individuals. Based on the Bloom and Summey conceptualization, we have illustrated that the doctor is in fact a representative of the medical profession and, in this capacity, acts on behalf of, and within the confines of sick-fund and state regulations. Some sociological studies have pointed out the fact that the doctor, acting on behalf of society, is indirectly fulfilling the function of social control.

For example, Parson's model of the sick role (Segal, 1976) is based on the very assumption that too much illness or exploitation of the illness situation, is detrimental to society. For this reason, in order to avoid social sanctions, either direct or indirect, the sick individual has to obtain certification from the doctor that he is indeed indisposed and unable to fulfill his normal social roles. In order to escape social sanction, the sick person is expected to fulfill a number of conditions related to the sick role which will consequently entitle him to a number of benefits. Benefits related to the sick role are exemption from normal duties and absolution of the responsibility for becoming sick or for getting well. In order to enjoy these benefits, the patient has two obligations: the first is to view the condition of sickness as undesirable and make visible efforts to recuperate, and the second is to seek competent medical help. In this manner, the doctor has a social as well as a medical obligation. He is not only expected to extend medical advice and treatment, but also to protect the patient from negative social sanctions which might result from inability to fulfill customary social roles.

This exemption usually takes the form of medical certificates which release the sick person from his normal roles for a stipulated time period. In this manner the doctor is also responsible to society in general for regulating the amount of illness admissible. The Parsons model has been criticized on a number of bases (Segal, 1976), the most important being that the model is really more suited to clear-cut episodes of short-term, curable illness in which the transition from health to illness and back again is clearly discernible. However, in the case of chronic, long-term illness, mental illness, and permanent disability, the model loses its effectiveness, as recovery is not expected. Moreover, in many cases, the patient is expected to resume his social roles after the initial period of rehabilitation, in spite of his disability. On the other hand, in the case of recurrent episodes of chronic disease, it is sometimes difficult to identify the difference between the state of illness and the state of health. Moreover, in the case of chronic illness, the patient sometimes becomes more of an expert on his condition than the doctor, which subsequently erodes the physician's unique position of authority.

A later study by Waitzkin 1991 provides further illustration of the doctor's position as an agent of social control. Studying taped recordings of consultations between doctors and their patients, Waitzkin found that doctors tended to ignore patients' cues or implicit requests, in order to maintain the smooth running of the normative social order. In an example of a consultation in which a female patient recovering from heart failure complained that she was feeling breathless and tired whilst performing her duties at home, Waitzkin shows how the doctor indirectly maintained the existing social order and the traditional definition of the woman's role. The doctor examined the patient, reassured her, and then congratulated her on her efforts to maintain a tidy home despite her illness. In this manner the doctor reinforced the traditional social role occupied by women in society, and did not sanction the underlying message which might be a request to be released, even temporarily, from these roles.

In the course of this chapter we have tried to illustrate the phenomena of health and illness as issues that are firmly embedded in the broader social context. In doing so we have shown how research traditionally concerned with the the patient–physician relationship can be employed to further understanding of the interaction between the patient and health professional.

References

Bloom, S, Summey, P (1978) Models of the doctor–patient relationship: a history of the social system concept. In Galagher, EB (ed) *The Doctor–Patient Relationship in the Changing Health Scene*, pp. 17–41. Washington, DC: US Dept of HEW.

Davis, DL (1984) Medical misinformation: communication between outport Newfoundland women and their physicians. *Social Science and Medicine* 18(3): 273–278

Goffman, E (1959) *The Presentation of Self in Everyday Life*. New York: Doubleday.

Good, BJ (1994) *Medicine, Rationality and Experience: An Anthropological Perspective*. Cambridge: Cambridge University Press.

Schaeffer, RT, Lamm, RP (1992) *Sociology*, pp. 133–134. New York: McGraw Hill Inc.

Segal, A (1976) The sick-role concept: understanding illness behaviour. *Journal of Health and Social Behaviour* 17: 162–169.

Shapiro, Y, Ben-Eliezer, U (1989) *Elements of Sociology*, p.49. Tel-Aviv: Am Oved Publishers Ltd.

Stimson, G, Webb, B (1978) The face to face interaction and after the consultation. In: Tuckett, D, Kaufert, M (eds) *Basic Readings in Medical Sociology*. London: Tavistock Publications Ltd.

Street, RL Jr (1991) Information giving in medical consultations: the influence of patients' communicative styles and personal characteristics. *Social Science and Medicine* 32(5): 541–548.

Szasz, TS, Hollender, MH (1956) The basic models of the doctor–patient relationship. *Archives in Internal Medicine* 97: 585–592.

Waitzkin, H (1985) Information giving in medical care. *Journal of Health and Social Behaviour* 26 June: 81–101.

Waitzkin, H (1991) *The Politics of Medical Encounters*. New Haven and London: Yale University Press.

Yehoshua, AB (1994) *The Return from India*. Tel-Aviv: Hakibbutz Hameuchad Publisher.

Zola, I (1980) Structural constraints in the doctor–patient relationship: the case of non-compliance. In: Eisenberg, L, Kleinman, A (eds). *The Relevance of Social Science for Medicine* pp. 241–252. London: D Reidel Publishing Company.

12

Bioethics

Jan Bruckner

Behavioral Objectives
•
Introduction to Beliefs, Values, and Moral Reasoning
•
Case 1: Dathan Smith
•
Case 2: Nancy Valencia
•
Case 3: Irene Patterson
•
Ethical Decision-Making
•
Casuistry
•
Conclusion

Behavioral Objectives

At the end of this section, the reader will be able to:

1. Define the following terms and concepts: belief, value, ethics, morality, law, normative ethics, and bioethics.
2. Describe the difference between law and ethics.
3. Define the following six ethical principles and explain their importance in bioethics: autonomy, beneficence, non-maleficence, honesty, respect for persons, and justice.
4. Define the term dilemma.
5. Define the term informed consent and explain its ethical basis.
6. Explain Pellegrino's concept of a state of 'wounded humanity'.
7. Explain Pellegrino's definition of a professional.
8. Describe Pellegrino's 'healing relationship'.
9. Explain the similarities and differences between a patient–healer relationship and a patient–treatment team relationship.
10. Define the term 'blow the whistle' and explain the ethical basis for this action.
11. Describe the Pellegrino–Thomasma model for ethical decision making.
12. Explain and differentiate between bioethical theories that are results-based, duty-based, and virtue-based.
13. Define the term *primum non nocere* and explain its importance to health care.

14. Define the term casuistry and explain how this method of ethical decision making differs from the theory-driven approaches.
15. Appreciate the value of learning bioethics.

Introduction to Beliefs, Values, and Moral Reasoning

Defining basic terms and concepts

Every day people make choices. People choose what clothes to wear, what to eat for breakfast, and how to spend their leisure time. We choose to obey or ignore traffic regulations. We make decisions about our personal finances and about our professional responsibilities. Some of these choices are matters of opinion. If decisions do not have right or wrong answers but are based on personal taste and temperament, they are amoral judgments. Moral choices reflect a value judgment that a certain idea or course of action is good or right. Health care professionals often make moral judgments as part of their daily routines. How aggressive should we be in treating this terminally ill patient? Should health care be rationed based on a patient's ability to pay? Should patients have the final say in what type of medical intervention will be done? Some of these questions are extremely difficult to answer.

Whenever someone asks. 'What should we do?', a value judgment is being requested. A value is an assessment of worth. If some object is worth a lot of money, we say that it has great value. If an idea has importance in defining good behavior, we say the idea is a moral value. Freedom of religion and freedom of speech are some of the moral values on which the United States was founded. A belief is a mental acceptance that something is true even though definitive proof may be absent. We can have some idea of what values people hold by asking them what they believe. People tend to agree with statements of their beliefs when asked and are inclined to act in ways consistent with their expressed beliefs. Of course, people can lie, and if we see that people act in opposition to their expressed beliefs, we tend to doubt their sincerity.

Ethics and law

Law and ethics are two different things. A law is a moral value that is defined by a duly authorized governing body and enforced by a legal and judicial system. When people do not comply with laws, they may be punished for the infringement.

Ethics is the study of morality. Morality encompasses concepts of right and wrong and principles for human behavior. The reasoned investigation into morality is ethics. Often people use the words morality and ethics interchangeably. They will be used interchangeably in this chapter. Ethical principles are not always explicitly defined nor are they legally binding. No retributive action will occur if people fail to act in accordance with ethical principles that have not been enacted into law. In general, laws are legally enforceable but moral principles are not.

A second difference between laws and moral principles is that a law may be immoral and a moral principle may have no legal basis. Many people thought that the laws that supported slavery were immoral. Some people think that laws that permit abortion or the death penalty are immoral. On the other hand, no law mandates that you must help a frail, elderly person walk across a street or treat your pets with kindness and compassion. We think that treating people and animals with consideration is good and meritorious behavior, but it is not legally obligatory.

How does someone know whether he or she has violated a law or a moral principle? You know when you are complying with or violating a law because the regulated behavior is explicitly defined. You can read the statue or regulation. How do you know if you have violated a moral principle? Moral values are not always explicitly stated. Sometimes we must rely on ethical reasoning to determine what is right and wrong.

People in ancient Greece worked out methods by which they could solve problems using reason and logic. These approaches proved so successful that they formed the foundations of such modern disciplines as science, mathematics, and philosophy. Problem solving using reason and logic can be found in a rigorous form within the field of philosophy. Philosophy is the study of wisdom and the search for knowledge. When we want to resolve some of the problems that we encounter in the clinic, we can use philosophical theories and techniques for assistance. One branch of philosophy that is particularly helpful is ethics, the study of morality. Normative ethics is a branch of ethics that seeks to define principles for human behavior (Barry, 1978). When we debate child labor laws, cleaning up the environment, or addressing the needs of homeless individuals, we seek to define the moral principles that govern our society. This is the realm of normative ethics. One sub-field of normative

ethics is bioethics. Bioethics applies the theories and methodologies of ethics to living things (Jameton, 1984). We can use bioethical principles to help analyze clinical problems.

In this chapter, we will examine six ethical principles: autonomy, beneficence, non-maleficence, honesty, respect for persons, and justice. These ethical principles were selected because they have direct relevance to the moral problems allied health professionals face in their clinical practice. The specific definitions of these ethical principles will be discussed in reference to the case studies presented below. A summary of these principles as they apply to health care professionals can be found in Table 12.1.

Table 12.1
Summary of Six Ethical Principles

The principle of patient autonomy
> Patients are the best judges of what should be done for them and should be granted final decision-making authority in their cases.

The principle of beneficence
> Health care providers have an obligation to act always in the best interests of their patients even if this involves acting against a patient's expressed wish.

The principle of non-maleficence
> Health care providers should avoid doing harm to their patients. A variation of this principle is *primum non nocere*, 'first, do no harm'. This principle has been attributed to the Hippocratic oath (see Purtillo and Cassel, 1981) though Veatch points out that the Latin formulation does not appear in the ancient Greek physician's writings (Veatch, 1981).

Primum non nocere gives primacy to the value that health care professionals should avoid causing harm to their patients before anything else.

The principle of honesty

Health care practitioners should tell the truth to each other and to the patients in their care.

The principle of respect for persons

Health care professionals should treat all people with respect, dignity, and compassion.

The principle of justice

The principle of justice charges health care professionals to treat colleagues and patients fairly. This principle also obligates society to allocate scarce resources equitably among the people who need health care.

All things being equal, clinicians should adhere to all ethical principles. Unfortunately, in the real world, all things are not equal and a conflict between ethical principles often forces clinicians to choose between equally unsatisfactory alternatives. A situation where someone must choose between equally unsatisfactory alternatives is called a dilemma. What follows are three case studies that illustrate situations where basic bioethical principles conflict and the clinician must resolve a moral dilemma. Real names have been changed.

Case I: Dathan Smith

Dathan Smith is a 23-year-old male who sustained a complete T7 spinal cord lesion from a motorcycle accident. Immediately after the accident, he was rushed to a trauma unit and underwent surgery to stabilize his spine. He was in acute care for eight weeks while his medical condition was stabilized. He was transferred to a rehabilitation facility and during his initial physical therapy evaluation in the rehab facility, Dathan told his therapist that he got injured while riding with a motorcycle gang. Dathan said that his injury was Divine punishment for being bad. He asserted that when he is forgiven for his evil ways, he will rIse up out of the wheelchair and walk the way he did before the accident. He does not think that physical therapy will help him. He wants to go to faith healers. During the course of his rehabilitation, Dathan attends therapy sessions only when brought by nursing or therapy personnel. If left on his own, Dathan sits in his room reading the Bible or gets someone to take him to the facility's chapel. He has found people whom he calls 'Good Christians' who take him to tent revival meetings and to faith healers. A conflict has developed between the therapy staff and the patient since Dathan has been attending these church meetings instead of his therapy sessions. The therapists have explained to Dathan that therapy will teach him how to become more independent in dressing, self-care, and transferring. They explained to him that without daily exercise, he will grow too weak to help himself and that he runs the risk of developing pressure sores, spasticity, joint contractures, and possibly urinary tract infections. The psychologist says that Dathan is suffering from a reactive depression and that Dathan is refusing to accept the reality of his situation. Dathan denies that he is depressed. He says that he wants the rehab team to leave him alone and that he will be fine as soon as he is forgiven for his evil behavior.

This case study illustrates a conflict between the principles of autonomy and beneficence. The principle of autonomy states that each person knows what is best for him or her and should be granted final decision-making authority. Within the health care arena, advocates of patient autonomy believe that health care providers are experts in the area of medical intervention but that the patient is the expert on what should be done in his or her specific case. Under the principle of autonomy, health care providers must give patients enough information about their condition so that the patients can make an informed decisions about the course of their own treatment. Patients must be rational adults, who can understand basic information and make reasoned decisions. When patients agree with health professionals to a set course of treatment based on reasoned decisions, we call this agreement informed consent for treatment. Health care providers can express their professional opinions about what they think would be the best course of action, but the principle of autonomy grants the final decision-making authority to the patient.

The principle of beneficence takes a different approach. Advocates of this principle assert that people have an obligation to improve the goodness in the world. Under the principle of beneficence, health care providers have an obligation to act always in the best interests of their patients even if this involves acting against a patient's expressed wish. For example, suppose a patient gets blinded in an industrial accident and decides that life as a blind person is not worth living. This patient refuses medical treatment. The principle of beneficence compels us to provide appropriate therapeutic intervention despite this person's protests. The underlying assumption is that the best interests of this patient are served if he or she can be helped to conceive of a meaningful life even without the ability to see.

Pellegrino points out that after a life-threatening accident or illness patients may not always be thinking clearly (Pellegrino, 1983). In this traumatized state, patients may be suffering not only from physical injury but also from mental anguish. These patients may be too overwhelmed by pain or grief to think rationally or to understand their own clinical situation. This agony compromises their ability to reason and diminishes their capacity to function as fully autonomous adults. Pellegrino says that these people are in a state of 'wounded humanity'. These patients need someone to care for them until they become sufficiently healed to regain their ability to think clearly. For some patients this state of wounded humanity is a temporary condition while other patients may never be able to decide about their own best interests. Examples of people who must have someone else make the crucial decisions about their care include patients who are brought into a hospital in a coma and never regain consciousness; Alzheimer's patients who suffer cognitive deficits as part of their disease; and adults with histories of mental retardation.

Dathan's situation represents a dilemma between the principles of patient autonomy and beneficence. If you believe that Dathan is a rational adult then you might believe that the principle of patient autonomy is the dominant factor here and let Dathan decide his own course of rehabilitation. If you believe that Dathan is clinically depressed and is not able to assess his own situation rationally, you may believe that the principle of beneficence is more important. At this stage, we can lay out the arguments on both sides of the case and see which are more compelling.

What are the arguments favoring patient autonomy? These arguments must prove that Dathan is a rational adult capable of making decisions in his own best interests. Dathan is chronologically over 21 years of age so he is legally an adult. His competency as a rational thinker hinges on his belief that only a faith healer can cure him. Is this belief an example of irrationality or a deeply held religious conviction? Adult Jehovah's Witnesses have the legal right to refuse blood transfusions even if this refusal will result in their death. Christian Scientists have the legal right to refuse medical treatment. Does Dathan fit into the same category of religious believers and their right to refuse medical intervention?

What are the arguments favoring the principle of beneficence? The spinal cord injury changed Dathan's life drastically. It is common for people to experience reactive depressions as a result of such life-changing experiences. There are no clinically documented cases of people with complete spinal cord lesions being miraculously cured by faith healers. Patients with spinal cord lesions who do not exercise appropriately do develop pressure sores, joint contractures, urinary tract infections, and become too weak to take care of themselves. Is Dathan's thought process so irrational that he should be compelled against his will to undergo therapy? How much coercion is warranted in such a situation? Should the rehabilitation team bargain with Dathan? For example, they could devise a contract stipulating that Dathan could attend a certain number of prayer meetings if he participates in a specified number of therapy sessions. If

Dathan refuses to make such a contract or fails to comply with such an arrangement, what do you think the rehabilitation team should do?

Case 2: Nancy Valencia

Nancy Valencia, a 19-year-old female with spina bifida, lived in a state-supported group home. The facility's rehabilitation team met to discuss her case. The physical therapist, Megan, reported that Nancy was non-ambulatory and had severe thoracolumbar collapsing scoliosis. Her spine compressed her left lung and kidney resulting in a history of lung and kidney problems. Megan recommended a plan including a spinal orthotic, exercises to strengthen her trunk muscles, and an hourly regime of wheelchair push-ups to help elongate her trunk. The nurse, Patricia, said that Nancy had frequent urinary tract and kidney infections owing to poor colostomy care. Nancy had skin breakdown where the scoliosis caused deep skin folds and creases. Patricia's plan was to teach Nancy proper colostomy and skin care. The psychologist, Tom, presented tests showing that Nancy was mildly mentally retarded and demonstrated little insight into the long-term implications of her actions. Tom said that Nancy had a long history of non-compliance with treatment regimes. He said that over the years the staff had tried various reward systems but none of them worked. Tom had noticed that Nancy was developing a crush on him and he decided to use her feelings as the motivator in a behavior modification program. Tom began spending more time with Nancy and started taking an interest in her daily activities. He tested her behavior. He told her that he liked a particular blouse and she began to wear it more often. He mentioned that he found a particular brand of perfume pleasing and Nancy started using it. Tom was now convinced that Nancy would do what he suggested. He proposed taking Nancy to lunch every time she performed well in physical therapy and that he would give her a small gift or take her out to a movie if she complied with the nursing program each week. Megan and Patricia were shocked that Tom would suggest such a program. They said that they would carry out their proposed treatment programs without Tom's help. As they tried to work with Nancy, she resisted. She found the spinal orthosis too uncomfortable and she did not like being taken away from her sheltered workshop job to attend therapy sessions. Nancy said that Patricia's inspection of her skin was a violation of her privacy and that the colostomy program was 'disgusting'. Nancy had a history of respiratory and kidney problems and, if her condition worsened, she could lose her left kidney. One option was surgery to stabilize her spine but the surgeon said that he would not operate on such a weak and non-compliant patient.

This case raises many questions. On what grounds is Tom's behavior modification program to foster Nancy's crush morally justified? What are the moral objections to Tom's program? If a member of the rehab team objects to the morality of Tom's program, what should happen? How are the moral obligations of a treatment team different than those in a simple two-person patient–healer relationship? Are treatment team members morally responsible for the professional behavior of all the members of the team? How can

we resolve conflicts when team members disagree?

To begin addressing these questions, we can look at the ethical principles of the case. Nancy has mild mental retardation and cannot be expected to view her situation as a mature, rational adult. The principle of autonomy does not apply if a person is not competent to make a mature, rational decision. Nancy does have strong feelings about her situation and patient advocates would argue that Nancy's wishes deserve to be heard and considered by the rehab team. Owing to her mental retardation, Nancy should not be granted final decision-making authority but a limited version of the autonomy principle is reasonable. To the degree that she is able to comprehend information, Nancy should be permitted to make decisions about her treatment program. Only when her decisions impact negatively on her health and welfare should her autonomy be suspended.

Tom can argue that Nancy's decision not to comply with the physical therapy and nursing programs demonstrates her lack of understanding of her own best interests. She cannot care for herself so she needs some assistance. Tom can justify his behavior modification program by the principle of beneficence. Tom's argument for promoting Nancy's crush on him is that this program will motivate Nancy to comply with the treatment programs that are in her own best interests.

Tom's behavior modification program may benefit Nancy in the short term but may cause her serious harm in the long term. The principle of non-maleficence states that people should avoid doing harm to others. Health care providers should avoid doing harm to their patients and Tom's program has the potential for causing Nancy serious emotional harm. How long can Tom maintain the pretext that he cares for Nancy? What will happen when Nancy discovers that Tom has no romantic interest in her but is merely using her feelings as a ploy to get her compliance with the rehab program? Normal reactions to such a manipulation include feelings of betrayal, anger and depression.

Tom's program also violates the principle of honesty. The principle of honesty says people should tell each other the truth. Health care practitioners are obligated to tell the truth to each other and to the patients in their care. Tom is not telling Nancy the truth. He is letting her believe that he cares for her romantically when he does not.

A third objection to Tom's program comes under the principle of respect for persons. This principle obligates people to treat each other with respect, dignity, and compassion. Respect can be defined by Kant's famous assertion that people are ends unto themselves, not a means to an end (Kant, 1977). Tom's program manipulates Nancy's feelings. Nancy's affections for Tom are the means by which he gets her to comply with the rehab programs. Pellegrino defines compassion as sharing some of the patient's experience of being ill (Pellegrino, 1983). Tom's program contains little compassion for Nancy's situation.

Nancy grew up in a state facility where overworked staff addressed most of her physical needs and little else. Nancy had no close friends. She was largely ignored unless she had a problem. As long as a problem existed, Nancy knew that she would have her caretakers' attention. Whenever the problem was solved, these people moved on to address the needs of other patients and Nancy was again

ignored. Tom's behavior modification program hinges on Nancy's need for companionship. Tom's time and attention would create the illusion that he was the friend that Nancy never had. Tom cannot maintain his deception forever and when Nancy discovers the truth behind Tom's actions, most probably she will experience a major psychological crisis.

What are Megan's and Patricia's ethical responsibilities in this situation? Are members of a health care team morally responsible for each others' actions? What is the basis for this moral responsibility? To answer some of these questions, we need to take a closer look at the relationship between the patient and the health care professional.

The English word 'professional' comes from two Latin words: *pro*, meaning 'before' and *fateri*, meaning 'avow or promise' (Compact Edition of the Oxford English Dictionary, 1971). Pellegrino explains that a professional is someone who promises the public that he or she has authentic skill and knowledge of a specific discipline (Pellegrino, 1983). Lawyers profess to have authentic skill and knowledge of the legal system and professional athletes are assumed to have the authentic skills and knowledge of the specific sport that they play. Before members of the public know anything else about the professional's background, they know that this professional has expertise in the specified discipline. Health care practitioners profess to have the authentic knowledge and skills to make patients healthy. Patients trust that health care practitioners will provide healing and submit themselves to their practitioners' care. Pellegrino argues that the healing relationship between a patient and a health care professional is founded on trust. The patient is in a weak and vulnerable state and comes to the healer to be made whole. To earn this trust, health care providers have a moral imperative to possess the authentic skills and knowledge of their professed disciplines, show compassion, uphold patient confidentiality and demonstrate personal integrity. While government licensure and regulation add legal sanction to the professionals' public promise, Pellegrino's healing relationship is a moral one.

Pellegrino's healing relationship involved one patient and one health care provider. In today's complex health care environment most patients are treated by a team of health professionals rather than a single health care provider. The need for team care arises from the fact that an increasing number of patients have medical problems that are too complex for a single health care provider to resolve. Since one person cannot know all of the knowledge from all of the health care specialties, we must rely on our colleagues from other disciplines to provide comprehensive care.

For example, a patient who suffered a stroke may have a primary care physician, consulting physicians from neurology and physiatry, a nurse, a physical therapist, an occupational therapist, and a social worker. The trust that served as a foundation for Pellegrino's healing relationship between a patient and a healer is now expanded to include all of the members of the health care team. All of the team members are morally obligated to possess the authentic skills and knowledge of their professed disciplines and professionally obligated to uphold the principles of bioethics and their professional codes.

How do we know if a professional colleague on a treatment team is behaving in a compe-tent and ethical way? This simple answer is that we cannot know for sure. We can only trust that our colleagues are competent and ethical professionals. Since we have neither the knowledge nor skills of our related disciplines, we must watch for our patients' improvement to get clues to the clinical competency of our colleagues.

Ethical behavior is even more difficult to assess. Each profession has its own unique code of ethics and individual practitioners usually have their own views on ethical standards. An area of agreement might be the tradition of *primum non nocere*, 'first, do no harm'. This principle has been attributed to the Hippocratic oath (see Purtillo and Cassel, 1981) though Veatch points out that the Latin formulation appears nowhere in the ancient Greek physician's writings (Veatch, 1981, *see* Coy, 1989). The principle gives primacy to the value that before health care professionals do anything else they should avoid causing harm to their patients. This idea is a variation of the principle of non-maleficence.

By extension, treatment team members are obligated to stop their colleagues from causing harm to their patients. Treatment team members may know that a colleague has a problem with mental illness, chemical dependency, or a cognitive disorder such as Alzheimer's disease. As this person's problem begins to impact on his or her professional duties, the team members, motivated by feelings of loyalty and friendship, may overlook, cover up, or attempt to correct mistakes made by their incompetent colleague. *Primum non nocere* charges the team members to prevent their patients from being harmed by their colleague's incompetence. They have a moral obligation to report their colleague's actions to the appropriate authorities before anyone gets injured (Bayles, 1981). The process of reporting a colleague's professional misconduct or 'blowing the whistle' on incompetent behavior usually has serious repercussions (Purtillo, 1990). The treatment team stops functioning as the focus of attention moves from the patient to the accused professional. The public accusation of misconduct destroys the trust that binds the treatment team together and the result can impact negatively on the accused, on the accusers, and on the patients entrusted into the team's care.

Megan and Patricia have an obligation to prevent Nancy from harm. Tom's behavioral modification program violates a number of ethical principles and has a real potential for causing serious psychological trauma to Nancy. Megan and Patricia have a moral obligation to 'blow the whistle' on Tom's program and stop him from carrying it out. Nancy is already developing feelings of affection for Tom. What are some strategies that Megan and Patricia could employ to protect Nancy's feelings and resolve the original problem of getting Nancy's compliance with the nursing and therapy programs?

Case 3: Irene Patterson

Irene Patterson is a two-year-old child with spastic cerebral palsy. Irene's mother, Jill, would like her daughter to receive physical therapy services but there are none available in the rural area in which they live. Jill discussed the problem with Irene's pediatrician who recommends that they send Irene to live in a group home in the closest city 150 miles away. At the group home, Irene would receive the full range of rehabilitative services. Jill is reluctant to send her daughter so far from home and wonders what kind of care Irene will receive in an institution. Jill calls the state Office on Developmental Disabilities and tells her daughter's story to Diane, a physical therapist in the early intervention programs. Diane tells Jill that she can see Irene in their home once a month. Diane says that she has a six month waiting list and she would be happy to put Irene's name on the list. Jill asks what she should do in the meantime. She thinks her daughter is becoming more spastic and her joint contractures are getting worse. Diane offers to send Jill information on how to manage Irene at home. The information contains suggestions on positioning, feeding, dressing, and self-care. Jill tries to follow the instructions but worries that her interventions are not adequate. Jill calls Diane back and asks for advice. After an emotional plea from Jill, Diane let herself be persuaded to see Irene on her way back from treating another patient in the area. Diane does not feel good about this. She will be driving three hours out of her way to see Irene and Irene is not the next patient on the waiting list. When Diane arrives at Irene's house, she finds a delightful two year old with a concerned and supportive family. While doing her evaluation, Diane realizes that Irene is developing joint contractures that will soon become permanent deformities if not treated. Irene responds well to Diane's handling and Diane sees that Irene has great potential for developing head control, sitting balance, and possibly, independent ambulation. Diane watches Jill handle Irene. Jill's touch increases Irene's tone and Jill is not able to position Irene so as to adequately stretch out the joint contractures. Diane believes that Jill could learn how to better handle her daughter but this would entail intensive training for a couple of months. Diane does not have the time to provide this training. She asks Jill if she would be willing to take Irene to a developmental center in the city for a few months. Both Irene and Jill would stay at the developmental center. Irene would get the therapy she needs and Jill would learn how to handle her. Jill says that this would pose a financial and emotional burden on their entire family. She would have to take a leave of absence from work and pay privately for all of the expenses in the city. Her husband would have to take care of their home and the other children while she was away. Jill wondered if somehow Diane could not squeeze Irene into her schedule. Diane wonders what to do.

This case raises the fundamental issues that come under the principle of justice. Rawls defines justice as fairness (Rawls, 1971). The principle of justice charges health care professionals to allocate scarce resources equitably among the people who need this care. Inherent in Rawls' Theory of Justice and Veatch's Theory of Medical Ethics (Veatch, 1981) is the recognition that some people have greater health care needs than others. Veatch and Rawls believe that justice means that patients with greater needs should get greater care. The criterion for allocating health care resources should be necessity rather than some other attribute such as wealth, status, influence, or geographical location. If we distribute health care resources based on necessity then all of us have an equal share in the process since all of us have the potential for getting sick or injured and requiring the services of a health care provider. To allocate health care resources

based on inequalities, such as wealth or social status, violates the principle of justice.

We can agree that health care resources should be allocated fairly but problems arise when we try to adhere to the principle of justice. All of the ethical principles described so far concern the actions of individuals. The principle of justice concerns an aspect of society (Stone, 1988). Veatch and Rawls describe justice arising from a social contract. They would have all members of a society agree to provide an equitable distribution of health care services to all people in need. They would tell Jill that it is unfair that Irene be denied physical therapy services because of where she lives. The social contract should include access to rehabilitation services and our society should provide them, but Veatch and Rawls are talking about a theoretical ideal. Jill already knows that in the real world, things are not always so fair.

Diane wants what is best for Irene but she must choose between equally unsatisfactory alternatives. If she insists that Irene wait her turn on the waiting list, Irene will develop contractures and possibly permanent joint deformities. These problems will interfere with Irene achieving head control and the rest of the normal developmental milestones. If Diane begins treating Irene then she is denying her services to some other needy child. She set up the waiting list so every child who needs therapy services could be seen in turn. Diane does not think it is fair that the child whose parent makes a stronger emotional appeal gets services sooner than an equally needy child who has been waiting patiently for six months. Diane could see Irene after her normal workday but the idea of the three hour drive to Irene's house sounds exhausting. Diane thinks that if she makes a special exception for Irene she should make a special exception for all of the children and she realizes that she could not possibly squeeze in all of the children who need her services. Diane knows that Jill has the option of placing Irene in a group home but that Jill is reluctant to place her child in an institution so far from the family. The short stay at a developmental center is another option. Diane can see where this would pose a hardship for the entire family.

To resolve Diane's dilemma, bioethicists use a process called ethical decision-making. The process will not provide Diane with an ideal solution but will enable Jill to choose an alternative that she can accept. The process allows Diane the opportunity to look at the dilemma logically and rationally and to seek a resolution based on reason. When confronting a true dilemma, an ideal solution is not always possible. Sometimes, the best we can achieve is to apply reason and logic to a difficult situation and find a solution with the least number of objections.

Ethical Decision-Making

What is the process of ethical decision-making? The traditional method begins with the study of ethical theories. These theories guide our thoughts when considering ethical issues and help us to develop coherent, consistent approaches to the moral dilemmas in our clinics.

Ethical theories usually fall into three categories: results-based theories, duty-based theories, and virtue-based theories. Results-based theories are concerned with outcomes. Duty-based theories are concerned with people following ethical principles, and virtue-based theories are concerned with the character of the person making the decision. A summary of these theories is provided in Table 12.2.

Table 12.2
Summary of Ethical Theories

Results-based theories
- Judgments are based on consequences and outcomes
- Three variations of these theories are seen in health care:

  Universal egoism This theory states that everyone should act in a way that results in the greatest good for himself or herself.

  Utilitarianism This theory states that everyone should perform that act or follow that moral rule which results in the greatest good for the greatest number.

  Patient egoism This theory states that health care practitioners should perform that act or follow that moral rule which results in the greatest good for their patients.

Duty-based theories
- Judgments are based on how well one does one's duty or follows ethical principles.
- Duty-based principles include the principles of honesty, autonomy, and respect for persons. According to these principles and regardless of the outcome, people have a duty to deal with each other truthfully, promote each other's autonomy, and treat each other with respect, dignity, and compassion.

Virtue-based theories
- Judgments are based on the character of the person doing the action.
- Emphasis is placed on the pursuit of ideals with the realization that attainment is not possible. Pellegrino uses a virtue-based approach when he describes a healer as someone who is competent in the authentic skills and knowledge of the healing professions and compassionate in sharing some of the patient's experience of being ill.

Results–based theories judge an action to be good to the degree that it produces the greatest ratio of long-term good to evil for a person or a group. Universal egoism states that everyone should act in his or her best interests (Hobbes, 1968). Utilitarianism states that everyone should perform that act or follow that moral rule which will result in the greatest good for the greatest number (Mill, 1962). Health care professionals often use a form of patient egoism and judge an action to be good to the degree that it produces the great-

est ratio of long term good to evil for the patient (Graber, 1988).

Tom's argument for promoting Nancy's crush on him was a results-based approach. He thought that he could improve her health status by getting her to comply with the nursing and physical therapy treatment plans. He balanced her health status against the fact that he had to lie about his feelings towards her and he concluded that his treatment program was justified. Tom's argument also points up a weakness in results-based theories. We are never sure if they will produce the long-term good results that we anticipated. In Nancy's case, if she finds out about Tom's manipulation of her and suffers a major emotional crisis, the case has a negative outcome and Tom's actions are morally wrong even by his own standards.

A second group of ethical theories are called *duty–based theories* and they judge a person's actions to be morally good to the degree that the person follows his or her duty (Graber, 1988). Several of the principles described above define duties to be followed. Duty-based principles include the principles of honesty, auton-

Figure 12.1 Calvin and Hobbes

Calvin and Hobbes — by Bill Watterson

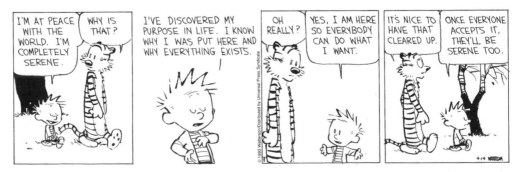

omy, and respect for persons. According to these principles and regardless of the outcome, people have a duty to deal with each other truthfully, promote each other's autonomy, and treat each other with respect, dignity and compassion. The difficulty with the duty-based theories is that we do not always know what our specific duties are and we do not have an easy way of resolving the problem if our duties conflict.

Figure 12.2 Patty the PT.

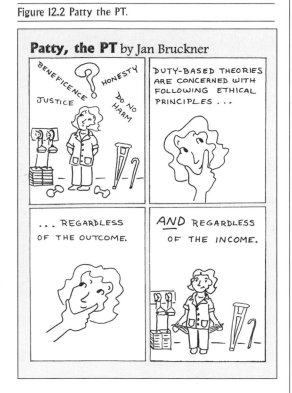

Patty, the PT by Jan Bruckner

A third set, the *virtue–based theories* are based on virtues or ideals. These theories emphasize the character of the person doing the action (Graber, 1988). Pellegrino provides us with a virtue-based picture of a health care practitioner (Pellegrino, 1983). This person is a healer: competent in the authentic skills and knowledge of the healing professions and compassionate in sharing some of the patient's

experience of being ill. These ideals are things to strive for but perfection in them is unattainable. Like the principle of justice, virtue-based theories require that we seek a theoretical ideal. This search for virtue serves as an excellent basis for classroom discussions and scholarly papers but is hard to use in a real world.

After learning about ethical theories, we can utilize a decision-making model to resolve specific dilemmas. Pellegrino and Thomasma (Pellegrino and Thomasma, 1984) described a six step model for ethical decision-making (Table 12.3).

Table 12.3
The Pellegrino–Thomasma Model for Ethical Decision-Making

Step One – Define the problem.
What are the facts of the case? List all of the relevant medical and social facts. include input from the patient, the patient's significant others and all of the members of the treatment team.

Step Two – Describe all relevant values
Input should come from all the members of the treatment team, the patient, the patient's family and anyone else involved.

Step Three – Determine whether any of the ethical values conflict
This process reveals the ethical principles that are relevant to the case and yields a deeper understanding into the conflict.

Step Four – Develop possible courses of action
Generate as many alternative solutions as possible. Creativity is encouraged and all possibilities should be considered.

> **Step Five – Choose a course of action**
>
> Decide on a specific treatment plan. The decision may seem like a purely professional one but on closer examination we discover that every choice also involves a moral judgment.
>
> **Step Six – Justify the decision**
>
> Defend the decision based on the ethical foundations that we claim to profess. Answer relevant questions. Was the treatment plan good for the patient? On what grounds do we judge it to be good? Why should we care what is good for the patient? Is the patient entitled to care? Who is obligated to provide this care? How far does the obligation go?

Step 1 We begin by defining the problem. What are the facts of the case? We list all of the relevant medical and social facts. This process should include input from the patient, the patient's significant others and all of the members of the treatment team.

Step 2 Here we describe all of the relevant values from all of the people connected with the case. Again input should come from all the members of the treatment team, the patient, the patient's family and anyone else involved.

Step 3 This involves determining whether any of the ethical values conflict. This process reveals the ethical principles that are relevant to the case and yields a deeper understanding of the conflict. Sometimes when the issues are laid out explicitly, a clear course of action is revealed and the case can be easily solved. At other times, the examination of the values reveals a definite conflict. A dilemma is defined and a solution must be sought.

Step 4 Here we must determine a course of action. People should generate as many alternative solutions as possible. Creativity is important and exploration of the broadest spectrum of alternatives is encouraged. In this brainstorming session all possibilities should be considered. The proposals need not be limited to reality. Sometimes the idea that seems the most fanciful turns out to be not only possible but also the best solution.

Step 5 During this step a course of action is chosen. The health care practitioners must decide on a specific treatment plan. In choosing a treatment plan, an ethical theory or a moral principle is also being selected. The decision may seem like a purely professional one but on closer examination we discover that every choice also involves a moral judgment.

Step 6 Now we must provide the reasons for our actions. We must defend our decision based on the ethical foundations that we claim to profess. We ask ourselves numerous questions. Was the treatment plan good for the patient? On what grounds do we judge it to be good? Why should we care what is good for the patient? Is the patient entitled to care? Who is obligated to provide this care? How far does the obligation go?

This model for ethical decision-making enables us to examine clinical situations in a logical and rational way. It helps us understand the ethical foundations of our actions and reflect on the implications of our decisions. We can develop a consistent approach to cases of a similar nature and be better prepared for difficult situations in the future.

Casuistry

An alternative method to ethical decision-making has been proposed by Jonsen and Toulmin (Jonsen and Toulmin, 1988, Arras, 1994). Instead of beginning with ethical theories and ethical principles, Jonsen and Toulmin begin with specific cases. This approach, called casuistry, derives the ethical principles from specific cases. Jonsen and Toulmin argue that bioethicists may disagree on the large theoretical issues but agreement is easier to achieve when specific cases are examined. The casuistical method more accurately represents the way we actually solve problems in the clinic and enables an analysis of more complex problems. In this approach, ethical decision-makers examine a case study and derive the ethical issues from the specifics of the case. We can illustrate the casuistical method by looking again at Case 3 and trying to decide what Diane should do.

From the case study, we learn that Irene is a two-year-old patient with spastic cerebral palsy. Diane, Irene's pediatrician, and her mother Jill think that Irene could benefit from rehabilitation services. Unfortunately, Irene and her family live in a rural area where rehabilitative services are not available. The state's Office of Developmental Disabilities will pay for Diane to see Irene once a month but Diane has a waiting list and Irene will have to wait 6 months for an appointment. Diane gave in to Jill's emotional plea and did an evaluation on Irene. Her evaluation showed that Irene is high risk for developing joint contractures and deformities without intervention. With intervention, Irene shows good potential for developing head control, sitting balance, and possibly independent ambulation. Physical therapy services are indicated and under the principle of beneficence they should be provided.

The pediatrician can cite the principle of non-maleficence as a reason for sending Irene to a group home. Without rehabilitative services, Irene's spasticity will increase and her joints will contract. She can be expected to develop permanent musculoskeletal deformities without the appropriate intervention. Jill can also cite the principle of non-maleficence as a reason for keeping Irene with her. Institutional care is often cold and impersonal. Irene will be separated from people she loves and from the people who love her. Jill knows that no institution can provide Irene with the same level of love and care as her family can provide her at home.

Our moral reasoning supports the position that Irene should receive rehabilitative services but the problem is how to provide them. In the just society of Veatch and Rawls, society should honor its social contract and provide therapy services for all who need them regardless of geographical distances. Since we do not live in the ideal just society, people must make difficult choices. Diane wants to help the children who need her physical therapy services but she has neither the time nor the resources to treat all of the patients who need her care. She set up a waiting list as an equitable approach to the overload. Under this system, the children who have been waiting the longest get the first available treatment times. The system is fair because it treats all people equally but enforcing such as system requires a dispassionate perspective and a strong will. Unfortunately, Diane succumbed to Jill's emotional pleas and did a physical therapy evaluation of Irene. Diane knows that Irene needs regular physical therapy treatments and she knows that she has neither the time nor the resources to provide them. She can insist on strict enforcement of the waiting list even if this means that Irene will develop contractures and deformities. She can treat Irene after her regular workday even if this means exhaustion and burn-out for Diane. She can urge that Irene be placed in the urban group home even though institutionalization carries its own set of negative factors. She can strongly recommend that Jill and Irene spend some time at a developmental center even though this places a heavy financial and emotional burden on the entire family. All of the options have serious negative aspects but Diane must decide on a course of action.

Ethical theories can help. Using reason and logic, Diane can examine each option more closely and see which is the least objectionable. Skilled bioethicists could use any of the theories to support any of the options. The discussion that follows does not try to be inclusive of all possibilities but serves merely to illustrate how each theoretical approach can be used to justify a particular option.

Advocates of the results-based theories are concerned with outcomes. A utilitarian might argue that the best option is to send Irene to the group home. This option satisfies a number of people. Irene will receive the rehabilitative services that she needs with minimal disruption of the family. Diane will have one fewer patient on her caseload and not have to worry about Irene's care. As long as the outcome yields the greatest good for the greatest number of people, this option is the right thing to do.

Advocates of duty-based theories might not agree. They judge an action to be good based on the degree that the action complies with a principle or a duty. They could cite the principle of non-maleficence and say that two-year-old Irene would suffer harm if she was forced to separate from her family. The principle of beneficence says that people should improve the goodness in the world. Diane was acting out of a misplaced concept of beneficence when she initially agreed to see Irene. After doing the physical therapy evaluation Diane feels a sense of duty to help improve Irene's condition. One option is for Diane to convince Jill to take Irene to the developmental center temporarily. Irene could receive the rehabilitation services that she needs and Jill could learn from the health professionals how to better care for Irene at home. Irene's father and siblings should also act in a way that improves Irene's condition so they should support Jill taking Irene to the developmental center.

Virtue-based theorists are concerned with ideals and the character of the person. They would urge Diane to demonstrate compassion for Irene and her family. Diane could see Irene in the evenings on a limited basis. These sessions would enable Diane to teach Jill a few techniques to prevent Irene from developing joint contractures and deformities. Afterwards, Diane might introduce Jill to other parents of children with disabilities and suggest that the parents form a support group. For people living in rural areas, the group could utilize such resources as the world wide web and e-mail. Diane could serve as a physical therapy advisor. The support group cannot take the place of actual physical therapy sessions but it could provide some assistance until Diane has an opening in her schedule. Virtue-based theories present ideals that people must pursue. One ideal is to maximize Irene's independence and a second ideal is to empower Irene's family to help her achieve this. As Diane works towards these ideals she demonstrates compassion for Irene and her family. As a virtue-based health professional Diane must continue to improve her clinical skills and knowledge and be guided by a genuine concern for the people entrusted in her care.

Conclusion

In today's health environments health care practitioners confront complex problems. They are called upon to make choices that influence the health and well-being of their patients. Some of these situations represent ethical dilemmas. To resolve these dilemmas, health care professionals must choose between competing moral principles. Resolving these dilemmas is never easy but a background in bioethics can help. Ethical principles can assist by identifying the salient issues. Ethical theories can provide guidance in making judgements. Methods of ethical decision-making offer systematic approaches to analyzing problems rationally and logically. Bioethics does not promise to give us ideal solutions to every problem but it does serve to remind us of what is important. Pellegrino said that at the heart of every profession is a public promise and that the healing relationship is based on a foundation of trust. As members of health care professions, our challenge is to earn that trust. A knowledge of bioethics can help show us the way.

References

Arras, JD (1994) Getting down to cases: the revival of casuistry in bioethics. In: Monagle JF, Thomasma, DC (eds) *Health Care Ethics: Critical Issues*, pp. 387–400. Gaithersburg, MD: Aspen Pub Inc.

Barry, V (1978) *Personal and Social Ethics: Moral Problems with Integrated Theory*. Belmont, CA: Wadsworth Pub Co.

Bayles, MD (1981) *Professional Ethics*, pp. 140–141. Belmont, CA: Wadsworth Publ Co.

Compact Edition of the Oxford English Dictionary, Vol. 2, p. 2316. Oxford, England: Oxford University Press.

Coy, JA (1989) Autonomy-based informed consent: ethical implications for patient noncompliance. *Physical Therapy* 69:826–833.

Graber, GC (1988) Basic theories in medical ethics. In: Monagle, JF, Thomasma, DC (eds) *Medical Ethics: A Guide for Professionals*, pp. 462–475. Gaithersburg, MD: Aspen Publ Inc.

Hobbes, T (1968) Leviathan. In: Macpherson, CB (ed) *Leviathan*. Harmondsworth: Penguin Books Ltd.

Jameton, A (1984) *Nursing Practice: The Ethical Issues*, pp. 278–298. Englewood Cliffs, NJ: Prentice Hall Inc.

Jonsen, AR & Toulmin, S (1988) *The Abuse of Casuistry: A History of Moral Reasoning*. Berkeley, CA: Univ of California Press.

Kant, I (1977) Fundamental principles of the metaphysic of morals. In: Cahn, SM (ed) *Classics of Western Philosophy*, p. 865. Indianapolis, IN: Hackett Publishing Co.

Mill, JS (1962) Utilitarianism. In: Warnock, M (ed) *Utilitarianism and Other Writings*. New York, NY: The New American Library.

Pellegrino, E (1983) What is a profession? *Journal of Allied Health* 12: 168–176.

Pellegrino, E & Thomasma, D (1984) Case presentation to demonstrate method of analysis of clinical issue. In: Pisaneschi, JI (ed) *Health Care Ethics for Allied Health Faculty: 1983 Institute Proceedings*, pp. 460–501. Lexington, KY: Univ of KY.

Purtilo, R (1990) *Health Professional and Patient Interaction*, 4th edn, pp. 41–43. Philadelphia, PA: WB Saunders Co.

Purtilo, RB & Cassel, CK (1981) *Ethical Dimensions in the Health Professions*. Philadelphia, PA: WB Saunders Co.

Rawls, J (1971) *A Theory of Justice*. Cambridge, MA: Harvard University Press.

Stone, IF (1988) *The Trial of Socrates*, pp. 47–50. Boston, MA: Little Brown & Co.

Veatch, RM (1981) *A Theory of Medical Ethics*. New York: Basic Books Inc.

13

The Process of Making Judgments

Elsa Ramsden

Introduction
•
Inference Model
•
Summary

Introduction

This chapter will focus on several factors that contribute to the process of making judgments. We will draw on information in chapters 3 and 4 related to sensory experience and learning, add to it, and apply the information to the clinical environment. The science of cognitive processing is in its infancy, but the past few years of technologic development, and the research enabled by it, has added to our understanding of this extremely complex function.

A critical component of our professional behavior in health care is the ability to make clinical judgments, which are key to making decisions; yet the processes used are poorly understood (Kassirer and Gorry, 1978). For many years, this topic has attracted a great deal of attention from psychologists, neurobiologists, and behavioral neurologists, among others. If we can understand how the process works for making judgments, perhaps we can plan curricula to maximize the learning opportunities, and design teaching–learning experiences that are the most efficient and effective. The ultimate goal is to increase our capacity to improve patient care.

Traditionally psychologists believed that reasoning was a rational, conscious activity for which one could use formal logic, and tried to create mathematical computer models of reasoning in order to understand the process of inference or judging. Wason and Johnson-Laird (1972) came to the conclusion that we cannot understand logical thought through the analysis of formal logic. Gradually behavioral scientists came to realize that much more than logic is involved, such as cue acquisition, memory and retrieval, and contributions of the individual's personhood, such as self-concept and value systems. We have found that people use pragmatic 'rules of thumb' that give quick solutions with little thought involved (Basic Behavioral Science Task Force, 1996). The model presented in this discussion was developed in an attempt to organize a large amount of information from several different domains that bear on the process of making inferences. The Inference model is summarized in Table 13.1 (Ramsden, 1984). Each of the seven steps is discussed separately in the sections that follow, and illustrated with a clinical example.

Current practice in health professional education demonstrates that nurses, physicians, physiotherapists, and others sharpen their skills and improve their clinical judgment through the clinical internship experience. They have learned the theory and basics of practice in the classroom, and observe their supervisor in the clinical setting, and then perform the activity themselves. However, the

Table 13.1
Inference Model for Human Information Processing in Decision-Making.

Stage	Activity	Description
1	Receive	Arrival of data via the sensory systems and transmission to the brain.
2	Infer	Selection of data for attention; comparison with cognitive maps; meaning assigned
3	Feel	Feelings are aroused by the meanings assigned: primary affective state, and somatosensory experience
4	Feel-about-feelings	Feelings aroused are checked against values and self-concept
5	Judge	When more than one inference is possible based upon the data received, a determination may be made about which one to select as most likely
6	Decide	Prepare to take some form of action, either consciously or unconsciously, in order to achieve one's goals
7	Act	Automatic and spontaneous or strategic action is implemented producing the stimulus for another person's observation

process of clinical problem-solving is rarely made explicit by the instructors or clinical supervisors; it is usually transmitted implicitly (Kassirer *et al.*, 1982). The expectation is that the student will observe the behavior and assimilate the requisite knowledge and skill by mimicking the behavior of the experts at their work. When asked to talk through their thinking processes, most experts find it difficult to articulate all that is going on inside their head as they observe a patient, gather data, and arrive at a clinical judgment. As we look at the steps described below it will become more clear why this is the case.

Inference Model

Imagine that you are a health professional who is seeing a patient for the first time. As you enter the treatment area and face the patient you bring your personal and professional experience and skills to this encounter, including your experience of the world and your personhood, with all its cultural and emotional baggage. The patient comes with his own life's experience and personhood, and anxiety related to the problem that precipitates this meeting. At first sight, without any interaction between the patient and yourself, and no words exchanged, a great deal has taken place inside your head and the patient's. What you see, hear, and smell is taken in by your sensory apparatus. We will follow the trail of this data as it moves toward an inference or clinical judgment.

General principles

The end organs of the sensory systems are the remote outposts of the central nervous system, connecting the outside world to the brain, linking the physical world with the psychological world. The human experience of the world is limited relative to the phenomenal amount of information that exists in the physical environment. Only a small portion of the information is taken in. We have five sensory routes to bring some features of the world to our awareness: visual, auditory, olfactory, taste, and tactile. Within each of these we are again limited in the nature and amount of information the sensory system and our brain can process. For example, our visual spectrum is a very small part of the electromagnetic energy spectrum of the total radiation around us, estimated to be one trillionth. Of the spectra most familiar to us, infrared and ultraviolet energy are the nearest on either side of the visual spectrum below and above the visual, followed by radar and x-rays. In the human auditory system the same limitations apply, allowing access to only a small portion of the sound waves that exist. Dogs and other animals are capable of hearing sound waves of a much higher frequency than we are. Hence we have the dog whistles that call one's pet, but cannot be heard by the master, and the rodent deterrent that emits high frequency sound waves which are not detected by humans, and ultrasound as a treatment device. The same principle pertains to the other senses as well.

Simplification and selectivity

Sensation is a complex experience involving information from the physical world around us; it is brought into the central nervous system via sensory end organs, and transmitted to the brain by way of sensory nerves.

Perception is a complex analysis that takes place in the brain; it involves breaking the whole of the sensory information into parts, transmitting it to various parts of the brain for interpretation, and bringing it together again for meaning. The biological structure of the senses selects only a small portion of the real world, making it available to us through the five sensory mechanisms. A comparison of human and animal vision and hearing makes it very clear that the experiences of the world are very different for different species. The stimuli for each species are simplified based upon the needs for survival.

Without selection of stimuli, we would have a chaotic experience of the world. At any given time we are aware of only a small part of the stimuli around us. As one sits and reads a book we are unaware of the mechanisms that allow us to deal with what is important and ignore that which is irrelevant and confusing; nevertheless, they are still around us. One way the senses deal with the overload is to respond to beginnings and endings of events; they are less responsive to continuous stimulation. When one walks into a bakery, the powerful smell of the bread and cakes baking is a strong sensory and perceptual experience. When one works in the bakery, the odor of baking goods no longer triggers a sensory response, as if we do not smell it at all. This is an example of *sensory adaptation*.

Comparison is another attribute of how our senses simplify and organize the stimuli in the world around us. A sensory change occurs when there is a difference in a stimulus from one moment in time to the next. These changes must extend beyond certain *thresholds*, which are the smallest amounts of energy needed to alert us to a difference in a stimulus. This difference may be from zero to some amount, or between awareness of the stimulus to awareness that the intensity or amount of that stimulus had changed, either increased or decreased.

Physical energy is changed into experience

Each sensory system is capable of responding to a particular form of physical energy. The only mechanism available to the brain to receive and process information is through the firing of neural impulses. The senses function to transform physical energy, such as sound and light waves, mechanical pressure, or chemical molecules that form odors, to electrical and chemical action so the brain can deal with it. This process is called *transduction*. What happens in the brain is something of a miracle in that these electrical and chemical reactions are somehow translated into human experience. The flower we see, the song we hear, the cake we smell, the hug we feel, are only electrical and chemical activity until the brain makes something of it.

Recent developments in technology make it more and more possible to track electrical and chemical activity in the brain. Research on the visual system leads scientists to speculate that there are cells in the brain, organized into modules specific to one kind of analysis, like edges and solid bodies. Their use of the word 'module' means a fixed plan with component parts that are standard (Fodor, 1983; Gazzaniga, 1985; Ornstein, 1986). Considerable speculation exists about whether these functions are hard wired into the brain or are a result of heredity and environment alone.

For illustrative purposes we shall trace the

sequence in the visual system from the arrival of physical energy of light waves at the eye to analysis in the brain. When light waves strike the retina, this physical energy is transduced into electrical energy that travels as neural firings toward the brain by way of the optic nerve, optic chiasm and tract, thalamus, and the lateral geniculate body. There axons transmit to the occipital lobe, where nerve cells of the visual cortex construct an image. The image we have before us in the form of the patient has shape and arrangement of parts that are configured in a particular way. We recognize some patterns that are familiar so it is not a totally new experience for us.

With these general principles in mind, we move on to describe the steps in the model for the process of making inferences. We could also use the words 'judgment' or 'impression'. The first step in forming and inference involves one or more of our sensory systems, bringing information from the environment to the central nervous system. In this heuristic model that step is called *receive* (Table 13.1).

Stage 1: Receive

The neuroanatomy and neuropsychology of the sensory system activity in bringing information into the brain were discussed briefly above in the section on General Principles. The quality or capacity of the sensory apparatus may introduce variations in the information that are not part of the real world data. For example, without my corrective lenses, my presbyopia renders the entire world a blur. The data entering my brain by way of my visual system is very different from the very same data seen by someone with 20–20 vision. Any physical or neuropathologic impairment along the pathway will have an impact on the accuracy of the data transmission. We all have a tendency to believe that everyone perceives the data in the same way that we do ourselves. That obviously and logically is not the case; but illogically we do not make accommodations in our behavior for that reality. In the clinical situation with people who are compromised by illness and disability, it is especially important to observe behavior for signs of disrupted sensory system function so we may modify our own behavior accordingly.

Stage 2: Infer

In addition to the simplification and selection of data that is biologically determined in our sensory apparatus, we have neuropsychologic mechanisms that help to focus attention on figure and ground, and organize the complex data into patterns that may be encoded. The needs and interests of the person receiving the data influence this focus and cause other data to recede into the background. For example, the patient we see for the first time may present with disheveled clothes and a strong odor to which we have a reaction based on our inferences. A variety of inferences is possible about this person – that he is a derelict, incompetent intellectually, emotionally challenged, a victim of an accident, or socially inept. We draw on the cognitive maps created over time and stored in memory to lead us to the closest approximation of meaning. Because the context is that of a treatment situation, we do not have the freedom we would have as a citizen on the street, where we could ignore him if we chose. As a professional in the health care environment we have a duty that carries with it responsibilities.

The cognitive maps allow comparison, consciously or unconsciously, of the data we have before us with that which is stored, in order to assign a meaning. If the data is vague or unclear we may focus attention on particular aspects and under-attend to others in order to find a 'fit' with meanings stored in memory. In addition, if the exactly right cognitive map is not available, we may alter the data to force it to fit one that is stored. Our psyche seems to resist dealing with uncertainty and the unknown, seeking to fill the vacuum with something, even if incorrect. Distortions are common in situations of uncertainty, and when people come from different cultures and subcultures, or are of different ages and sex. A brief discussion of the processes of memory follow to expand upon the information in Chapter 3, and increase our understanding and appreciation of this very complex function.

The processes of memory   Psychologists have no problem describing the functions of memory, but how these functions take place continues to be the focus of research and debate. The two primary processes of memory are the *memory cycle* and the *memory system*. The former describes the process through which we experience an event, retain it in some manner, and retrieve it later. The memory system identifies different components of memory that range from momentary visual impressions to retention of an event for the duration of our lives (Ornstein and Carstensen, 1991).

The memory cycle depends upon three processes that need to occur first: perception, which is the assignment of meaning to data brought to the brain; retention, which is a storage mechanism; and retrieval, which is a process by which stored information is brought back into consciousness as needed.

The process of perception was discussed above; retention and retrieval need further explication. The theory of retention suggests that we remember things for as long as we need them, ranging from a few seconds to a lifetime. Of course students taking an exam might want to dispute that, but other factors, such as the emotions, enter into that test-taking situation, affecting retention and retrieval.

Two types of retrieval have been identified: recognition and recall. Recognition is the ability to identify an object or event when presented with it among other detractors. The word recognition in this sense means 'to know again'. Recall is the capacity to bring up from storage information about an object or event without the actual object or event before us again. Recognition is more readily accomplished than is recall. For example, multiple-choice tests are easier to perform and do well in than are tests that require recall, such as short-answer or essay types.

The memory system includes short-term and long-term memory. For short-term memory we can use the analogy of making a note of a telephone number on a piece of paper, which we then throw away. The capacity extends to about seven numbers and the memory of it lasts a few seconds at most. We might be interrupted while dialing by someone with a trivial piece of information. The number we had in our head is gone and we have to look it up again. On the other hand, the storage capacity for long-term memory is enormous. Information committed to long-term memory may include almost any kind of material, from stories and songs heard in childhood, names and addresses of friends, old phone numbers no longer in use, to a broad spectrum of more important material. The research in this field is aggressive in the quest to push out the boundaries of our understanding of this all-important function.

In research, testing the brain's capacity to remember frequently utilizes individuals with known deficits which have been localized anatomically. While this is very interesting and useful in the long run, we still have a long way to go in understanding how long-term memory really works. Mishkin and his colleagues suggest that memories are stored at some higher level processing areas of the several sensory systems within the brain (Mishkin and Aappenzeller, 1987). The hippocampus and amygdala also seem to be involved in the processing of information; the hippocampus seems to be responsible in remembering the location of things while the amygdala deals with the formation of associations of many types of memory and emotion. Mishkin suggests that the sensory impressions travel from the sensory areas of the cerebral cortex to these two bodies in the complex process of recall.

Remembering is so important a cognitive function and so much a part of our thinking and doing, that we are usually unaware of its capacities until we encounter a failure to perform. A wide variety of illness, head trauma, and high emotional states have a profound impact on memory. The study of aging and memory has attracted keen interest among geriatricians and psychologists in recent years. An increased understanding about memory, how it works, and what interferes with its functioning, will help health professionals deal with some of the difficulties we all encounter in conditions of stress, illness, and aging.

Returning to the patient we have before us, our inferences, based on the data taken in by our eyes and nose, will be a direct result of earlier experiences stored in long-term memory. A collection of experiences may constitute one or more cognitive maps that provide meaning for the new date, and bring with the meaning associated feelings.

Stage 3: Feel

Neuropsychologists increasingly believe that experience is stored along with the feelings engendered by that experience. The cognitive maps that develop over time include the experience, the meanings, and the emotions aroused by them. When a meaning is assigned to the data, the feelings may range in strength from positive to negative, and may be very strong or very weak. The feelings in this stage are identified as primary and somatosensory. Primary feelings are basic affect states, with such words as happy, sad, angry, and pleased to describe the state. Somatosensory feelings use words such as warm, cold, tense, tight, or relaxed to describe them.

The feelings aroused by the inference may have an effect upon the inference, especially when the feelings are strong. In this case the strong feelings may cause a particular focus on part of the data and may affect the accuracy of the perception. For example, research has consistently demonstrated that high anxiety reduces one's accuracy in perception, and moderate anxiety enhances awareness of important information. Let us return to our patient with the disheveled clothing and strong odor. We could imagine that a young, inexperienced health professional might feel a high degree of fear and anxiety with this encounter. The focus of attention of the therapist is on the odor and disheveled clothing which leads to a narrowing scope for gathering further information and results in heightened emotions. With a shift from that focus to the face, voice and body movement, the inferences arrived at may be quite different. The feelings would be different as well. In general, the inferences we make are consistent with the feelings elicited by the experience, and are limited in accuracy to the extent that our focus for gathering information is limited.

Stage 4: Feel-about-feeling

The previous steps followed the incoming information from the sensory apparatus to the brain where it is matched with cognitive maps stored in long-term memory to produce both a meaning and feelings of primary and somatosensory type. In stage 4 the psyche becomes involved by comparing the inference and the associated feeling against the self-concept and values of the individual. The question dealt with in this stage is 'How do I feel about feeling this way?' and 'Is it OK or not OK for me to feel this way?'. The patient referred to earlier may elicit an inference that he is dirty, perhaps dangerous, and is not concerned about offending or causing discomfort to others. This inference might cause feelings of anger. Or we might infer that this person is homeless, and has kept his appointment in spite of his problems. This inference might result in feelings of sympathy and concern. Can the same data result in two such different inferences? Absolutely!

At this point a brief discussion of values will highlight their importance in the inference process, presented in the form of a model. The Values model is a way of organizing a great deal of information to aid our understanding. It is not possible to go into great detail about values, just as it is not possible to go into detail about the process of analyzing electrical impulses as they are converted into inferences.

Values: the 3–M model Values are an integral part of our daily lives, though we are usually unaware of the influence they have on our behavior. They enter into conversation in casual ways, guide the way we set priorities, influence problem solving and the decisions we make. We use the word 'values' frequently without giving it much thought. Just what do we mean when we talk about values? We need to separate this word from some others that may be confused with it such as attitudes, preferences, beliefs, and ethics. All these words have casual use in our languages, and more formal use in the context of psychology, philosophy, and sociology. In order that we may have common understanding of the use of the word 'values' in our discussion here, we define it as *a set of principles held to be important by an individual or group.* Certain criteria have been described by Rath (1966) to delineate values from attitudes and preferences. To qualify as a value, the principle must be chosen freely from among alternatives, must be thought to be important, and must be acted upon in a consistent fashion. The fact that I choose strawberry frozen yogurt nine times out of ten does not qualify as a value, but as a preference. There is an underlying value, however, related to nutrition and fat consumption that influences the choice of frozen yogurt over ice cream. The taste of strawberry is clearly a preference.

Values evolve slowly from childhood, are strongly influenced by the environment in which we grow, the culture and ethnic groups in which we have membership, and by learning experiences throughout childhood and adulthood. Values are not fixed permanently, but shift subtly as we become more independent, and broaden our experiences of life and others who have different values. They become increasingly more complex as we grow older. Values influence the way information is received and interpreted, and influence the strategies we use to arrive at decisions, a key component in the process of making inferences. Values are so integral to all that we do that it is often difficult to discuss them with others without becoming defensive. The following model is designed to identify the different kinds of values we hold, and to explain how differences exist among individuals, how conflicts arise between two or more people, and how conflict may exist within ourselves under certain circumstances. Figure 13.1 summarizes the main points discussed below.

The 3-M Values model by Ramsden is composed of two environmental *contexts* and three *levels* of individual involvement for each. These are arbitrary divisions for purposes of discussion and are not intended to represent actual boundaries. The two environmental contexts are called *social* and *professional*. The social

Figure 13.1 The 3-M model of values of individual involvement.

Social context levels	Professional context levels

Macro
    Society
	Macro
	    Profession

Mezzo
    Family
	Mezzo
	    Department (organization)

Micro
    Individual
	Micro
	    Individual

context represents the environment in which we live and encounter much of our informal interaction with others. The professional context refers to the specialized environment of health care in other professional situations in which we work. The levels of individual involvement are called *macro*, *mezzo*, and *micro* (the three Ms). We will look at these first within the social context.

The macro level This includes those values held by the society as a whole, and includes those things that most all individuals in that society agree are important in general. Of course these vary from one country to another. So, for example, in the United States of America, a set of amendments to the Constitution called the Bill of Rights, are particular values held dear by citizens of that country. They include the rights of citizens to freedom of speech, to worship in a manner of one's choosing, to education, to bear arms in defense of the country, and so on. Citizens of other Western countries have similar values, but may not have them codified in the same manner.

The mezzo level This includes those values that are learned within the family and held collectively by members of the family. These are transmitted from parents to children as explicit and implicit 'rules' which form the basis for getting along together. For example, in some families, children learn to speak in particular ways to adults, as a way of showing respect. The rule or value is to 'be respectful toward adults or one's elders'. This rule involves a very complex set of behaviors that includes specific words to be used, tone of voice (paralingual) and other non-verbal behavior including eye contact and body movements. Children learn these rules through direct instruction: 'Say please when you ask for something!' and through indirect messages, as in 'good' behavior being rewarded and 'poor' behavior being ignored or punished.

Values are also expressed through role functions within the family. How do the 'jobs' of running a household get assigned, and who does them? Values guide how the members of the family interact with one another, and the activities engaged in. Who does the laundry? Who prepares the food for meals? What are the expectations about shopping for food? Who makes the beds, cleans the house, takes out the garbage, repairs the equipment when something breaks, or cleans up after meals? Who brings money into the household to support the family? How do decisions get made about who spends money for what kinds of things? Does the family eat meals together? How do they celebrate holidays? Do they engage in religious observances? Each family develops its own system of values that organizes behavior around important issues; the structure of this system varies from one family to another.

The micro level This takes the discussion of values to the individual who has achieved some independence from the family. With increasing autonomy we find that some values that guided behavior within the family become modified. We have new priorities that shape what we do and how we do them, which may be quite different from those adopted when we were younger. School and the influences of peers have a strong effect on some values. A visit home during college years frequently brings a collision of values between parents and almost adult children. We may

have modified some of our values after only a few months away from home. Young people often hear statements like: 'As long as you are living under my roof, you abide by my rules' from parents who object to this evidence of new behavior they perceive as disrespectful of their family values.

We can trace a single value through all three levels to illustrate how a discussion of values using this model might happen. In many countries there is general agreement that individuals have the freedom to worship in a manner of their own choosing. This is a society or macro level value. This value is generally held in countries with a State-supported religion, and in the United States of America is codified under the Constitution in the Bill of Rights. In these nations, family members may have this value for all citizens, but as members of this family, hold the additional commitment that this family shall worship in a particular way. The value is expressed in particular observances, at particular times, with expectations of obedience for all in the household. This is the mezzo or family level expression of the value related to religious expression. At the micro level a single member of this family may grow into adulthood developing somewhat different values, leading to an expression of faith that varies from that of other family members.

The potential for conflict between individuals exists at each level in the system. It is a human characteristic for us to function in our interpersonal relationships as if the other person holds values and beliefs similar to our own. When their behavior suggests otherwise, we may need to pause. It is uncommon for people to question basic values that lead to specific behavior in an open and accepting manner.

Such questions frequently appear in a challenging tone, in a confrontational style which adds further discomfort to the situation that precipitated the discussion.

We can apply this model to the discussion of values within the professional sphere of our lives as well, to illustrate how conflicts may occur, and how conflicts may exist between our professional role and our role as a member of society. At the macro level, our professional organization has a code of ethics that serves as a guide to behavior in our practice. This is expressed differently in different professions and in different countries, but have many common features that derive from the fundamental ethical principles in Western societies which grow out of a branch of philosophical thought. One of these is stated in terms of the duty of the professional to respect the individual who is the recipient of care.

The example used here applies this value, expressed in our professional code of ethics, to a situation in the work environment. At the mezzo level, the department within which we work has policies and procedures that govern work in that clinical facility. When we accept a position in the facility, we agree to abide by those policies and procedures. One of the policies probably relates to timeliness of evaluating and treating a patient following referral. As an example, we may use a common policy that stipulates that when referral is received by four o'clock in the afternoon, the patient will be seen that day for evaluation and initial treatment.

An individual therapist, working in this department, has the value of respect for patients. On this day she or he has a full schedule throughout the day. Upon receiving the referral at four o'clock this therapist is confronted with a dilemma – how to add one more patient for evaluation and treatment to an already full schedule. The therapist does not want to 'cheat' the patients on the roster by cutting down on their scheduled treatment time, nor disappoint the new patient who places hope in the health care professional for relief of pain and distress. The situation may precipitate a complex set of emotions. Emotions are not logical, but they surely impact on our behavior. Some of these feelings might be anger at the supervisor for the referral, anger at the policy because it seems unreasonable, anger at the new patient for being there, anger at the physician for the unreasonable timing of the referral and insistence on treatment today, guilt about the anger, frustration because of the need to compromise another strongly held value – quality of treatment for all the patients, in order to comply with the rules.

This is a situation involving a conflict of values and complex emotions. We encounter these situations repeatedly throughout our working days. Usually we do not stop to consider the competing values, but move directly into problem solving. Frequently the feelings are left unresolved so that at the end of the day we have some sense of discomfort that all was not as it should have been.

Life is rarely simple, so let us compound the dilemma with an additional dimension. At the end of this particular day, the health care provider has a very special engagement that they are anticipating with some excitement. Feelings are strong about being on time for this engagement, so permission was received several days ago to leave work a few minutes early, in order to get home to shower and change and travel the distance to the event. The referral of the new patient means the health professional will have to give extra time, because the regularly scheduled patients will use all the time available. It will be impossible to leave early. In fact, it will be necessary to stay late to do justice to all the patients involved. All other staff already have a full roster as well, so it is unlikely that they will want to take on an additional patient. A conflict of values exists at the micro and mezzo levels for this persons' role in the social and professional contexts.

To summarize, the model described in Figure 1 outlines a framework within which one may examine values at the three levels of involvement in society (macro), the family (mezzo), and with the individual (micro) within the environmental contexts of our social roles. It serves also to scrutinize the values within our professional roles at the three levels of the profession, the working environment (department or office), and as an individual health professional.

We now return to stage 4 of the Inference model, regarding the disheveled patient. The values we hold as an individual in the social context and as a professional, as well as our self-concept, have a profound impact on the inferences we assign to the data we receive. We may have strong values about how people should dress and behave when visiting a health care professional – neat and clean at a minimum. We have strong values as a professional that we have a duty to treat, and that all patients are equally deserving of care. If the feelings aroused were angry feelings along with disgust in response to the odor, we may find a collision of values between the two contexts, social and professional, at the micro

level, with a negative impact on our self-concept. It is not OK to feel angry and disgusted when in the role of a health professional dedicated to providing care to those in need. We will feel disappointed and perhaps angry in ourselves for this reaction, and perhaps angry at the patient for precipitating the situation. The complexity is obvious, the outcome is uncertain.

Stage 5: Determine

The activity at this stage focuses on determining what is being perceived and the nature of the feelings; each contributes to the basis upon which an action is taken in response. The result of the preceding stages may come into awareness at this point, or we may continue to be unaware of the psychological and cognitive processes. When confusion exists because there are multiple possible inferences, the puzzlement and uncertainty might cause conscious awareness that can lead to consideration of the situation. If one inference has aroused very strong feelings, it is quite possible that a spontaneous reaction will dominate all logical thought. For example, if the disheveled appearance and odor emanating from the patient have aroused very strong feelings of anger and disgust, it may not be possible to pause and consider other possible inferences that exist in our mind. If we accept the conscious or unconscious determination or inference based upon these strong feelings we run the risk that the distortions will go undetected and lead us into a spontaneous action that is both unthinking and unjust.

Stage 6: Decide

Based on the previous step, the determination has been made, the inference drawn. The question to be dealt with at this point has to do with the effect one wishes to achieve through one's action. This process may also take place either at the conscious or unconscious level. If one is aware of some part of the process at earlier stages, more options are possible. For instance, if one is conscious of feeling not OK about the feelings of disgust, one can decide to covertly recheck the internal processing of the data to be sure that the determination was correct. One does this by reflecting on the original data received, the feelings triggered, the feelings-about-feelings, and the determination. This process of reflection, by its very nature, will provide additional time and consideration of the situation to allow a more deliberate decision on a course of action. If confusing aspects of the data continue to exist, this reflection would allow one to decide to clarify that data with the patient. Recall that as the situation was posed at the outset, we have not yet spoken with this person.

This brings us to another order of decision options having to do with overt response. If the process has occurred out of awareness, the overt response is spontaneous and beyond our control. Or parts of the process may contribute to a larger collection of behavioral cues about the patient that will lead to a clinical judgment. For example, the manner of dress and the odor may go together with body posture, facial expression, and characteristic movement that leads us to hypothesize about a clinical diagnosis in addition to a social diagnosis. Earlier in Chapter 3 on learning, this process was called insight.

Now would be a good time to talk with the patient, before rejecting him based upon a spontaneous reaction to the limited data received. Careful observation of the behavior of the patient's verbal and non-verbal behavior will contribute to validation or reformulation of earlier inferences. A variety of communication skills can be used to collect further information from the patient; some of these are discussed in Chapter 14.

Stage 7: Act

As mentioned above, the action may be the result of conscious or unconscious determination. The entire process from the time of receiving the data to the time of responding may consume no more than a fraction of a millisecond. To capture the process and freeze-frame it for analysis takes practice and time to develop. The incentive to do so is that we would like to be deliberate and thoughtful about our actions with patients whom we have a desire and duty to help. A conscious strategy of response would include considering different courses of action beginning with an attempt to elicit more information from the patient through careful interview technique.

Your response provides the stimulus data received by the other person, who then processes it in a similar manner to the one described in this chapter. The mental processes of another are not available to us; even our own are frequently not available to us. We may draw inferences about the other person based upon non-verbal behavior, such as facial expression and posture. But we must be alert to the reality that those inferences are based upon our own life experiences and cultural heritage, and may have little to do with the current situation and the other person.

Even as we try to verbalize our observations of the other person, it is very difficult to remove the inferences from the description. For instance, we may say that the patient sits quietly and attends to the words of the therapist. How do we know that they are attending? That is an inference based upon posture, eye contact and eye movement, head nods, and so forth. We do not know about the psychological processes going on inside the head of another, we do not know whether they are attending. We attribute these psychological processes through inferences related to their behavior and the analogy of our own behavior (Mason, 1997). We may describe a person's behavior as threatening when he moves into the personal space of another. How do we know that the behavior is threatening? The inference is based upon our own cultural norms for personal use of space that has rigid boundaries for distance between strangers. To be objective in our descriptions of behavior we need to use language that others can agree on. In the latter example we might say that the person moved toward another, stopped, and stood less than two feet from him, and began to speak using sweeping arm motions. All of this is laborious and time consuming in describing a person's behavior or a situation to others. In Western languages the tendency is to include the inferences we have drawn into the description, for example 'The man moved toward the other person in a threatening manner, as if to assault him'. Our inferences may be entirely incorrect, particularly if the individuals involved are of Near Eastern or southern European origin.

Summary

We began with a brief discussion of general principles that govern the process of data analysis, from receipt of information by the sensory apparatus to perception of meaning in the brain. A conceptual model was described to explain how inferences develop as part of this analysis in the brain that leads to a course of action. Each individual processes the data in a highly personal manner. A model to describe values was presented to highlight the contributions from psychological processes of affect and self-concept, values, and cultural heritage in making inferences.

References

Basic Behavioral Science Task Force of the National Advisory Mental Health Council (1996) Basic behavioral science research for mental health: thought and communication. American Psychologist 51: 181–189.

Fodor, J (1983) The Modularity of Mind. Cambridge: MIT Press.

Gazzinga, M (1985) The Social Brain. New York: Basic Books.

Kassirer, JP, Gorry, GA (1978) Clinical problem solving: a behavioral analysis. Annals of Internal Medicine 89: 245–255.

Kassirer, JP, Kuipers, BJ, Gorry, GA (1982) Toward a theory of clinical expertise. The American Journal of Medicine 73.

Mason, WA (1997) Discovering behavior. American Psychologist 52: 713–720.

Mishkin, M, Aappenzeller, T (1987) The anatomy of memory. Scientific American June: 80–89.

Ornstein, R (1986) Multimind. Boston: Houghton Mifflin Company.

Ornstein, R, Carstensen, L (1991) Psychology: The Study of Human Experience, 3rd edn. New York: Harcourt Brace Javanovich.

Ramsden, E (1984) Bases for Clinical Decision Making: Perception of the Patient. In Wolf, S (ed) Toward Excellence in Physical Therapy Practice. Philadelphia: FA Davis.

Rath, LE (1966) Values and Teaching. Columbus, Ohio: CE Merrill Publ Co.

Wason, PC, Johnson-Laird, PN (1972) Psychology of Reasoning: Structure and Content. Cambridge, Mass: Harvard University Press.

14

Communication in the Therapeutic Context

Elsa Ramsden

Introduction
•
Role of the Health Professional
•
Therapeutic Context
•
Talking with Patients
•
Summary

Introduction

This chapter develops the argument that it is necessary to think about communication in the therapeutic context differently than we do about communication in our everyday, social context. The paradigm shift in interpersonal communication suggested here explains the need for specific kinds of communication behavior to deal more effectively with the different needs in the health care treatment relationship.

The role of the health professional is described and contrasted with the role of the individual in society. The special nature of the therapeutic context is described and contrasted with

the social context. I suggest that the role of a health professional in the therapeutic environment requires communication that is both deliberate and skillful. Communication processes commonly found in health care settings are identified and organized into five categories:

1. Establish rapport.

2. Orient to the clinical environment.

3. Clinical performance or health behavior.

4. Individual behavior.

5. Personal problems.

Five different kinds of intervention strategy used by health professionals are described as providing:

1. Information.

2. Feedback.

3. Coaching.

4. Counseling.

5. Referral.

I suggest that these interventions are specially designed to respond to a different content that ranges from the superficial and objective to that which deals with increasing amounts of personal and subjective material. We have learned some of these intervention strategies in informal learning experiences through modeling and observation without careful examination of the form and intent. This discussion is aimed at providing some increased awareness and understanding about the appropriate application of these communication strategies.

For many years communication in the therapeutic relationship has been thought of as an intuitive process. Either one can 'do it' or one cannot; people used to believe it was not something one can learn. Here we argue that indeed one can learn about deliberate and strategic communication behavior and one can become skillful in applying these interventions. To do so involves acquiring knowledge and practicing the skills. Through thoughtful and deliberately skillful communication we can avoid many of the interpersonal problems that result in disrupted relationships.

Little attention is given in health professional curricula to the role of the health professional in communication with a patient. It is little wonder that we proceed based on the rules we've learned prior to that educational and socialization experience. In fact the dynamics

of the patient–health professional relationship are dramatically different from our role in society. These dynamics are described as the rationale for a *paradigm shift*, suggesting that the communication behavior in the social role, learned in family and school, is not adequate to accommodate the special role functions of health care practitioners. (Wherever the term health professional is used, one may substitute any health professional identity such as nurse, physical therapist, occupational therapist, or physician.)

The therapeutic context is described as the setting within which the interpersonal interaction takes place, because it has important implications for the communication process. Finally, a model is presented that addresses different kinds of communication need that can arise in relationship with patients. The specific interpersonal interventions are explained, and the relationship of the interventions to these issues is explored.

Role of the Health Professional

We are socialized to our role as health professional through a long process of education and training that is distinctive in each of the several professions. In its simplest form, role theory looks on individual behavior as a function of both self and function in a group or society (Sarbin, 1956). Role theory has been discussed by many social scientists for more than a century. This construct provides an understanding of how one becomes socialized to a particular function in society (Archer, 1889; Parsons, 1951; Lindzey, 1956). The theory is interdisciplinary in nature because it draws upon studies of culture, society, and personality.

For example, sociolinguists maintain that we learn about how to behave under certain circumstances, otherwise known as our roles, through the process of communication. Our first social role is culturally transmitted, initially learned in the family, and then modified as we grow older by our age and peer group, the school we attend, and by the nature of our work and its environment. The role that is shaped and evolves for each of us results from our experience in life that includes a complex process of coding language that controls both how specific meanings are created and organized in our heads, but also the conditions under which they are sent and received (Bernstein, 1975).

The anthropologists view social roles within the framework of culture and suggest that we develop expectations and behaviors that are associated with particular roles (Stewart and Bennett, 1991). For example, middle-class Europeans and Americans characteristically separate their roles at home from their roles at work. For each of these roles, specific functions are assigned to particular people trained or specialized to deal with the activities and the problems. Of interest to this discussion is Parsons' work on the cultural phenomenon related to the roles of health professionals and the sick role of the patient, in his classic treatise *The Social System* (Parsons 1951). The past 30 years has seen a consumer movement in health care that accompanied the growing need of patients to know more about their health care. These events have brought about changes in the health care environment that has led to an evolution in the education and practice of health professionals.

Ramsden (1962, 1995) found that health professionals hesitate to respond to the psychological needs of normal patients while treating physical problems. Their hesitation is understandable when a review of course lists and outlines from many health professional academic curricula indicate they have a low priority for behavioral science content (Ramsden, 1991). Without education in fundamental social science principles and training in professional interaction skills, health professionals feel ill prepared for an important part of their professional role. The absence of both the knowledge and the skills leaves the professional ill prepared, and leads to feelings of inadequacy in stressful situations that demand responsible behavior. As the health professional tries to cope with feelings of inadequacy, it is common to distance one's affect from the patient when there is stress in interpersonal communication. In some situations a health professional may feel so ill at ease that they retreat from the patient entirely. Imagine the following situation, if you can.

A professor of social work had spent several days in the hospital owing to complex and severe symptoms characterized by fatigue and weakness. This was the second hospitalization for the problem, which had not been diagnosed on the previous admission. The patient had prepared to leave the hospital after all tests were completed, and was waiting for the physician to explain the test results and provide the diagnosis. The physician entered the patient's room and said: 'You have ALS (amyotrophic lateral sclerosis or Lou Gehrig's disease). It is universally fatal. You have maybe three years to live. There's very little we can do for you except try to keep you comfortable. Call my office if you have any questions'. He then left the room. The patient felt devastated. He was overwhelmed by feelings of dismay and had many questions to ask, but the physician had retreated (Hanlon, 1972).

Diagnosis and treatment pose problems for physicians that are both cognitive and social in nature. Over time social practices have developed to guide a physician's behavior in diagnosis and management of patient problems resulting in an occupational ritual (Bosk, 1980). In some very difficult situations the ritual is not well developed, as in this bad news scenario. This physician had a poor understanding of his role and responsibility in providing 'bad news' to a patient and exercised no skill in his communication with the patient. He should not have retreated from the patient at this time, abandoning him in a time of great distress. Perhaps he felt inadequate to the task and perhaps his own feelings were beyond his understanding and control. These possible explanations do not excuse the behavior.

We all bring the skills in social interactions that we have learned over a lifetime to our relationships with patients (Hanlon and Ramsden, 1972). Without information to the contrary, and at least at a subconscious level, most professionals assume that these social skills apply directly to therapeutic situations as well. Much of the time these socially learned skills do apply. Patients regularly place health professionals in roles that are not common in social relationships.

A patient looks to the professional as *caregiver*, *informant*, and *advisor* because of the interpersonal dynamics of *authority*, *trust*, and *power* (Szasz and Hollender, 1956; DiMatteo and DiNicola, 1982; Stoffelmayer *et al.*, 1989). The professional who is unprepared disrupts the trust and the authority by failing the patient

in times of great need. The health professional also risks misusing the power to the detriment of the patient. Both patient and health professional bring expectations about their own and the other's roles to the interaction. Patients' minimum expectations are that the health care professional will be caring, will listen, and will be helpful.

Therapeutic Context

The health professional perspective

The dynamics of the communication process between two people depends on three primary factors:

1. The physical setting where the interaction takes place.

2. The experience or personal history of each.

3. The relationship of each person to the other.

In the social context between peers, interactions may be negotiated more freely; the communication process is worked out and determined by the individual participants as they engage with one another. In the therapeutic context the interactions are not freely negotiated because the patient is dependent upon the health provider and in that relationship is not a peer. Both the patient and the professional implicitly understand that the health professional is the authority figure; she or he has specialized knowledge and expertise to deal with the patient problem. In addition, the health professional has a responsibility to provide services (treatment) to the patient, and intends to bring about improvement in the condition of the patient that would not normally accrue without the intervention. These attributes are not true of peer or friendship relationships.

The role of the health professional in interpersonal interactions within the therapeutic relationship has some distinctive features that contrast it from the role of that same person in a social context. Five important distinctions appear, with regard to the health professional:

1. They are the explicit authority, with responsibility to structure the relationship and set limits.

2. They are the content expert for the duration of interaction.

3. They provide highly specialized and technical services to the consumer.

4. They are implicitly responsible for caregiving behaviors.

5. They have access to the intimate body space of the patient, to make physical contact with the patient in the absence of an intimate interpersonal relationship.

Some similarities exist among the first three factors in traditional authority relationships in the social context, such as a school or a business. It would be unusual to find caregiving in these social environments, but access to intimate body space would rarely if ever apply.

Differences exist between social and therapeutic interactions by virtue of unwritten 'rules' about our roles that have evolved within the culture of health care, and are tailored by each professional group. Each individual learns the rules as part of the socialization process of becoming a health professional in the academic training program, and during early exposure in clinical training and later during early years of employment.

The professions share some common features in these implicit rules, as well as having distinctive features of their own. For example, physicians are socialized to believe that they are ultimately responsible for the condition of the patient; if anything happens, either good or bad, they are accountable. This places a premium on being correct in all decisions made in relation to the care of the patient. The problem-solving approach used in medicine encourages a highly targeted list of potential problems, identifying the data needed to arrive at a conclusive diagnosis, and selecting the appropriate treatment interventions. The disease entity is the focus of attention of the communication between the physician and the patient, and between the physician and other health professionals. On the other hand, social workers are socialized to work with the patient in terms of the patient's support system, focusing on the long-term outcomes of treatment in the context of relationships with significant others who provide support, and the community resources available. Theirs is the 'big picture' view of the patient. Social workers and physicians frequently have difficulty understanding one another in problem-solving discussions about patients because their worldviews of patient care are so different, and because the rules related to communication are so different.

The patient perspective

The person who becomes a patient has learned vicariously something about the patient role as a member of society through the various forms of media, such as television, newspapers, and magazines, as well as from friends and family who have had experience as a patient. Through these experiences, we all learn indirectly about the implicit rules that exist in the health care environment, such as the expectation that the patient will do what the health care provider recommends without question. When one enters the system and becomes the patient one learns more specific rules about that role. Some behaviors are positively reinforced and others are negatively reinforced by the health professionals giving care. The patient discovers that the social-role behaviors commonly used in daily life do not work very well in the health care institution (Ramsden, 1980).

For instance, a very accomplished professional person slipped and fell downstairs, grabbing the railing at the last moment to stop the descent. This had the effect of pulling the head of the humerus away from the joint quickly and sharply. The result was a tearing of all muscle and ligamentous structures around the joint, while preserving the nerves. The physician, a specialist in orthopedics, recommended a passive range of motion to preserve the range until active motion could be initiated, and an anti-inflammatory medication by its brand name. The patient asked for information about the side effects of the medication and then said: 'I can't take that because ...'. With increasing irritation two other prescription medications were suggested with a similar response. The physician became visibly irritated. It was unusual to have a patient pose such questions, and he was irritated about the need to provide answers. This patient was quite able to make his own decisions in concert with the advice of the physician. The patient needed to

understand the intent of the medication, and match the potential hazards against what he knew, and the physician did not know, about his body. The physician was unaccustomed to this level of involvement by patients in decision making, and resisted the participation of the patient in a solution that was not the physician's alone.

Some of the implicit and explicit rules that guide behavior in health care are formal rules, while others are informal rules left to a discovery process, such as trial and error (Goffman, 1974). Rules exist to guide conduct and activities so that an environment is conducive to the work of everyone. When a patient 'breaks' these explicit or implicit institutional rules and the rules about role behavior, interpersonal stress develops. A patient on sterile precautions may not leave the floor of the hospital where assigned unless accompanied by a member of the staff. That is an explicit rule to protect both the patient and the public. When the patient repeatedly turns on the 'call light' and calls out for a nurse to come to the bedside, a variety of non-verbal negative reinforcement routines may be used to discourage that behavior. The implicit rule is that to be a 'good patient' one does not call for help except in extreme necessity.

These rules in the therapeutic context vary depending upon the three primary factors identified earlier: the physical setting, the personal history each brings, and the relationship each has to the other person. We will take a brief look at each one of these factors.

Physical setting

The nature of the physical setting has the potential for a strong impact upon the patient–provider interaction. These environmental factors include all the non-human elements that surround the interaction, such as the physical space, the contents within that space such as furnishings and how they are arranged, color, temperature, sounds, and smells.

We can contrast the physical characteristics of an acute care treatment facility such as an emergency room with those of the bedside treatment space in a hospital, a rehabilitation gym, a community health care clinic, and a home care setting, to name just a few. Each setting has unique features that influence the communication taking place within it. The subculture of the institution provides specialized rooms, furniture, technical equipment, and stylized interior decorations, which are familiar turf for the health professional but sterile looking and harsh to the outsider.

The patient's room in the hospital has more flexibility, though it is still very limited. Greeting cards may be displayed on some surfaces, the bedside stand may be moved to the more advantageous side of the bed. Flowers may grace the room and add some color and softness to the otherwise harsh appearance. Whereas the home care setting is a reflection of the owner with features that represent the culture and socioeconomic status of the patient. The observant health professional may learn a great deal about the patient and family system; an unobservant one will leave having learned very little (Ramsden, 1993).

Consider the following scenario. A student physical therapist, together with her supervisor, visited the residence of a client in a poor neighborhood of a large city. The residence was a one-room apartment located in a large house. Most of the space in the room was occupied by a double bed and a large overstuffed chair; the kitchen alcove was off to one side. The bathroom was located down the hall, and shared with others on that floor. Clothes were spread everywhere, some apparently cast aside after removing them. The alcove was a clutter of dirty dishes with an unwashed pot and opened tin cans everywhere. The room was dominated by a very large television set, much larger than the room needed, and much larger than the graduate student could have afforded. The patient was reclining on the bed, eyes on the screen.

When leaving the apartment, the student inquired of her supervisor how this patient and his wife could afford such an expensive television set. She knew there were days when they did not know where the next meal was coming from. She was told that they paid an exorbitant rent per week to have the set. Next week they might not be able to pay it, so they would lose the set until they could again pay the fee. However, if they rented it for a year it would cost them twice the regular selling price of the set.

It seemed a strange set of values to the student, a misplaced priority. The supervisor pointed out that the television was the only opportunity these people had to escape the rigors of their poverty. It took them out of their desolate lives for periods of time each day. The high rate per week to an unscrupulous agent was worth the price because it gave them a release from their problems. No reputable firm would sell them a set unless they paid for it with cash. The patient, of course, had no way to obtain credit to purchase the set over a period of time.

The living accommodation told the graduate student more about the patient and his wife than she could have surmised from many conversations with the patient himself. Their life was so different from her own; words alone could not convey the essence of their existence. Her value system had developed in a middle-class suburban community: she always knew where the next meal was coming from; she had a bank account and could save money to make important purchases. Things that were beyond her budget had to wait. Having a budget was a foreign concept to this patient. Money was spent as soon as it was obtained. Tomorrow was not a problem today; there might not be a tomorrow. They worried about the present, the moment they were experiencing now. It would have been entirely unrealistic for the student to expect that this patient could do a home exercise program without supervision from a visiting therapist. This patient was able to think about the future in terms of a few hours, at most, not days or weeks.

Individual identity

The health professional and the patient enter the treatment relationship, bringing their life experiences to influence the rules they select and how they choose to play them out. All the demographic and cultural details of age, sex, nationality, race, and religion have a strong impact on the way we perceive events and the behavior of others (Gudykunst and Kim, 1984). The many socioeconomic and environmental factors contribute to our individuality and to our ability to judge one another. The socioeconomic factors include the several group memberships we hold, as in age group, ethnic group, cultural subgroup, minority group, occupational group, and so forth. The environmental factors include those having to

do with rural or urban lifestyle, formal education, travel, and experience with people who are different from oneself.

In the example above, the apparently naive graduate student had been raised in an affluent suburban community that really only had a single class. Her first contact with poverty was this home visit with her supervisor. Yet she was highly educated, had traveled to foreign lands, and spoke three languages. One might have expected that she would understand the circumstances of the poor. Such was not the case.

The needs and motivations of each of the parties in the encounter, in addition to the psychosocial maturity of each, bear upon the relationship and affect how it develops (Hofstede, 1979). Other important ingredients in the dynamics of the interpersonal relationships are the separate but parallel reality roles and responsibilities in each person's day-to-day life that contribute to who they are, such as that of family member, lover or mate, or parent, or caregiver to a parent.

Imagine for a moment seeing the rehabilitation gymnasium through the eyes of an elderly woman who immigrated to the United States from Sweden. She came to visit an aunt, met a young German immigrant with whom she fell in love, and decided to stay. They married, both worked on Wall Street, then moved to upstate New York where both were employed while they raised a family. They lived in an upper-middle class suburb of a medium sized city, and subsequently the children all completed college and postgraduate training. When she and her husband retired, they built their retirement home in a well-to-do community in the south-western part of the country where they lived in good health for 12 years. After her husband's death she moved back east to live near her children. She sustained a hip fracture which was surgically repaired, and was referred to a rehabilitation facility for physical therapy. We might speculate about how this woman sees her role as a patient, and how she views the role of the therapist in the rehabilitation gymnasium. What are her needs and motivations?

We might also consider our approach to a male patient who has a very different background, and imagine how he perceives the rehabilitation gymnasium, and what his needs and motivations are. This gentleman left South Korea to escape political persecution, leaving behind all his family and possessions. He came to the United States and found his way to a large city in the North-East where he worked as a dishwasher in a restaurant until he could speak English. He lived in an ethnic neighborhood with distant relatives from his homeland. He married and had three children. When he had acquired a few basic language skills, he rented space in a city center farmers' market and set up a vegetable stand, stocking it with the fruit and vegetables he recognized. As clients asked for things he did not have, he learned the names for them and bought them the next day at the food distribution center. In this way he acquired words in his vocabulary, and increased the stock at his fruit and vegetable stand. The whole family worked in this business. Not long ago, his wife took over the first stand while her husband opened a second business in a suburban farmers' market. He has come to the rehabilitation facility because he sustained a serious injury to his right leg through a fall, and had difficulty walking and standing for any length of time.

How do we gain an appreciation of how these people see the world, and most particularly the rehabilitation gymnasium? Social psychologists have suggested that the more like another person we are, the better able we are to understand their values and behavior. How does someone who is very different from this woman or this man learn about the patient's internal frame of reference in order to plan a treatment program most effectively? The patient's chart and the patient him or herself can provide a wide variety of information about age, national heritage, and financial security. Some of that information should lead one to pause, to inquire about their perceptions of the current situation, their goals, the impact of the experience on their daily lives, and how they perceive the environment in the gym. These are only a few of the issues that can be raised in the course of interviewing the patient prior to treatment, during the evaluation, and during treatment itself. The more differences that exist between the health professional and the patient, the greater the likelihood of misunderstanding and drawing inaccurate inferences from the patient behavior.

To penetrate beneath the surface of these apparently self-evident issues one can reflect on the following questions:

- How do these factors exist together within the individual?

- Do all the different factors and roles come together into a comfortable sense of self that is identifiable?

- Do the values and beliefs that come together seem to exist in harmony within the human being?

- If not, how does the disharmony express itself?

Relationship history

Most of us approach an interpersonal situation assuming the other person perceives the circumstances and the relationship in a manner similar to our own. This common human tendency can easily lead to trouble, because the perceptions of each person may, in fact, be very different, as we learned earlier in Chapter 3 (Elliot *et al.*, 1991). Our impressions of another person evolve over time through the interactions taking place in the relationship, through earlier associations, or through information about the specific person, or people who are similar to this person.

Patients hear about physiotherapy, for example, from other patients who have experienced it, and may describe it as wonderful or a torture chamber. The patient approaches the new experience with a mindset based upon heresay, but influential nevertheless. Health professionals frequently hear about a patient through impressions handed on by others before seeing them. The 'crock' or 'complainer' has a reputation that precedes them. The expectation created in the mind of the health care provider is based upon the experience of others with that patient, not their own experience leading to their own judgments. The human tendency in this circumstance is to prepare oneself for a bad experience, revealed not so much in words but in the non-verbal behavior. Anticipation of a difficult interaction usually leads to increased tension in the facial muscles, a restrained manner in the initial greeting, and voice quality that suggests defensiveness. Such behavior may provoke the expected behavior in the other, even if it was not forthcoming on its own.

The information we have acquired and personal stereotypes, prejudices, and biases we hold strongly influence the dynamics of a relationship and affect the course of the current meeting and the development of the relationship (Reusch and Bateson, 1968; Fallon 1990). For instance, the social structure of the country, transmitted by individuals through time in cultural traditions, places limits on minority group members that effectively limits access to education, and imposes socioeconomic disadvantage. Membership in these groups predisposes individuals to restricted opportunities, limits resources and role models, and reduces prospects for advancement in any field, no matter how capable they are (Steele 1997). A practical application of this effect is seen in the lives of many women entirely equal to men in math ability, who find hurdles and road blocks to academic advancement and career development opportunities because they are female. The cultural traditions of many Western nations have discriminated against women who have competence in previously male dominated disciplines. Math and engineering, law and medicine, and many others have until recently been male dominated professions. At the very least, health professionals must have awareness of their own prejudices and biases that will interfere with evaluation, treatment planning, and working with the patient to achieve common objectives.

Talking with Patients

We realize that the interpersonal dynamics in the therapeutic context are very complex. The chapters in this book have described many different factors that contribute to the individuality of each one of us, from genetic heritage and early home environment, to sociocultural standards and psychosocial development throughout the life cycle. With this amazing complexity of factors that impact on human personality and cognitive ability we are seriously challenged to understand human behavior and plan health care interventions that are appropriate to the needs of patients.

One might try to argue that it is impossible to do so. In fact that was the argument until the 1960s, when behavioral science began to make meaningful contributions to our understanding of communication processes in patient care. If we are dealing with people with actual psychopathology, we have reason to doubt our ability to meet the patient's needs, but most people with physical illness and disability do not have psychopathology. Their behavior usually can be explained in terms of lost independence, increased dependence, feelings of loss, hopelessness, helplessness, and reactive depression that is entirely realistic, given their circumstances.

The following section describes a model designed to identify and organize the communication agendas characteristically found in treatment, and explain the different intervention strategies appropriate to deal with each. The underlying assumptions were developed earlier in this chapter, that is:

1. The role of the health professional in the therapeutic context is different from the role of that person in the social context.

2. This difference results in demands for different kinds of behavior, including communication behavior.

3. This communication behavior has rules and form that are different from those used in the social context.

4. This behavior can be learned, though it requires some practice and skill to be effective, as does any skill.

The objective of the communication is to be strategic rather than spontaneous, deliberately trying to meet specific needs rather than reflexively responding in terms of personal reactions. We call this a paradigm shift for communication in the therapeutic context.

Agendas in communication

The communication between health professional and patient may be organized into several interpersonal agendas or themes:

1. Establishing rapport.

2. Orientation to treatment.

3. Clinical performance.

4. Individual behavior.

5. Personal problems.

The first items in this list are more objective in nature and deal primarily with impersonal material. As one moves from point 2 to point 3 and on down the list the items become progressively more subjective, and deal with highly personal material in point 5. We will describe each of these.

To *establish rapport* is the first step in becoming acquainted, in which the health professional invites the patient to be involved in a treatment program. The health professional is the authority figure and is both responsible and in control of how the session is conducted. To do this one introduces oneself and may engage in casual conversation briefly to provide the patient with some experience of the health provider; the topic of this early discussion may be unrelated to treatment. This rapport agenda also includes seeking information from the patient about their current status, along with expectations and goals for treatment. Although this step seems informal and straightforward, it is very important. It sets the stage for what is to follow.

Orientation to the treatment identifies who is to do what, under which circumstances, and how to go about it. This is an opportunity for the health care provider to explain the nature of the treatment in this department or clinic and give the patient an opportunity to ask questions about it. The health professional identifies the implicit and explicit 'rules' of the process. Little emotional content is expected in this discussion because it is primarily factual. However, this step may also include values, such as 'physical therapy is a place to work hard' and 'this department is oriented to improvement and to the future'. Occasionally a health professional may approach this kind of discussion with highly charged emotions because personal preferences, self-concept, and self-esteem are involved, rather than the presentation of the information alone. For example, if the health professional does not like to work with obese patients, or if the patient somehow causes the therapist to feel intimidated and threatened, the emotions of the professional may enter into the interaction unwittingly.

In the third theme, labeled *clinical performance*, discussion of how the patient has performed in treatment has an objective component, but potentially is laden with emotional material as well. This focus on performance may convey good news, bad news, or both to the patient.

Commonly, in the face of criticism, an individual has an emotional response designed to protect themself from what feels like an attack. The patient may feel defensive and act defensively to the perceived attack. In treatment, the health professional's purpose in making this kind of comment is to identify a specific 'performance' problem in order to bring about a change that will lead to improvement in the future. Although this sounds simple enough, it is rarely a simple matter in practice.

The fourth theme deals with *individual behavior*. Health professionals sometimes need to comment on behavior that is considered unbecoming or inappropriate, such as particular language that is vulgar or profane, or gestures and touching that are offensive. The content of such an encounter invariably involves a conflict of personal values. The discussion in Chapter 13 describes how each of us has a set of personal and professional values and beliefs that includes guidelines about how we relate to others in our role in the therapeutic environment. These are learned and modified throughout our lifetime, are extensive and durable, are compatible with one another in the healthy individual, and are dependable and consistent.

Sometimes reduced control over one's behavior results from conditions such as head injuries, other central nervous system disorders, and metabolic disturbances. On occasion the injury may cause serious insult to the patient's identity. Patients may feel the need to test the health care professional to determine whether they are perceived as attractive. These are very real problems for the patient and call for sensitivity when responding. Sometimes the cultural values of the patient are at variance to such a degree that appropriate behavior for the patient in his cultural group is considered inappropriate in our culture. The accuracy of our perceptions and assumptions may need to be validated before challenging behavior that violates our expectations.

The patient's apparent failure to follow through on a course of treatment is especially bothersome to health professionals. Both parties in the relationship may profit from a discussion of the specific 'offending' behavior, the reasons for the behavior, and the rationale for the expected behavior. When the patient appears not to be following through on a recommended treatment regime, sometimes referred to as non-compliance, the health professional may need to assess how this can happen if the patient is participating actively in the planning and goal setting processes.

When a patient approaches the health professional with a *personal problem* the dynamics of the relationship and the role functions shift from those of traditional treatment to that of counseling, except perhaps in the case of the social worker. The roles of the patient and the health professional are explicitly the same, but implicitly the patient is seeking a counselor – someone who will listen and advise, someone who may engage in solving a problem that appears to be more a personal matter than a treatment matter. The patient risks both status and reputation when seeking the help of a personal nature from the health professional giving care (Ramsden, 1993). The health professional faces a conflict of interest, and risks becoming personally involved when trying to help in this way. The role functions of counselor are different from those of the

health professional providing direct physical care. It is useful to identify the *real* problem and clarify the needs in order to identify the best possible resources and the most appropriate resolution. For example, a patient may express mental anguish in the course of a treatment session. Further discussion reveals serious concerns about the need to return to work to provide financial support for the family. The nurse or physical therapist may feel ill equipped to deal with this situation. While accepting the validity of the patient's concerns, a referral to an appropriate resource is needed.

The interpersonal strategy we choose to deal with the communication presented by the patient depends on how the issue is defined. The more subjective the issue, the more interpersonal skill we need to assess the situation and provide an intervention that meets the need. Even when the issue appears on the surface to be one of giving information, one must be alert for potential emotional content that requires sensitivity and skill when responding.

Intervention strategies

When we talk with patients in the clinical setting, the form of response should match the issue being raised. If the patient is asking for information, it seems axiomatic that information would be provided in response. It would be nice if life was really that simple. Several circumstances may immediately come to mind where providing information may not be the best strategy. Before we look for the exceptions, let's explore the different strategies identified in this model and the patient agenda or theme to which it is targeted.

The forms of the response may be identified as providing:

1. Information.

2. Feedback.

3. Coaching.

4. Counseling.

5. Referral.

A particular communication event may call for one or more of the intervention strategies. Figure 14.1 provides an illustration of the relationships among communication agendas and intervention strategies.

Providing information This is a common feature of the health professional's role. We don't often think about the need for specific training to do it. Learning theory suggests there are 'better' or more successful ways to provide information. Information statements may take one of several forms. Empiric statements are factual, either true or false. Ethical statements identify a value and frequently contain a 'should', as in 'You should do …'. Aesthetic statements reflect appreciation, as for art, cre-

Figure 14.1 Relationships among communication agendas and intervention strategies in the therapeutic context.

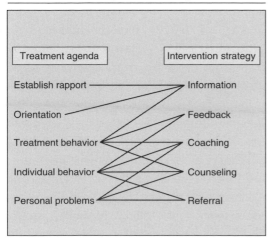

ativity, or beauty, such as 'That was a creative way to get your shirt on'. Personal values may appear in even the most objective forms of information, as it is difficult to omit our values, even from these statements. The selection of what information to provide, under which conditions, and to whom it will be provided are all a function of personal choice and values.

Feedback This is a process in which one person sends information about behavior back to the source of the behavior. It is a term borrowed from the field of electronics (McLuhan, 1964). In the treatment setting feedback is a useful tool to reward desirable behavior, comment on the current situation, provide corrective comments about a behavior, and redirect energies to achieve more appropriate behavior. Seven benchmarks characterize effective feedback (Ramsden, 1987). It must be:

1. Given promptly.

2. Agreed to between the parties in advance.

3. Intended to be helpful.

4. Specific in detail.

5. Described in a non-judgmental manner.

6. Provided in a balanced manner.

7. Personal.

The following vignette illustrates these points.

[The feature of both parties agreeing to feedback in advance is implicit in the treatment relationship.] The patient was executing a transfer procedure in the clinic. The health professional approached him and said, 'Just a moment ago I observed you do the transfer from your wheelchair to the mat [given promptly]. Basically you managed the procedure well but you need to modify the way you are lowering yourself from standing to sitting [balanced manner]. Your intention here is to protect yourself from injury. You let yourself drop down to the mat rather than using a controlled descent [specific in detail] [non-judgmental manner]. We don't want to develop a carelessness that could cause you harm [intended to be helpful]'. [All comments are directed to the specific patient in the form of 'you …', so the seventh criterium that the statements 'must be personal' is also met.]

Each of the seven benchmarks is important to achieve the goals of feedback. When we identify the behavior specifically and objectively in a constructive manner, along with our impressions of it, the implicit message is that we care and we are trying to be helpful. We do not intend to censure or blame.

Coaching   This is well known in athletic pursuits, and may be applied readily in the health care environment. It evolves naturally when a specific behavior has been identified in feedback with encouragement to try a new way of doing something. It is a useful tool to affirm a behavior, or to identify one in order to alter it. When a feedback message is given effectively, there can be an easy progression to coaching, to guide the patient into new behavior with constructive statements.

The patient may respond to feedback with an emotional response, and may be unable to follow the coaching suggestions. The appropriate strategy in this circumstance may be a *counseling* intervention when this occurs. The key criterion to determine a need for a counseling response is that the objective of the intervention is related to treatment and to the patient–health professional relationship. The emotional component interferes with the treatment or the relationship. The following vignette provides a situation in which a need for a counseling type of response is used.

> The health professional was working in the area and saw her patient applying an elastic bandage inappropriately to his stump. She approached the patient and suggested that he rest for a moment. She identified what she had observed in the specific bandage wrapping behavior using a well-formed feedback message, and identified the precise changes needed to correct the error. She then demonstrated the correct method on the patient, then unwrapped and rewound the bandage so the patient could try again. The patient said he understood. As the health professional left, she noticed that his face was red, his forehead had beads of perspiration, and his facial expression appeared angry. She saw from a distance that the patient repeated the incorrect wrapping pattern. A short time later the health professional spoke with the patient again. This time her feedback message was specific to his non-verbal response to her earlier statements and his repeated use of the incorrect bandage wrapping pattern. Then she said, 'I have the impression that you didn't like the revision I recommended.' The patient replied, 'I was doing it the way they taught me at the other hospital. They said that was the right way to do it. They were very careful that we learned to do it that way.'

Several possible explanations come to mind. The patient may have forgotten how to do the procedure, may have learned the procedure incorrectly or, in fact, may have been taught incorrectly. There is no use in debating those issues. It is also possible that the patient has difficulty dealing with divided loyalties, resolving in his own mind the question of which authority to trust – the former well-known health professional or the present new one. Conflict with the current authority may lead to uncomfortable feelings of embarrassment and anxiety, with possible anger toward the professional in front of him for creating these circumstances.

The health professional can identify the apparent differences in method, accept his feelings about the discrepancy, and then in a congenial manner try to resolve the problem. It might seem easier for the health professional to say, 'I know what I'm talking about. Do it as I have told you while you are here'. That kind of response diminishes the patient by ignoring his emotional reaction and denies his cognitive and motor abilities. Counseling responses are potentially powerful tools that require practice to develop skill. But, like other skills, when developed to a high degree the behavior becomes automatic.

Referral may be the action of choice when a health professional believes that a patient has a personal problem and needs counseling. When the problem appears to be primarily related to something beyond the current treatment situation, or when it seems to be complex, the health professional may feel inadequate to deal with it. For example, when a patient complains of being depressed and the discussion indicates that this is not a single nor a new event, the health professional naturally may feel perplexed. Depression is a common experience of patients with illness and disability, and for those of advanced age. Does this situation warrant expert advice? If the health professional is not trained in counseling, it is advisable to seek assistance and refer the patient. Even those who are trained may choose to refer to a professional counselor when the problem extends beyond the realm of their traditional professional practice. Some alternative resources include social work counseling, rehabilitation counseling, clinical psychology or neuropsychology, psychiatry, or

pastoral counseling. It is probably inappropriate for the health professional to develop a serious counseling relationship with the patient within the framework of ongoing treatment. The roles will inevitably conflict.

When the patient has a problem in the 'individual behavior' and 'personal problem' areas, they cannot be addressed adequately by responding with information alone. For example, when someone's behavior is offensive or inappropriate, orienting the patient to rules of the department does not address the fundamental aspects that focus on feelings and relationships. When the patient expresses fear or anxiety about a symptom, pain, or treatment procedure, simply telling the patient what is happening or what to expect is not enough to allay those feelings. The behavioral medicine research literature is growing exponentially with studies documenting the effects of psychological support on physiologic mechanisms during episodes of stress imposed by physical illness. Choosing the appropriate communication intervention strategy to meet the specific need of the issues raised by the patient is the responsibility of the health professional. Knowing when to apply the strategy is the next decision. Knowing how to apply that intervention takes practice to be skillful.

Figure 14.2 provides a visual representation of the model of communication in the therapeutic context discussed in this chapter and developed throughout the book. The figure indicates that the therapeutic context is the focus of our attention, identifies the three primary factors that determine the nature of the communication: physical setting, individual identity, and relationship history, and identifies the treatment agendas and intervention strategies. The model also depicts the relationships

Figure I4.2 A model of communication in the therapeutic context.

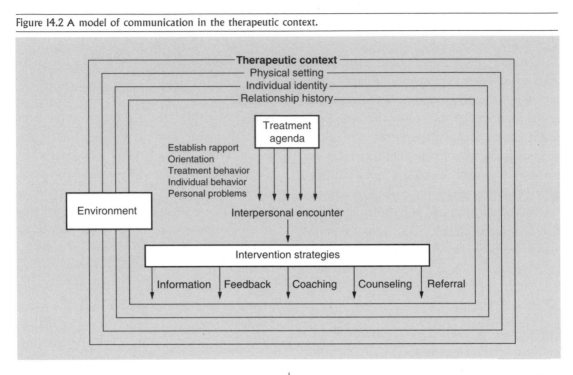

among the several components involved in the communication process

Evaluate results

This discussion has focused on steps to be taken in deliberate communication to effect an intervention that has a particular objective. We would be remiss if we omitted the final step of evaluating the results of the intervention. This step is frequently omitted in interpersonal interaction where subjective impressions are the common measure. When one achieves one's stated objectives, it is common to move on quickly to the next piece of business without reflecting on what was good and what could have been better about what just transpired. Qualitative research methods may help us to understand some of these dynamics better. The caveat rests in the fundamental requirement that the health professional has

respect for the human being and considers this person worthy of care.

Summary

In this chapter the role of the individual in society was contrasted with the role in a therapeutic relationship in the health care environment. The role dynamics of the therapeutic relationship call on different communication rules, suggesting the need for a paradigm shift from casual communication to that which is deliberate and skillful.

Environmental factors are identified that affect the dynamics of interaction between the health professional and the patient. These are the context that brings two people together, the physical setting in which the interaction takes place, the multiple psychosocial factors that contribute to the personal identity of each, and the knowledge they have of one another preceding the current encounter.

A heuristic model was discussed that identifies communication issues in treatment: rapport, orientation to treatment, clinical performance, individual behavior, and personal problems. These issues are related to particular intervention strategies requiring thoughtful and deliberate behavior. These intervention categories are separated in the model for the purposes of discussion though in reality the margins are blurred. The most objective strategy is to provide information, followed by feedback, coaching, counseling, and referral with increasing subjectivity. Communication in the therapeutic relationship is not merely an intuitive process, though insight and intuition are very useful. In the therapeutic context, communication requires knowledge and skills, both of which can be learned. We can avoid some of our communication blunders by not leaving our communication behavior to chance. We can learn and develop our communication skills to function even more effectively in the treatment of patients.

References

Archer, W (1889) *Masks or Faces*. New York: Longman and Green.

Bernstein, B (1975) *Class, Codes and Control: Theoretical Studies Towards a Sociology of Language*. New York, NY: Schocken Books, Inc.

Bosk, CL (1980) Occupational rituals in patient management. *The New England Journal of Medicine*, 303(2): 71–76.

DiMatteo, RR, DiNicola, DD (1982) *Achieving Patient Compliance*. Elmsford, NY: Pergamon Press Inc.

Elliot, TR, MacNair, RR, Herrick, SM, *et al.* (1991) Interpersonal reactions to depression and physical disability and dyadic interaction. *Journal of Applied Social Psychology* 21: 1293–1302.

Fallon, A (1990) Culture in the mirror: sociocultural determinants of image. In: Cash, TF, Pruzinsky, T (eds) *Body Image: Development, Deviance and Change*, pp. 80–109. New York: Guilford Press.

Goffman, I (1974) *Frame Analysis: An Essay on the Organization of Experience*. New York: Harper & Row, Publishers Inc.

Gudykunst, W, Kim, Y (1984) *Communicating with Strangers*. New York: Random House Inc.

Hanlon, A (1972) Notes of a dying professor. *Pennsylvania Gazette*. Philadelphia, PA: University of Pennsylvania.

Hanlon, A, Ramsden, EL (1972) Interview with a colleague. University of Pennsylvania, personal communication.

Hofstede, G (1979) Value systems in forty countries. In: Eckensberger, L, Lonner, W, Poortinga, Y (eds) *Cross–Cultural Contributions to Psychology*. Lisse, The Netherlands: Swets & Zeitllinger.

Lindzey, G (ed.) (1956) *Handbook of Social Psychology*. Cambridge, Mass: John Wiley and Sons, Inc.

McLuhan, M (1964) *Understanding Media: The Extensions of Man*. New York: McGraw-Hill Book Co.

Parsons, T (1951) *The Social System*. Glencoe, Ill: Free Press.

Ramsden, EL (1962) The effectiveness of a clinically oriented seminar in interpersonal communication for physical therapy students. Boston, MA: Boston University, unpublished doctoral dissertation.

Ramsden, EL (1980) Values in conflict: hospital culture shock. *Physical Therapy* 60: 289–292.

Ramsden, EL (1991) Psychosocial aspects of illness and disability: course structure and content. *World Confederation for Physical Therapy Proceedings*. London, UK.

Ramsden, EL (1993) Cultural considerations. In May, B. (Ed). *Home Health and Rehabilitation Concepts of Care*. Philadelphia, PA: FA Davis.

Ramsden, EL (1995) Communication skills of five health professions as measured by the Cartoon Listening Test. *World Confederation of Physical Therapy Proceedings*. Washington, DC.

Ramsden, WE (1987) *Managing for Improvement*. Philadelphia, PA: Medical Education Systems.

Ruesch, J, Bateson, G (1968) *Communication, the Social Matrix of Psychiatry*. New York: WW Norton & Co Inc.

Sarbin, TR (1956) Role theory. In: Lindzey, G (ed) *Handbook of Social Psychology*. Cambridge, MA: John Wiley and Sons, Inc.

Steele, CM (1997) A threat in the air: how stereotypes shape intellectual identity and performance. *American Psychologist*, 52(6): 613–629.

Steward, EC, Bennett, MJ (1991) *American Cultural Patterns: A Cross-Cultural Perspective*. Yarmouth, ME: Intercultural Press, Inc.

Stoffelmayer, B, Hoppe, RB, Weber, N (1989) Facilitating patient participation: the doctor–patient encounter. *Primary Care*, 16: 265–278.

Szasz, TS, Hollender, MH (1956) A contribution to the philosophy of medicine: the basic models of the doctor–patient relationship. *Archives of Internal Medicine* 97: 585–592.

Glossary of Terms

Accommodation – a process of modifying a mental scheme to account for new information taken in, that alters the dimensions of the scheme.

Adaptation – the ability of an organism to change or adjust in order to survive in its environment.

Amoral judgment – decision based on personal taste or temperament without right or wrong values, for example, preferences in food, use of leisure time.

Anxiety – a feeling of painful or apprehensive uneasiness of some unclear threat.

Apathy – absence of emotion; absence of interest and enthusiasm.

Assimilation – the integration of information into an evolving set of structures, of both biological and intellectual dimensions.

Attitude – a predisposition having emotional, belief, and behavioral components that determines a person's reaction toward a particular social stimulus.

Authoritarian – strict adherence to the rules.

Automatic behavior – well-practiced behavior that allows performance without conscious thought.

Autonomy – the ethical principle of the freedom to make a decision and choose a course of action, based upon the requirement of access to information in order to do so, and respect for the autonomy of others.

Belief – acceptance that something is true, though proof may be lacking.

Beneficence – the ethical principle to do good.

Bioethics – a branch of philosophy devoted to the study of morality in the health care environment.

Casuistry – a method of ethical reasoning that derives ethical principles from a case study.

Classical conditioning – the association of two or more stimuli with a particular response.

Cognitive dissonance – incoming data triggers two or more cognitive maps with disparate meanings, both of which cannot be applied to the data.

Cognitive map – mental schema that organizes information and events around common themes and carries in them expectations and emotions.

Comorbidity – the presence of more than one disease process in an individual.

Compliance – the extent to which a person's behavior coincides with medical or health advice.

Concept – a label, an abstraction to classify a complex set of features in nature as well as empirical observations.

Conformist – one who adheres to standards of behavior and dress of a particular group.

Consciousness – a state of awareness in which we are cognizant of mental processes and can describe what is going on.

Construct – refers to something intangible, that which cannot be seen or felt.

Coping – dealing successfully with circumstances and managing to move on with life.

Crisis – a crucial point in the course of events.

Culture – customs, beliefs, values, and norms for behavior shared in common by a group of people.

Debilitation – enfeeblement.

Deconditioning – the multiple changes that occur in organ systems that are induced by inactivity and restored by activity.

Dementia – an acquired impairment of intellectual and memory functioning caused by organic disease of the brain.

Deoxyribonucleic acid (DNA) – molecules that are the chemical building blocks of chromosomes found in the cell nucleus.

Depression – an emotional state characterized by feelings of sadness and lethargy, which frequently leads to withdrawal from social contacts.

Developmental task – a new behavior that arises at expected and periodic intervals in the life cycle and leads to increased physical and social accomplishments.

Dialectic – relates to a discussion and logical disputation.

Disability – as defined by the World Health Organization, is any restriction or lack of ability to perform an activity in the manner or within the range considered normal for a human being.

Duty – an obligation.

Duty–based ethics or deontology – ethical theories that describe the judgment of behavior based upon fulfillment of a duty or obligation; includes, for example, principles of honesty, autonomy, justice.

Ecology – a sub-field within biology that deals with relationships between living organisms and their environment.

Efficacy expectancy – the belief that one can successfully execute the behavior necessary to produce the outcome.

Elderly – somewhat old, past middle age, retired, senior citizens, pensioners.

Epidemiology – a branch of medical science concerned with the occurrence, transmission, and control of epidemic diseases.

Episodic memory – a function of memory in the brain for retention of specific episodes in one's life.

Ethics – a branch of the discipline of philosophy devoted to the study of morality.

Ethnic – shared experience that includes racial similarities as well as religion, social structure and definitions of gender roles.

Existential – a variety of philosophical thought that emphasizes personal experience and responsibility.

External control – a person's expectancy that outcomes in life are the result of fate or powerful others who have ultimate control.

Feedback – information back to the source about how the message was received.

Gender – the manner of behavior culturally defined for males and females in a society.

Generativity – the final stage of Erikson's psychosocial theory of development.

Genes – the basic components of heredity in all living things, made up of deoxyribonucleic acid (DNA).

Holistic – the philosophical position that the whole is greater than the sum of its parts.

Honesty – the ethical principle to tell the truth.

Imitate – repetition of a behavior that one has observed in another.

Impairment – as defined by the World Health Organization, is any loss or abnormality of psychological, physiological, or anatomical structure or function.

Individuation – Levinson's theory that deals with the change in a person's relationship to himself and the external world.

Inference – the process by which meaning is assigned to data coming into the brain.

Informed consent – the requirement that patients have sufficient information to give consent to a procedure, provided in an environment free of coercion.

Insight – the integration of two or more pieces of information to create a problem solution.

Interaction – people behaving towards one another in a face-to-face situation.

Internal control – a person's expectancy that outcomes depend upon one's own actions.

Justice – the ethical principle to be fair.

Latent – potential (or energy) exists but has not been activated.

Latent learning – a change in one's ability without an obvious change in behavior immediately.

Law – a moral value that is established by an authorized governing body, and enforced by a legal and judicial system.

Leadership – a role within a group of two or more that acts to promote the actions of others in accomplishing a task and maintaining effective interactions within the group.

Learned helplessness – a term popularized by Seligman, attributed to animals and humans who encounter inescapable conditions of discomfort, and 'learn' that no action of their own can lead them out of the painful situation.

Learning – a change in behavior as a result of experience.

Legitimation – the degree to which something is stigmatized.

Locus of control – a person's beliefs about whose actions affect outcomes: his own (inner) or that of others (outer).

Memory cycle – the process through which we experience an event, retain it in some manner, and retrieve it later.

Memory system – the components of memory that range from momentary visual impressions to lifelong retention.

Mentor – a knowledgeable person who provides guidance and advice.

Message content – the level, detail, and sincerity of the information being provided.

Middle old – individuals between the ages of 75 and 85.

Mid–life crisis – a period of time in the late thirties and forties characterized by thoughts of past years, the remaining time for accomplishments being limited, and emotional distress.

Model – an analogy for the real thing.

Modeling – demonstration of particular behavior for others to observe and emulate.

Morality – concepts of right and wrong related to human behavior.

Moral judgment – a decision that reflects a value of good or right.

Morphology – rules that govern how words are formed.

Mutuality – a relationship within which each of the two individuals is responsive to the behavior of the other, and regulates his own behavior in accordance with that of the other.

Neurosis – behavior characterized by agitation and anxiety, which may be highly targeted to an activity or person.

Non–maleficence – the ethical principle to do no harm.

Normative ethics – a branch of ethics that defines principles for human behavior.

Nosocomial infection – hospital acquired infection.

Nurture – to give care and promote the development of another.

Objective career – a series of social statuses and clearly defined offices.

Observational learning – one acquires information through the experience of others.

Old old – individuals older than 85.

Operant conditioning – the law of effect states that we select behavior that will obtain pleasure and avoid pain.

Orthostatic hypotension – a sudden decrease in blood pressure when changing to the standing position.

Paradigm – a change in the way we see things, a change in our view on how to deal with a situation or problem.

Perception – a complex process that involves analyzing sensory information and assigning meaning to it.

Performance accomplishments – one of the factors that influences self-efficacy through one's own experience of success.

Personhood – the quality or condition of being an individual person.

Phonology – a system of sounds that are coded to provide meaning.

Physiologic status – one of the factors that influences self-efficacy based on a person's perception of their physiologic state as well as their actual physiologic state.

Primum non nocere – 'first, do no harm' attributed (probably erroneously) to the Hippocratic oath; the ethical principle that maintains that before health care professionals giving any care, they should do no harm.

Principle – a rule or an axiom.

Procedural memory – a function of memory in the brain that holds and organizes a wide variety of rules that make it possible to function in our world.

Psychosocial theory – studies human behavior across the span of life.

Psychosomatic illness – physical illness resulting from stress and emotional response to stress.

Ptophobia – fear of falling.

Rapport – the initial step in developing a relationship with someone, identifying oneself to the other, and beginning to exchange information.

Reinforcement – any stimulus that is more likely to result in repetition of a desired behavior, both positive and negative in nature.

Respect (for persons) – a principle stating that people relate to other people with dignity and compassion.

Results–based ethics (consequentialism) – ethical theories that posit judgment of actions as good or bad based upon the long term effect or outcome upon a person or group.

Role – expectations concerning the behavior and obligations of an individual occupying a social status; the metaphor is borrowed from the theater and denotes the conduct or behavior of a certain 'part' rather than to the players in them.

Self–concept – the ways in which an individual perceives themself; a set of self-schemas that provide a clear set of beliefs about oneself.

Self–efficacy – the belief in one's capabilities to organize and execute the course(s) of action required to accomplish a given objective.

Self–esteem – the evaluation one makes of oneself and usually maintains over time indicating the extent to which he believes himself capable, significant, successful, and worthy.

Selfhood – personality, separate and conscious existence.

Semantic memory – a function of memory in the brain that stores the symbol we use to represent our thoughts and language.

Semantics – a system of meanings.

Sex – biologic description.

Social attachment – patterns that evolve through a process of building emotional bonds with a significant other.

Social cognitive theory – explains human behavior in terms of the three factors of cognitive, social, and environmental influences in one's life.

Social psychology – a behavioral science discipline which studies human behavior in the context of its relationship to others; a combining of psychology and sociology perspectives.

Status – a term used to define a position in a group or society; conceptualization of high as opposed to low status can differ from one group or society to another in accordance with values.

Stigma – an aspect of an individual which elicits a negative response from others that disqualifies them from full social acceptance.

Subjective career – the moving perspective in which an individual sees their life as a whole and interprets the meaning of their various attributes.

Symbols – words, objects, or gestures which communicate significance or sentiment beyond the literal meaning or use. For example, a sports car is not merely a means of transportation, but also communicates something about the owner's financial position. In this sense it functions as a status symbol.

Syntax – rules of sentence structure.

Theory – a logically interrelated system of concepts that provides a framework for understanding observations in nature.

Timing – the psychosocial and neurophysiological readiness of an individual to accept the intended message content successfully.

Trajectory – the total organization of work over the period of the physiological course of a chronic disease, plus the impact on those involved with the patient.

Transduction – transformation of physical energy to electrical and chemical action for activation in the brain.

Type A personality – a theory describing certain characteristics of a person that include impatience, aggression, high energy and productivity.

Values – a set of principles held to be important by an individual or group.

Verbal persuasion – one of the factors that influences self-efficacy through the encouragement or discouragement of others.

Vertigo – a sensation of whirling and a tendency to lose balance.

Vicarious experience – one of the factors that influences self-efficacy through the observation or awareness of another individual performing the task.

Virtue–based ethics (aretaic ethics) – ethical theories based on ideals, emphasizing character, motives, and intentions of the person acting.

Workaholic – a person who spends more than the usual number of hours working, and is dependent on work for satisfaction.

Young old – individuals between the ages of 65 and 75.

Index

Accommodation *see* Adaptation, behavioral;
    Cognitive maps
Activity theory, 127-128
Adaptation
    behavioral, 25-26, 49-50
    biological, 12
    plastic, 12, 70, 92
    sensory, 233
Adolescence
    case studies, 67-68, 74-75, 76-77, 79-81
        see also patients' experiences
    challenges of, 72-78
        physical growth and development, 72-75
        self in relation to world, 77-78
        self-creation, 75-77
    patients' experiences
        compliance, 82-84
        perceptions of own resources, 84-89
        respect and reciprocity, 79-82
    principles of practice, 89-97
        holism, 69-70
    South African context, 70-71
Adulthood
    development theories, 100-102
    developmental tasks, 102-112
    health problems in, 112-117
Aging, 123-125
    aspects of, 132-133, 135
        physical, 135-136
        psychological, 136-142
        social, 143-145
    biological theories of, 125-126
    case studies, 126-127, 128, 131-132, 136, 140-141

in developed world, 149-151
in developing world, 151-153
health issues, 145, 150
myths, 165-166
'normal', 132-133
psychosocial theories of, 126, 127-128, 129-131
research issues, 133-136
'successful', 133, 148
wisdom, 138-139, 166-167
see also Chronic disease, older people
Alzheimer's disease *see* Dementia
Assertive behavior, 86-87
Assimilation *see* Adaptation, behavioral; Cognitive
    maps
Association, 30, 31, 32
    sensorimotor causality schemes, 49-51
Attachment patterns *see* Social attachment
Authoritative control, 60
Automatic behavior, 29-30
Autonomy
    principle of, *214*
        case studies, 215-217, 218
    versus shame and doubt, *14*, 58-59

Bandura, A, 39, 112, 189-190
Behavior modification, 33-34
    ethical issues, case study, 217-221
Behavioral adaptation, 25-26, 49-50
Belief systems, 20-21
    see also Values
Beneficence, principle of, *214*
    case studies, 215-217, 218, 228
Bereavement, 142

Bioethics *see* Ethical principles
Biographical work, 176, 177-178, 179
Biological system, 11-12
    major components, *12*
Biological theories of aging, 125-126
Bloom, S & Summey, P: social interaction model,
        205-208, 209
Body language *see* Non-verbal behavior
Buehler, C: life stages, 129-130

Cardiovascular disorders, 153-154
    and personality type, 114-115
Care
    versus rejectivity, 100-101
    work as expression of, 105
Caregivers *see* Families, as caregivers;
Parenthood
Casuistry, 227-229
Causality, sense of 50-51
Cerebrovascular accidents, 154-155
Child development
    in adversity, 70-71
    case study, 56, 57, 61-65
    emotional development, 53-54
    imitation, 55-56
    language development, 56-58
    motor development, 49
    mutuality with care giver, 54-55, 118
    object manipulation, permanence and categories,
        51-52
    prenatal, 44-45
    psychosocial agenda, 58-61
    sensorimotor schemes and early associations,
        49-51
    sensory/perceptual interconnectedness,
        48-49
    social attachment, 45-47, 52, 53-55, 57
Chronic disease
    coping strategies, 106-107, 180-182
    initial disruption, 176-178
    living with, 179-182
    management, 178-179
    role theory approaches
        functionalist, 170-175, 210
        interactionist, 175-182
        reconciliation and comparison, 182-184
    trajectory of, 175-176

Chronic disease in older people
    cardiovascular disorders, 153-154
    and caregivers, 166
    cerebrovascular accidents, 154-155
    dementia, 162-164
    developing countries, 153, 154-155
    hospitalization and institutionalization, 161-162
    physical disability, 145-146
        and depression, 154, 155, 158-159, 159-160
        incontinence, 160
        loss of mobility and function, 156-157
        pain, 157-159
        and sleep disorders, 160-161
    treatment, 164-166
Classical conditioning, 31-33
    versus operant conditioning, *33*
Clinical judgment *see* Inference model
Clinical skills development, 30
Coaching, 258
Cognitive competencies, 36
Cognitive development, 27-29
Cognitive function in older people, 136-139
Cognitive learning, 36-39
Cognitive maps, 36-37, 234-235, 236
Communication
    agendas in, 254-256
    intervention strategies, 244-245, 256-259
        evaluation, 260
        model, 259, *260*
        physical setting, 249-251
    see also Health practitioner–patient relationship
Compliance, 82-84
    sick role theory, 174
    see also Non-compliance
Conditioned pain behavior, 158
Conditioning *see* Classical conditioning; Operant
        conditioning
Consciousness, 29
    levels of, 30
Consent, informed, 208-209
Consumerism, 173, 198
Coping strategies, 36
    activating, 118-120
    adolescence, 78
    case study, 76-77
    chronic disease, 106-107, 180-182
    in extreme adversity, 71

Coping strategies (continued)
  older people, 139-140
    case study, 140-141
    pain, 159
  problem solving focus, 113
  sense of humor, 84-85
Corbin, J & Strauss, A: chronic illness, 175-176, 177, 178, 179
Counseling, 256, 258-259
Cultural context, 26-27
  adult developmental tasks, 102-103
  doctor-patient relationship, 205, 206
  emotional development, 53-54
  gender-role identification, 60
  language development, 57-58
  non-compliance, 199
  older people, 142, 143, 150-151
  perception, 28-29
  shaming response, 59
  see also Developing countries; Ethnic subcultures
Cultural determinism, 19
Culture, 19, 20-21
  and subcultures, 206-207
CVA see Cerebrovascular accidents

Decision-making see Ethical decision-making; Inference model
Deductive process, 3-4, 6
Dehumanization see Integration and humanization model
Dementia, 162-163
  psychosocial aspects, 163-164
Depression, 116-117, 165
  cerebrovascular accidents, 154-155
  chronic pain, 158-159
  physical illness and disability, 159-161
Developing countries, 151-153, 154-155
  South Africa, 70-71, 155
Deviance, illness as, 170-171, 172, 184
Disability
  definition, 145-146
  initial disruption, 176-178
  models, 7-8
  see also Adolescence, case studies;
    Cerebrovascular accidents;
    Chronic disease in older people, physical disability

Disengagement theory, 126-127, 128
Dissociation, 181
Doctor see Health practitioner
Duty-based theories, 223, 224-225, 228

Ecological system, 6-7, 21-23
  biological system, 11-12
  psychosocial theory, 13-18
  societal system, 19-21
Education level and health, 150, 165
Emotional development, 53-54
Erickson, Eric, 13-18, 55, 72, 78, 100-101, 130-131
Ethical decision-making, 225-226, 226
  casuistry, 227-229
Ethical principles, 214-215
  case studies
    non-compliance, 215-217, 217-221, 224
    resource allocation, 221-223, 227-229
Ethical theories, 223-225, 228
Ethics and law, 213-214
Ethnic subcultures, 27, 207, 251-252
  definition, 19-20
Ethnocentrism, 20
Exchange theory, 128-129
Expectations, 36, 39, 189-190
  role, 201-202
  unrealized, 199-200

Falling, 156-157
  risk factors, 187
  treatment, physical therapy, 187-188
Falling, fear of, 187
  case study, 191-194
  self-efficacy
    assessment tools, 194-195
    factors in case study, 193-194
    ideal therapeutic environment, 195-196
Families
  as caregivers
    mutuality and coordination, 54-55
    and older people, 166
  one-parent, 109
  as source of values, 238-239
  structure and ethos, 27
Fantasy, activating inner resources, 119
Feedback, 257-258

Feeling *see* Emotional development; Sensation and perception
Fetal development, 44-45
Functional limitation model, 7-8
Functionalism *see* sick role theory

Gender differences
    adult development, 101-102
    doctor-patient relationship, 208-209
    life expectancy, 149-150
    life patterns, 107-110, 111
    muscle stength in older people, 157
    parenthood, 103-104
Gender-role identification, 59-61
Generativity
    versus stagnation, *17*, 100-1
    see also Parenthood; Work
Genes and inheritance, 11-12, 43-44
Goffman, E, 144, 172, 178, 181, 182, 183, 204-205, 249

Handicap, definition, 146
Harm, avoiding *see* Ethical principles
Hazan, H: integration and humanization model, 143-145
Health care resource allocation, case study, 221-223, 227-229
Health practitioner
    perspective, 247-248
    role, 245-247
Health practitoner—patient relationship
    co-operative partnership, 90-92, 96
    elements
        interactive, 204-208
        structural, 201-204
    history, 253
    individual identity, 251-252
    patient perspective, 79-84, 248-249
    problems in, 82-84, 198-201
    role theory, 170-171, 173, 202-204
    trust in, 219-220
    see also Communication
Holism, 69-70
Hollender, M *see* Szasz, T & Hollender, M
Honesty, principle of, *215*
    case study, 219
Human Genome Project, 11, 44

Humor, sense of, 84-85

ICIDH *see* International Classification of Impairments, Disabilities and Handicaps
Identity *see* Self-concept
Imitation, 55-56
Incontinence, 160
Inductive process, 3
Infancy *see* Child development
Inference model, 231, 232-243
    principles, 232-234
    stages, *231*, 234-243
Information, providing, 208-209, 257
Inheritance and genes, 11-12, 43-44
Insight, 37, 242
Institutionalization, 144-145, 150-151
    and hospitalization, 161-162
Instrumental conditioning *see* Operant conditioning
Integration and humanization model, 143-145
International Classification of Impairments, Disabilities and Handicaps (ICIDH), 7-8

Jung, C, 130
Justice, principle of, *215*, 222

Labeling, 173
Language development, 56-58
Latent learning, 37
Law *see* Ethics and law
Leadership, 105-106
'Learned helpessness', 40, 117, 182
Learning, 29-30
    in older people, 138
    theories
        cognitive, 36-40
        conditioning, 31-35
    ways of, *36, 39*
Legitimation, chronic illness, 171, 172-173
Life expectancy, 149-150
Lifespan development theory, 129-132
Lifestyle and health, 112-113
Locus of control, 112, 165, 195

Memory processes, 40-42, 235-236
    in older people, 137-138, 162-163
Menopause, 111-112
Mid-life crisis, 110-112

Mobility
    loss of, 156-157
    treatment, 164
'Model', definitions, 5, 8
Modeling, 38, 159
Moral reasoning, 213
    see also Ethical decision-making
Motivation, 86-87, 188-189, *191*
Motor development, 49
Musculoskeletal problems, 115-116
Mutuality, development of, 54-55, 118

'Nature of nurture' debate, 11-12
Neuromuscular plasticity, 69-70
Non-compliance
    ethical issues, case studies, 215-217, 217-221, 224
    health practitioner–patient relationship,
        198-199
    Non-maleficence, principle of, *214*, 218-219, 220,
        227, 228
Non-verbal behavior, 205
Normalization, 181

Object manipulation, permanence and categories, 51-
    52
Observational learning, 38
Occupational health *see* Work, health hazards
Older people *see* Aging; Chronic disease in older
    people
Operant conditioning, 33-35
    versus classical conditioning, *33*

Pain in older people, 157-159
Paradigm shift
    communication, 245
    health care, 96-97, 118
Parenthood, 103-105
    metaphor, health practitioner–patient
        relationship, 202-204
    and work, 107-110
Parsons, T: sick role theory, 170-175, 209-210
Passing, 181
Patients *see* Health practitioner–patient relation-
    ship
Pellegrino, E, 216, 219-220, 225, 229
    and Thomasma, D: ethical decision-making
        model, *225–226*, 226

Perception
    and interpretation, 28-29
    see also Sensation and perception
Personality
    health practitioners, 204
    in older people, 139-140, 142
    theoretical approaches, 5-6
    type and heart disease, 114-115
    see also Coping strategies
Physical setting, 249-251
Physiological status, 189, 190, 193
Piaget, J, 25, 26, 27, 49, 50, 52
Plastic adaptation, 12, 70, 92
Post-traumatic stress disorder (PTSD), 40
Primum non nocere, *215*, 220-221
Professional values, 240, 241
    see also Ethical principles
Psychosocial crises, 17-18
Psychosocial development, 7
    adaptation, 25-26
    childhood, 58-61
    cultural context, 21, 26-27
    Erikson's stages of, 13-18
        major components, *18*
Psychosocial theories of aging, 126-132
Ptophobia *see* Falling, fear of
PTSD *see* Post-traumatic stress disorder
Punishment, 34, 35, 60

Reciprocity *see* Mutuality, development of; Respect
    and reciprocity
Referral, 259
Reflex activity *see* Sensorimotor causality
    scheme
Reinforcement, 33-35, 92
Rejectivity versus care, 100-101
Research designs, older people, 134-135
Respect for persons, principle of, *215*, 219
Rrespect and reciprocity, 79-82
Respondent conditioning *see* Classical
    conditioning
Results-based theories, *223*, 228
Retirement, 141-142
Role theory *see* Chronic disease, role theory
    approaches; Health practitioner–patient
    relationship, role theory; Sick role theory;
    Social roles and status

Scientific process, 2-4
Self-care *see* Self-efficacy
Self-concept
    in adolescence, 72-78
    in chronic illness, 177-178, 179-180, 181-182
    definition, 188
    in older people, 166-167
    and society, 20, 77-78, 184
Self-confidence, 58, 97
    building, 90-91, 92, ,190, *191*, 195
    definitions, 188, 189
Self-efficacy
    corollary concepts, 188-189, 190, *191*
    definition, 112
    model, 189-190
    older people, 164-165
    see also under Falling, fear of
Self-esteem *see* Self-confidence
Self-image, disrupted, 177-178
Sensation and perception
    inference model, 232-234, 236-237, 241, 242
    interconnectedness, 48-49
Sensorimotor causality schemes, 49-51
    clinical application, 51
Sexuality and aging, 141
Shame, 59, 180
    versus autonomy, *14*, 58-59
Sheehy, G: passages in adult life, 107-110, 110-111
Sick role theory, 170-171
    criticism, 210
    exemptions, 171-172
    obligations, 171, 172-174
    patient–health practitioner relationship,
        200-201, 209-210
Skinner, B F, 33, 34
Sleep disorders, 160-161, 165
Social attachment, 45-47, 52, 53-55, 57
Social cognitive theory, 39-40, 112, 189-190
Social control agents, 209-210
Social isolation, 180
Social roles and status
    older people, 143-145, 151-152
    patient–health practitioner relationship, 201-202,
        245, 247
Socialization, to chronic illness, 181-182
Societal systems, 19-21
    major components, *21*

Stigmatization, 172, 180-181
Strauss, A *see* Corbin, J & Strauss, A
Stress, 40, 113-114
    in older people, 141-142, 148
Summey, P *see* Bloom S & Summey, P
Szasz, T & Hollender, M: interaction model,
    202-204

Theory
    components, 4-6
    development, 2-3
    testing, 3, 6
Therapeutic principles
    activating psychological resources, 118-120
    co-operative partnership, 90-92, 96
    excellence versus perfection, 93-96
    holism, 69-70
    paradigm shift, 96-97, 118
    'practice makes perfect', 92-93
Therapist *see* Health practitioner
'Total institutions', 144-145
Trust, 219-220
    versus mistrust, *14*, 54-55

Uncertainty, 176-177

Values, 36, 213
    3-M model, 237-241
    conflicting, 239-241, 250-251, 255-256
Verbal persuasion, 190, 194, 195-196
Vicarious experience, 190, 194, 196
Virtue-based theories, *224*, 225, 228-229

'Whistle-blowing', 220-221
Wisdom, 138-139, 166-167
Women
    health problems, 115, 116, 117
    menopause, 111-112
    motherhood, 103-104
        and work, 107-110
    older, 152-153
Work, 105-107
    health hazards, 114, 115-116
    retirement, 141-142
    unemployment, 113